Clinical Perspectives on the Supervision of Psychoanalysis and Psychotherapy

D1569061

CRITICAL ISSUES IN PSYCHIATRY
A Series for Clinicians

Series Editor: **Sherwyn M. Woods, M.D., Ph.D.**
University of Southern California School of Medicine
Los Angeles, California

THE INTERFACE BETWEEN THE PSYCHODYNAMIC AND
BEHAVIORAL THERAPIES
Edited by Judd Marmor, M.D., and Sherwyn M. Woods, M.D., Ph.D.

LAW IN THE PRACTICE OF PSYCHIATRY
Seymour L. Halleck, M.D.

NEUROPSYCHIATRIC FEATURES OF MEDICAL DISORDERS
James W. Jefferson, M.D., and John R. Marshall, M.D.

ADULT DEVELOPMENT: A New Dimension in Psychodynamic Theory
and Practice
Calvin A. Colarusso, M.D., and Robert A. Nemiroff, M.D.

SCHIZOPHRENIA
John S. Strauss, M.D., and William T. Carpenter, Jr., M.D.

EXTRAORDINARY DISORDERS OF HUMAN BEHAVIOR
Edited by Claude T. H. Friedmann, M.D., and Robert A. Faguet, M.D.

MARITAL THERAPY: A Combined Psychodynamic–Behavioral Approach
R. Taylor Segraves, M.D., Ph.D.

TREATMENT INTERVENTIONS IN HUMAN SEXUALITY
Edited by Carol C. Nadelson, M.D., and David B. Marcotte, M.D.

DRUG AND ALCOHOL ABUSE: A Clinical Guide to Diagnosis
and Treatment
Edited by Marc A. Schuckit, M.D.

CLINICAL PERSPECTIVES ON THE SUPERVISION OF
PSYCHOANALYSIS AND PSYCHOTHERAPY
Edited by Leopold Caligor, Ph.D., Philip M. Bromberg, Ph.D.,
and James D. Meltzer, Ph.D.

MOOD DISORDERS: Toward a Psychobiology
Peter C. Whybrow, M.D., Hagop S. Akiskal, M.D., and
William T. McKinney, Jr., M.D.

A Continuation Order Plan is available for this series. A continuation order will bring delivery of each new volume immediately upon publication. Volumes are billed only upon actual shipment. For further information please contact the publisher.

Clinical Perspectives on the Supervision of Psychoanalysis and Psychotherapy

Edited by

Leopold Caligor, Ph.D.
Philip M. Bromberg, Ph.D.
James D. Meltzer, Ph.D.

The William Alanson White Psychoanalytic Society
New York, New York

PLENUM PRESS · NEW YORK AND LONDON

Library of Congress Cataloging in Publication Data

Main entry under title:

Clinical perspectives on the supervision of psychoanalysis and psychotherapy.

(Critical issues in psychiatry)
Includes bibliographical references and index.
1. Psychoanalysis—Study and teaching—Supervision. 2. Psychotherapy—Study and teaching—Supervision. I. Caligor, Leopold, date-   . II. Bromberg, Philip M., date-   . III. Meltzer, James D. IV. Series. [DNLM: 1. Clinical competence. 2. Organization and Administration. 3. Psychoanalysis—Education. 4. Psychotherapy—Education. WM 19.5 C641]
RC502.C55   1983   616.89′17   83-22939
ISBN 0-306-41403-1

© 1984 Plenum Press, New York
A Division of Plenum Publishing Corporation
233 Spring Street, New York, N.Y. 10013

Printed in the United States of America

Dedicated to
The William Alanson White Institute
of
Psychiatry, Psychoanalysis, and Psychology
in this, its fortieth year

Contributors

PHILIP M. BROMBERG • Supervising Analyst, William Alanson White Institute of Psychiatry, Psychoanalysis and Psychology, New York, New York and Assistant Clinical Professor of Medical Psychology, College of Physicians and Surgeons, Columbia University, New York, New York

LEOPOLD CALIGOR • Training and Supervising Analyst, William Alanson White Institute of Psychiatry, Psychoanalysis and Psychology, New York, New York and Clinical Professor of Psychology, Adelphi University Postdoctoral Program in Psychotherapy, Garden City, New York

GERARD CHRZANOWSKI • Training and Supervising Analyst, William Alanson White Institute of Psychiatry, Psychoanalysis and Psychology, New York, New York and Associate Clinical Professor of Psychiatry, Psychoanalytic Division, New York Medical College, New York, New York

ALLAN COOPER • Director of Curriculum, Fellow, Training and Supervising Analyst, William Alanson White Institute of Psychiatry, Psychoanalysis and Psychology, New York, New York

RALPH M. CROWLEY • Fellow Emeritus and Training and Supervising Analyst, William Alanson White Institute of Psychiatry, Psychoanalysis and Psychology, New York, New York and Past President, American Academy of Psychoanalysis, New York, New York

AMNON ISSACHAROFF • Fellow, Training and Supervising Analyst, William Alanson White Institute of Psychiatry, Psychoanalysis and Psychology, New York, New York and Attending Psychiatrist, New York Hospital-Cornell Medical Center, New York, New York

ROBERT J. LANGS • Program Director, Lenox Hill Hospital Psychotherapy Program, New York, New York

RUTH M. LESSER • Clinical Professor, Training and Supervising Analyst, New York University Postdoctoral and Doctoral Programs in Psychology, New York, New York and Guest Lecturer, William Alanson White Institute of Psychiatry, Psychoanalysis and Psychology, New York, New York.

EDGAR A. LEVENSON • Fellow, Training and Supervising Analyst, William Alanson White Institute of Psychiatry, Psychoanalysis and Psychology, New York, New York and Clinical Professor, Graduate School of Arts and Sciences, New York University, New York, New York

ZVI LOTHANE • Clinical Assistant Professor of Psychiatry, Mount Sinai School of Medicine, City University of New York, New York, New York; Training Analyst, Institute for Psychoanalytic Training and Research, New York, New York; National Psychological Association for Psychoanalysis, New York, New York

JAMES D. MELTZER • Teaching Faculty and Supervisor of Psychotherapy, William Alanson White Institute of Psychiatry, Psychoanalysis and Psychology, New York, New York and Chief Psychologist, The Roosevelt Hospital of the Saint Luke's-Roosevelt Hospital Center, New York, New York

RUTH MOULTON • Fellow, Training and Supervising Analyst, William Alanson White Institute of Psychiatry, Psychoanalysis and Psychology, New York, New York and Life Member, American Psychoanalytic Association, New York, New York

ROY SCHAFER • Training and Supervising Analyst, Columbia University Center for Psychoanalytic Training and Research, New York, New York and Adjunct Professor of Psychology in Psychiatry, Cornell University Medical College, New York, New York

JOHN L. SCHIMEL • Associate Director, Fellow, Training and Supervising Analyst, William Alanson White Institute of Psychiatry, Psychoanalysis and Psychology, New York, New York and Clinical Professor of Psychiatry, New York University-Bellevue Medical Center, New York, New York

ROSE SPIEGEL • Fellow, Training and Supervising Analyst, William Alanson White Institute of Psychiatry, Psychoanalysis and Psychology, New York, New York and Consulting Psychiatrist, Saint Luke's-Roosevelt Hospital Center, New York, New York

EARL G. WITENBERG • Director, Fellow, Training and Supervising Analyst, William Alanson White Institute of Psychiatry, Psychoanalysis and Psychology, New York, New York and Past President, American Academy of Psychoanalysis, New York, New York

MILTIADES L. ZAPHIROPOULOS • Director of Training, Fellow, Training and Supervising Analyst, William Alanson White Institute of Psychiatry, Psychoanalysis and Psychology, New York, New York and Associate Clinical Professor of Psychiatry, College of Physicians and Surgeons, Columbia University, New York, New York

Foreword

In order to complete training successfully, every psychoanalyst has to be a supervisee. This experience leads each analyst to want to become a supervisor. Until recently, very little has been discussed about what supervision is, how it is done, and how it is related to the various theories of psychoanalysis that are held as articles of faith.

The 1980–1981 program of the William Alanson White Psychoanalytic Society was devoted to supervision—with representatives of various "schools" demonstrating their ways of doing consultations with analysts about patients. This book is an extension of that endeavor. In it, supervisors of various persuasions discuss this topic.

The editors—Leopold Caligor, Philip M. Bromberg, and James D. Meltzer—are to be congratulated for the high level of discourse represented by the various chapters. They are to be commended as well about the eloquent statement this book makes—namely, there are many answers and approaches and no final answer to the questions raised by the volume.

This book will be valuable to a number of different groups. For supervisors, it will offer an opportunity to see what other supervisors are thinking, and it will enable them to sharpen their own perceptions and help them to formulate their own ideas. For practitioners, it is a grand opportunity to clarify what kinds of people they would want as consultants. For beginners, it will enable them to ascertain the thinking of different individuals before selecting them as supervisors. For the field as a whole, it is another giant step toward making the discipline more open and less a trade guild. The editors are to be congratulated for the dedication, thoughtfulness, and fair-mindedness this volume represents.

Earl G. Witenberg

Preface

In 1979, the editors of this volume became the core members of a Study Group on Supervision formed under the auspices of the William Alanson White Psychoanalytic Institute.

As the study group members became more familiar with some of the controversial issues surrounding psychoanalytic supervision—for example, should supervision be pedagogic or therapeutic, to what degree should the supervisory relationship be explored, does the supervisor focus on the patient or the training of the candidate, who has the ultimate responsibility for the case, and so forth—we realized that we would need to study the actual supervisory process. We were fortunate in being able to obtain tape recordings of supervisory sessions from experienced supervisors at several psychoanalytic institutes representing a wide range of theoretical orientations. These tape recordings became our first "data base."

When one member of our group (Leopold Caligor) was elected president of the William Alanson White Psychoanalytic Society in 1980–1981, he and the program chairman (James Meltzer) developed a program of scientific meetings about the supervisory process. We asked five senior psychoanalysts (Chrzanowski, Schafer, Lothane, Lesser, and Langs) to supervise a candidate in front of the William Alanson White Society in much the way they would in their offices. These live supervisory sessions stimulated a great deal of interest and excitement in the supervisory process. The present volume is an outgrowth of that interest and enthusiasm. It seeks to bring together representative exponents of a broad range of clinical styles in analytic supervision. Just as no single perspective guided our thinking in choosing the participants for the 1980–1981 meetings, no attempt was made to establish a common language unifying the following chapters. What mattered was the openness and expertise of each contributor and the relevance of the material each had to offer. To whatever extent theoretical synthesis or a search for communality between viewpoints is of interest to the reader, we hope that the clarity and candor of the individual positions expressed here will provide a useful data base.

The supervisory study group continues to meet. Much of our understanding of supervision remains tentative and untested at this point. However, a number of general observations or patterns have begun to emerge from the data.

First, each supervisor has a very personal supervisory style that is identifiable when he or she is working with different supervisees. It is not based on the supervisor's theoretical orientation, which is in fact extremely hard to discern from listening to or observing a supervisory session. Instead, a supervisor's "signature" seems to result in large part from those particular analytic events or issues in which he is interested or knowledgeable. For example, a supervisor may consistently single out dreams, or the patient's first comments in the hour, or transference issues. He may consistently make his focus patient centered or analyst centered. Or the supervisor may focus on the supervisory relationship itself, and so forth. There are also clear differences in the supervisor's attitude as to whether he sees himself or the supervisee as having ultimate responsibility for the case. Stylistic variability is also striking in the degree of formality with which the supervision is conducted and in the level of activity that the supervisor feels comfortable in bringing to the process. This includes the degree to which he is confrontational, the freedom he appears to feel in presenting his own ideas or giving alternative formulations, and how much a supervisor will tend to say—overall. While it is difficult to be more than speculative about stylistic variables and their sources, there is some degree of evidence from our observations that a certain supervisor will adopt a manner with the supervisee that he hopes will be a model of identification for the supervisee as an analyst.

Second, an ever-present liability in the supervisory process is that the supervisor is seen by the supervisee as both an educator and as an authority. This may make it difficult for the candidate to question or contradict the supervisor and to explore other possible ways of understanding with the knowing expert.

When, in reality, the supervisor is responsible for the supervisee's continued progress at an analytic institute, the pressures of evaluation can excessively burden the supervisory relationship. Under some circumstances, the pressure for a good evaluation can potentially become intense enough to distort severely the primary educational functions of supervision. The candidate may become more concerned with pleasing the supervisor than with increasing his own capacity to understand and experience.

This overly great concern with evaluation may lead a candidate to choose a supervisor whose style or area of analytic interest is familiar to him and poses no threat. An example here is the empathic candidate who chooses a supervisor who works with dreams, and avoids supervisors who demand close theoretical reasoning. It is commonplace that candidates become quite anxious when a specific supervisor is recommended to help remediate an obvious deficit in their education.

Third, as a result of many hours of listening to recordings of our own and other supervisory sessions, our study group has arrived at a rather general working definition of effective supervision. It is our strong impression that good psychoanalytic supervision encourages the supervisee to attend to the *process of the analysis*. That is, there is a recognizable, progressive, structural, unfolding process that is the hallmark of psychoanalysis. The particular content and shape of the process cannot be precisely defined or predicted, but it is marked by the emergence in both participants of an increasingly reflective, nonobsessive sensitivity to the multiple levels of interpersonal communication. The analyst-in-training must become an expert in this process, and be highly attuned to its nuances.

With a talented person, the supervisor can encourage and facilitate this way of listening and participating. If there are difficulties in the supervision, they can be discussed and resolved because both supervisee and supervisor feel basically competent and valued. However, when the supervisee is not talented in this type of work, or when his capacity to learn from supervision is limited because he is too guarded, defensive, or remote, the supervision becomes problematic.

Fourth, as the psychoanalytic community shifts away from emphasizing parochial theoretical interests to a greater concern with the data of clinical processes, the close study of supervision will assume greater importance. Supervisors will become more comfortable in revealing their work to colleagues. Other models of supervision will be explored.

For example, we have found that having two advanced supervisees share a supervisory hour can be a most valuable experience, provided that they are already skilled psychotherapists with considerable one-to-one psychoanalytic supervision. This supervisory context seems to diminish regression and unthinking obeisance to the authority of the supervisor and to enhance creativity on the part of all participants. It is humbling for the supervisor when the supervisees develop insights and approaches to the material that are as cogent and compelling as his own views. Finally, it teaches the student to be constructively critical of another's analytic work—a helpful education for his own later work as a supervisor.

We also see great potential in the growing interest in supervisory peer groups. Our study group itself has forcefully demonstrated to us

the value of peer supervision. Being a talented analyst does not necessarily make one a talented supervisor. Most of us have had little formal
training in doing supervision. Participation in ongoing or periodic peer
supervision can be both invigorating and enlightening.

It is a pleasure to conclude this preface by acknowledging our deep
appreciation to all those who in various ways made this volume possible. First, a debt is owed to the following participants in the 1980–1981
White Society scientific program, who by their willingness to share
openly with their colleagues a firsthand, unedited view of their work,
set the tone that led to the idea behind the present book: supervisors
Gerard Chrzanowski, Robert J. Langs, Ruth Lesser, Zvi Lothane, and
Roy Schafer; candidates Elizabeth Goren, Ellen Loefler Waldman, Ann
McMahon, Jeffrey Sachs, Kathleen P. White, and Joseph K. Younger-
man. We would also like to express our gratitude to the 1980–1981
members of the board of directors of the William Alanson White Psychoanalytic Society for their immediate and unanimous endorsement of this
endeavor under the aegis of the society. The board, during Dr. Caligor's
tenure as president, consisted of the following members; Albert Bryt,
Lawrence Epstein, Elaine Grimm, Murray Krim, James Meltzer, and
Robert B. Shapiro. In addition to the preceding, we wish to thank the
members of the training committee of the institute for their moral support and unfailing open spirit of scientific inquiry that has been the
hallmark of their identity.

We would also like to acknowledge our indebtedness to those
whose time and effort concretely helped to ease the completion of this
task. Thanks are due to Arthur H. Feiner, editor of *Contemporary Psychoanalysis,* and to Martin P. Levin, trustee of the William Alanson White
Institute, for generously sharing their expertise in matters literary and
their knowledgeability in the world of publishing. Our particular gratitude goes to Sondra Wilk, director of administration and development
of the institute, whose sensitivity to issues and uncomplaining responsiveness to our need for advice and guidance was invaluable at every
stage of the project. Finally, we are indebted to the clerical, typing, and
organizational assistance of Helen Ekstein and Joan Friedman, who repeatedly went out of their way to assure that what we needed was
provided.

To the Reader

We believe that the issues discussed in *Clinical Perspectives on the Supervision of Psychoanalysis and Psychotherapy* are germane to the supervision of psychoanalysis and dynamic psychotherapy in the disciplines of psychiatry, psychology, social work, counseling, and psychiatric nursing.

It is also our conviction that an in-depth understanding of the supervisory process is of relevance to students, teachers, and practitioners of psychoanalysis and dynamic psychotherapy, as well as supervisors.

Leopold Caligor
Philip M. Bromberg
James D. Meltzer

Contents

1

Parallel and Reciprocal Processes in Psychoanalytic Supervision

Leopold Caligor

The question of what comprises psychoanalytic training—how best to teach a candidate how to become an analyst—has had a long and checkered history. Much has been written over the last 70 years. It is apparent that major shifts have occurred in the definition of supervision, the model for learning in supervision, the use of the analytic versus the didactic teaching method between student and supervisor, and how the supervisor uses himself with his student. These issues remain central and unresolved. I believe they reflect current changes in our understanding of how the analyst can best use himself with his patient. Concepts such as Langs's (1976) *bipersonal field* and H. S. Sullivan's (1954) *participant-observation* come to mind.

Perhaps a brief overview of the history of supervision is in order. Before psychoanalytic training was formalized, the model was that of master-apprentice. "In the early days, small groups that gathered around Freud analyzed, taught and supervised each other" (Gustin, 1958, p. 63). One's personal analysis was seen as the foundation of the future analyst's training (Eckstein & Wallerstein, 1958).

In 1922, formal standards were set—along with course work and one's own psychoanalysis—by the International Psychoanalytic Society

This chapter was delivered as the Presidential Address to the William Alanson White Psychoanalytic Society on May 28, 1980, and was first published in *Contemporary Psychoanalysis*, 1981, 17(1), 1–27. It is reprinted by permission of the William Alanson White Institute.

Leopold Caligor • Training and Supervising Analyst, William Alanson White Institute of Psychiatry, Psychoanalysis and Psychology, New York, New York 10023 and Clinical Professor of Psychology, Adelphi University Postdoctoral Program in Psychotherapy, Garden City, New York 11530.

that called for the treatment of several patients under supervision (Eckstein & Wallerstein, 1958).

In the 1930s there was considerable debate about how supervision could best be accomplished. One group, from Budapest, believed that supervision—called "control analysis"—was a continuation of the candidate's personal analysis, and that therefore both should be done by the same analyst. The emphasis would fall on transference in the candidate's own analysis and on countertransference in supervision. "Such a philosophy indeed would make it very difficult to differentiate between the personal therapeutic experience and the supervisory experience. One grew out of the other, and could not be seen apart from it" (Eckstein & Wallerstein, 1958, p. 244).

The opposing view, as expressed by Bibring (1937) and centered in the Viennese school, opted for complete separation of personal analysis and supervision, with supervision emphasizing didactic teaching. It was believed that countertransference difficulties should be dealt with in the candidate's personal analysis.

It was Eckstein and Wallerstein (1958) who first focused on the supervisor–therapist relationship in the learning process and its impact on the therapeutic process. Theirs was a process-centered model with emphasis on the interaction between patient, analyst, and supervisor. The student's problems about learning in supervision often reflect the problems that exist between the therapist and his patient. Thus, the supervisor utilizes ongoing processes that are observable in the therapist–supervisor relationship to clarify difficulties the student has in the patient–therapist relationship. This permits the student to use his own experience of emotional difficulties in coping with his supervisor to facilitate his understanding of the patient's situation with him. The therapist's "learning problems" in supervision often reflect the problems that exist between a therapist and his patient. Thus, a "parallel process" exists in which the therapist's problems in supervision and the patient's problems in psychotherapy are related to each other.

Eckstein and Wallerstein (1958) point out that the observing and understanding of the interplay of the forces in the parallel process of therapy and supervision make for effective supervision. The supervisor, in their model, actively participates in a helping process that focuses on learning and personal growth rather than on psychotherapy for the student.

Actually, very little has been reported in the literature on the parallel process. Searles, it is interesting to note, reported on the phenomenon in 1955, four years earlier than Eckstein and Wallerstein. In his article "The Informational Value of the Supervisor's Emotional Experiences," Searles (1955) states:

> But when the supervisor finds himself experiencing some emotion during the supervisory hour, he should be alert not only to the possibility that the source of this emotion may lie chiefly in his own repressed past, in which case he is experiencing a classical countertransference reaction to the therapist; he should be alert also to the possibility that the source of this emotion may lie chiefly in the therapist–patient relationship and, basically, in the patient himself. If the latter is found to be the case, then one may say that the supervisor's emotion is a *reflection* of something which has been going on in the therapist–patient relationship, and, in the final analysis, in the patient. This reflection process is by no means to be thought of as holding the center of the stage, in the supervisory situation, at all times. Probably it comprises, in actual practice, only a small proportion of the events which transpire in supervisory hours. Yet its part is a vital one, for it may offer clues to obscure difficulties besetting the patient–therapist relationship. (pp. 136–137)

Dealing specifically with the parallel process, Doehrman (1976), at the Psychology Clinic of the University of Michigan, utilized a clinical analysis of the interview data of each supervisor and each student therapist working together after each hour of supervision. She concluded:

> If there is any one conclusion all these findings add up to, it is that the parallel process phenomenon occurs and recurs in a remarkable multiplicity of forms. At the very least, one comes away from this material with a sense of humility about the complexity, subtlety, and depth of human relationships. One is struck by the multifaceted nature of what on the surface seems to be a simple and even limited relationship. Having discovered this order of complexity in a seemingly limited relationship, one wonders about the complexitites that must infuse other human affairs. (p. 82)

THE PRESENT STUDY

I should like to state at the outset that my hope in studying the parallel process in supervision is not to diminish the importance of didactic teaching nor to imply that the supervisory process is in any sense a substitute for, or diminishes from, the centrality of the candidate's own analysis. Rather, I believe that parallel processes are much more frequently operative than is recognized and that not recognizing them can have unfortunate implications for the teaching–learning process called supervision.

Rather than studying the process from above, which would be an intellectual exercise one step removed from the clinical and supervisorial reality, I would like to present portions of two taped supervisory sessions as a basis for discussion so that what we would discuss clinically or theorize would never go beyond the observable data.

I would like to think that what I am doing is clinical research. The design of the experiment, as rudimentary as it is, would go as follows. First, there is a unit of two candidates, one male and one female, who have been in cosupervision with me for more than a year. Second, there is a peer supervisory study group of which I am a member. The taped supervisory sessions were replayed and discussed in the peer supervisory study group, and those proceedings were also taped.

One candidate—Fred—is a very bright, well-read, empathic, very competent, soft-spoken, somewhat reticent, and verbally talented young therapist. He does have a tendency to keep his distance, tends to avoid intense affect, and shows considerable intellectual constraint. He has worked well with a variety of patients, both male and female. He tends, in brief, toward the obsessive-cognitive.

In supervision, he has been able to listen and learn, and yet not blindly accept my observations. He has been able to share his thoughts and feelings openly. I have enjoyed working with him and watching him grow as a therapist and as a person.

The other candidate—Madge—is bright, energetic, and rather verbal and affective. She is emotional, warm, and can be playful. She is somewhat affect dominated, though clear thinking. In brief, she tends toward the hysteric-affective. She is as talented as Fred, but she has a different style of perceiving and responding—understandably so. Each has selected the other for supervision with me.

I find that having two candidates share supervisory sessions can be most valuable as a later supervisory experience; a threesome makes for less transference on the part of the candidate; there is less probability of countertransference to any one student by the supervisor; there tends to be greater criticality operative on the part of all; and different affective perceptual and cognitive grids examining the same data tend to make for a broader perspective. Also, there tends to be less regression than can occur in the one-to-one situation because the supervisor is perceived much less as God the authority, and the candidate therefore feels freer to be critical of his contributions and to verbalize his own. It is humbling for the supervisor when the candidate comes forth with superior insights and recommendations that are frequently better than his own. All this makes for the analytic ethos of equality and dialogue leading to insights broader than are available to one person. Finally, it teaches the student how to be constructively critical of another's work and how to be engaged actively as a participant in the supervisory process—a helpful education for his own future work as a supervisor, and hopefully, someday as his own supervisor.

THE PEER SUPERVISORY STUDY GROUP

If the candidate's work is to be studied with him by a peer and a supervisor, then it stands to reason that the supervisor should have a place where his work can also be studied with him. Philip Bromberg, James Meltzer, and I decided to meet for a double lunch hour at the institute once a week to study the supervisory process. This sprang from our need for peer-group dialogue. We have enjoyed the intellectual stimulation and have shared honest dialogue and camaraderie. I want to thank them for their collaboration and encouragement to use data of the peer supervisory study group in this chapter.

We became aware of the need for live tapes to study in our peer group. Since these were hard to obtain, I asked Fred and Madge to permit me to tape their supervisory sessions for our study group to peruse. Both were not (or minimally) threatened, and they agreed to have their work studied. It was emphasized that I and the supervisory process were to be primarily examined, rather than they as therapists. And, of course, all our discussions would be confidential.

Please note that neither the peer supervisory study group (Philip, Jim, Lee) nor the two candidates (Fred, Madge) had any idea of the materials being used for publication, since this possibility arose after all the data had already been collected.

In brief, the model espoused permits evaluation of resonances between the ongoing therapy process and the supervisory process—and also evaluation of the supervisory process itself. The three dyads to be studied and their impacts upon each other are the patient–therapist, the therapist–supervisor, and the supervisor–peer supervisory group.

THE FIRST SUPERVISORY HOUR

Since we are focusing on the parallel process in supervision and in psychotherapy, I will present vignettes that depict the patient–therapist relationship (Helen and Fred) and the supervisory relationship (Fred and Lee).

First, a few words about the patient. Helen is about 35 years old, has never married, and is overtied to her mother, who is quite hysterical, sacrificing, and overprotective. It has been a struggle for Helen to separate from her mother physically and emotionally. Helen was adopted at birth and never knew her real parents. She lost her father at age 7 (he had been invalided at home for several years, and she had been quite close to him). Helen has always had difficulties in making relationships with men—in trusting that they would be there for her. Prior to beginning analysis, the patient had the following dream: She is in her mother's house. There is a man who has no face. Helen is involved with him, she gets close to him, he has power over her. She awakened feeling deep fright and a sinking sensation. Helen has a need to keep her distance from men by avoidance or infrequent contact. When intimacy cannot be avoided, she can be erratically compliant, clinging, helpless, demanding, easily upset, teary, enraged; she can deny and distort the facts—and see herself as the victim. Helen is currently in a relationship of two years' duration with a married man who has been described variously as warm, self-centered, and unevenly available.

Fred came into the supervisory session apparently upset. He felt that Helen and he were at an impasse and that he could not get through to her. The difficulty centered upon the relationship with her boyfriend, Mel.

A Summary of the Content of the First Supervisory Hour

Fred states that Helen has made considerable progress. "I think she has made considerable progress in a number of areas. She doesn't complain so much, she doesn't have some of the physical symptoms that she described many times before and they seem to be much less frequent. There is much less report of her getting panicky or having anxiety attacks or being terribly upset."

Fred focused on two upsetting issues. First, Helen wants to cut back on the number of her therapy sessions. She says the problem is primarily money. Fred is aware that he has not confronted her directly about this. The patient has a part-time free-lance job; she is skilled and can easily work a few more hours for the cost of therapy.

Second, Mel is currently less available and the patient is upset. She knows he is erratically available on a part-time basis. She sees herself as the victim. She is aware that in the beginning Mel was always there, available to her. But now that has changed. How can she trust a man? Yet Helen fears that without Mel she will be lonely and depressed.

Fred states:

I get frustrated now when she brings up the issue because I don't know what else to add to her. And sometimes it seems to me that there is no intent of leaving Mel. There's only the intent of complaining about it's not enough, he betrays me when he goes on vacation for two weeks, he wasn't available when I had vacation, now he's away, I could have spent more time with him. She gets pissed off, she gets frightened, she makes noises about it. Should I leave? This is crazy, what should I do, I'm getting older. But whenever it comes to making a decision, I can't make a decision. Why hasn't therapy helped her more so that she can make decisions, etc.

No matter how Fred attempts to get Helen to look at what transpires with Mel, he receives swirls of words, incoherence, unrelated responses, floods of affect, vacillation, and paralysis.

Again and again Fred *tires* (typing slip—I meant *tries*), but he is not heard. As he talks about this, it is apparent to me that he feels quite exasperated and frustrated. As the supervisory session progresses, he depletes, ending up feeling frustrated, impotent, defeated, withdrawn, and avoidant. He is overwhelmed by her torrent of words. Finally, he feels as though he would like for himself or for her to just go away. *Yet all this is at best in partial awareness.*

About the issue of Helen's determination to cut back on the number of sessions, Fred soon succumbed, and he did not press the point. He described it all with muffled rage and defeatism.

When on several occasions I tried to get Fred to focus on what he was experiencing as he related the material, he responded with swirls of words, not quite hearing my questions nor responding to the content appropriately. When I would try to point out certain material, he would either interrupt me or say yes, and then go back to where he had been.

Again and again, I tried to get Fred to focus on Helen's way of relating to Mel—that rather than her being exclusively the victim, she, with her problems about intimacy, was relating in a way that could drive him away. But Fred could not hear, swirled with words, changed the topic, interrupted me.

When I tried to focus on the similarities between the patient's way of relating to Mel and to him, he again could not hear me. It was only toward the end of the session that he *began* to perceive that he and Mel were somehow in the same boat with respect to the patient. When I queried several times what he felt was going on between us, he veered off, as has already been described. The session ended with a frustrated feeling that some issues had been stated but that nothing had been resolved.

I want to emphasize that all the preceding is atypical of this promising therapist's previous work with this patient, with other patients, and his usual way of relating and presenting in supervision.

I should like to summarize the parallels in the relationships between patient and therapist, therapist and supervisor, and the supervisor–supervisory peer group.

Patient-Therapist. It was apparent that the patient was evasive with Fred—distancing, avoiding contact, nor hearing him—that every attempt he made to reach her was foiled, and that after a while he was just depleted. When he described what transpired with the patient, he sounded defeated, was often unduly silent, somewhat morose, not clearly focused, passive, and could not think clearly. He apparently felt muffled rage of which he was at best partially aware. There was a quality of loginess and stupor about him.

Therapist-Supervisor. In supervision, Fred managed, again without awareness, to communicate his unfocused state, defeatism, and paralysis.

When I attempted to engage Fred to discuss this with him, he related to me with the same evasion and inability to hear me as the patient did with him. After many attempts I gave in and stopped trying. I too joined somewhat in the stupor, the passivity, and defeatism, and I was enraged in a semiaware low-key way—as I think Fred was with his patient.

Supervisor–Supervisory Peer Group. When the group (Jim, Philip, Lee) heard the tape as it went on, Philip and Jim each individually felt the same apathy, loss of focus, impotence, and frustration as I had felt during the supervision. It was as if all three of us were one supervisor.

When Jim and Philip tried to probe and query, I became defensive and evasive—just as Fred the therapist had been with me. However, the peer group did not actively press me, just as I had not pressed Fred during supervision.

THE SUPERVISORY PEER-GROUP DISCUSSION

Figure 1 recapitulates or schematizes the parallel process by using several clearly observable variables as we observed them in our supervisory peer-group discussions. All this is modeled after the patient as evoker and the therapist as recipient.

It is noteworthy that the therapist and supervisor can switch roles and play either the evoker or the recipient. For example, the therapist is recipient with the patient, and is the evoker with the supervisor. The supervisor is the recipient with the therapist and the evoker with the

The Patient–Therapist Relationship (Form 1)	
Patient as evoker	Therapist as recipient
Resistive and evasive	Stuporous and depressed
Swirls of words	Unduly silent
Scattered thinking	Lack of critical thinking
Quite anxious and upset	Muffled rage
The Therapist–Supervisor Relationship (Form 2)	
Therapist as evoker	Supervisor as recipient
Resistive and evasive	Stuporous and depressed
Swirls of words	Unduly silent
Scattered thinking	Lack of critical thinking
Anxious and upset	Muffled rage
The Supervisor–Supervisory Peer Group Relationship (Form 3)	
Supervisor as evoker	Supervisory group as recipient
Resistive and evasive	Stuporous and depressed
Anxious and irritable	Unduly silent
(So Philip and Jim tell me)	Lack of critical thinking
	Muffled rage

FIGURE 1. Schematization of the parallel process.

peer supervisory group. These switches in roles are again modeled after the patient as evoker and the therapist as recipient.

When we discussed this in our supervisory peer-group, we were awed by the tug of the parallel process. We had a growing awareness that perhaps one can speak of contours based upon the original shape of the patient with the therapist that may be the patient's way of setting up transferential relationships in life. The shapes—like a ripple of concentric circles getting weaker toward the periphery—would go as follows:

1. The patient : therapist
2. The therapist : supervisor
3. The supervisor : supervisory group, of which the supervisor is a part

As I heard the supervisory session a second time in the peer supervisory group, I became more clearly aware of the rage, the helplessness, the irritability, defeatism, entrapment, and stupor that I had felt with Fred during the actual supervisory session. I also became more clearly aware of *his* rage, helplessness, defeatism, entrapment, irritability, and *his* stupor with his patient. I believe both Fred and I were peripherally aware of this—he in the therapy hour with his patient and I in the supervisory hour with him.

It was during the supervisory study group that all of this came into focus for me. Jim and Philip queried why I had not pressed the candidate, why I had not been in touch with my own rage, and why I had been rather passive in letting him continue to shut me out. I then felt caught—caught between Fred and the supervisory hour and pressures and queries from the peer supervisory group. In a sense, I was between Fred and the supervisory group in the same way that Fred was between his patient and his supervisor. At the end of the peer-group session, Jim shrieked, "My God, how is it possible to do therapy in the first place."

The supervisor is caught in the middle, as is the candidate—the supervisor having both an affective "inside" partially merged experience in supervision and a cognitive external view as part of the peer supervisory group. This affords an excellent opportunity to study how the processes of emotional learning and emotional communication transpire in therapy and in supervision.

THE SUPERVISOR'S SUBJECTIVE RESPONSES

I would like to tell you what my subjective responses were when I heard a replay of the supervisory hour during the peer-group session. As previously mentioned, I became more fully aware of how enraged, frustrated, and anxious I felt with Fred—but mostly at myself for feeling this way without full awareness during the supervisory session.

I could rationalize and say that my supervision was didactic-teaching and therefore I wanted to focus (explosively—typing slip!) exclusively on the patient and the therapist—but that is a rationalization.

Was this my countertransference? To some extent, yes, because of a family history of the men being overprotective of the women. But I have little difficulty in venting rage or exasperation and in taking strong stands in supervision—with Fred and in life. So at best, my countertransference is a partial explanation.

What was I being sucked into (in this parallel process)? Fred was relating to me as the patient had to him. I was experiencing Fred's anxieties, frustration, and the like—*not* primarily my own. Why? It was *not* a logical process, nor was it consciously "in the service of learning."

Rather, it felt toxic. I was taking over Fred's feelings, perceptions, and so forth—or, rather, they were taking me over. I was experiencing his dilemma firsthand, his impasse that was, as he experienced it with his patient and I in supervision with him, beyond my control. During the peer supervisory group *replay* of the tape, I doodled and scribbled: "Why did I not see my rage??? I feel shut out . . . neglected . . . I feel irritable . . . I can't function, can't think . . . I can't get across to him . . . He won't listen to me." My BIG, BIG doodles: "Why did I *not* cope with his rage??? . . . My irritability."

I was *stuck in the situation,* just as he was. There was no resolution— just this exasperating, anxiety-laden, *unclear thinking process going nowhere.*

Why did this happen to me? Freud's Latin epigraph (1900/1954) to *The Interpretation of Dreams* came to mind, which, translated, reads as follows: If I cannot bend the Higher Powers, I will move the Infernal Region.

I felt that I could not move or alter the situation from above, and therefore I had no choice but to take the lower route, to be there, so as to grasp what the process was all about, to make cohesion out of *my confusion,* which mirrored or was bent to the shape of the therapist's confusion. It was as if *I* was in this bind with these feelings and perceptions in me and as if I had had to resolve this situation for myself.

I must reiterate: Had I not *reheard* the tape during the peer-group supervision, I am not sure if all this would have surfaced as effectively and economically in terms of time. My hunch is that Fred and I would have struggled for several more sessions—he with his feelings in therapy and I with his feelings in me in supervision, and that it would have surfaced but that it would have taken longer to do so. Also, the intensity and the immediacy of the experience would have been defrayed.

Having the peer supervisory group available allowed me to experience some of the candidate's bind-feelings-perceptions-responses in supervision with *my* "supervisors" (Philip and Jim). I was now in the learner's seat. I was experiencing the process simultaneously from the internal (from below) and external (the overview, from above) vantage points.

The internal view was affective, uncritical, or at best only partially aware of what was going on. Affective experience was high, and cognition lagged behind. The external view, supplied by the supervisory group, afforded the necessary criticality and cognition, some of which I had lost, hopefully, only temporarily.

The juxtaposition of the toxic, affective, and uncritical merged response with the supervisee and the criticality gleaned from the peer group (of which my latent criticality was a part) was discordant and anxiety provoking. I felt as if two conflicting forces were operating simultaneously on me or in me. I was now confronted with my anxieties, blind spots, and ineptness as the learner (the candidate's role) in relation to my "supervisors" (Philip and Jim). Of course, there is the question of how much of this is sheer induced parallel process and how much of this is my own countertransference.

PREPARING FOR THE SECOND SUPERVISORY HOUR

In anticipation of the second supervisory hour with Fred, I reviewed the contents of the previous session, his apparent countertransference impasse with the patient, and how to best proceed in supervision.

During the first supervisory session, I had focused on (1) Helen's way of relating to Mel; (2) Helen's way of relating to Fred (the same in general as with Mel); (3) attempting further understanding of the patient's history and repetition compulsion of fearing to trust the man and of being deserted by him; (4) attempting to help Fred see some countertransferential response in his way of coping with Helen—but with little success; and (5) Fred's limited awareness of his dissociated rage and irritability that he did not sufficiently recognize during the therapy session, with the result that he felt sullen, resentful, submissive, defeated—or needling and pressuring Helen as unaware expressions of his rage.

I formulated Fred's countertransferential response to Helen as follows:

1. The fear of upsetting the hysterical woman, therefore not challenging her and needing to take care of her. Similarly, the supervisory peer-group, fearing to upset me, protected me when confronted with my anxiety indicators and needed to take care of me by not "upsetting" me by questioning as to why I did not confront Fred.
2. The fear of being flooded by the hysterical woman.
3. The fear of being flooded by, or triggering off, his own rage or anxiety, which he fears will run away with him.

For myself, I realized I had not focused on or discussed Fred's relationship to me and his impact on me. I decided my task would be how to use the Fred–Lee (therapist–supervisor) relationship, which is the parallel process of the Helen–Fred (patient–therapist) relationship, for elucidating what transpired between them in therapy.

THE SECOND SUPERVISORY SESSION

In the service of brevity, I will focus primarily on the parallel process during the supervisory session. I will attempt to summarize the data with occasional verbatim vignettes interspersed to communicate the flow of topics and the flavor of the session.

Fred started the session with a review of the patient's gains and her current impasse: Whether to leave or stay in the relationship with Mel.

Fred then reviewed some aspects of the last supervisory hour: How he felt at an impasse to be heard by the patient, his increasing awareness of his anger at her, and his "too mild" confronting of her.

FRED: We then talked last session about how come I didn't do more confronting of her the first time around. We talked about how I had been very angry with her at the time and had sort of mildly confronted her but didn't confront her as rigorously as I ought to have, and we talked a little bit about why I might not have. I imagine it had to do with, as far as I could tell, probably my being afraid about not being caretaking, producing too much anxiety, impressing her, and—I have to take care of people, protect them so that they don't experience too much upset. We also talked a good deal about her impact on me. Well, Lee had mentioned also something about how whether or not I had discussed with her, her impact on Mel and whether she has done things or behaved in ways that caused him to spend less time with her. And I said, "Not really."

As Fred continued to present material, I tried to get him to focus on it. He would respond with "Yes, yes," interrupt me, and continue on his own way. During this time I was in touch with my frustration and irritability.

At this juncture I attempted to get Fred to focus on what was transpiring between Helen and him.

LEE: [*Summarizing*] What happened, though, was that she dropped one of her sessions. She's not interested in putting out and working to find the money for that session. She's unhappy in the past at the thought of your going on vacation. You are supposed to be there for her, but she's not supposed to be there for you. She wants you there in a holding position, but she wants to have her privacy. She needs time for herself. But the point is that something was going on between the two of you that was very similar to what was going on with Mel. In both cases, she starts off with enormous need, and she pulls back, and you're supposed to be there for her. But she's not supposed to be there for you. And then she comes in, she has a dream—she remembers having a dream.

Fred was momentarily flustered since he had forgotten the dream, and then he did recall it.

FRED: Oh, that's right. She said, "Oh, I have terrible news." I said, "What's that?" She said, "I had a dream, but I can't remember it." That's how we got into that thing about working. She said, "I have terrible news. I had a dream, but I can't remember it." Oh, by the way, I didn't really think anything about what we discussed last time, about the problems with Mel and—I just didn't feel like thinking about it. So I said something like, "You're telling me in no uncertain terms you don't feel like working."

LEE: In retrospect *now*, as you review this in your mind's eye, that session, and she tells you this, what did you experience?

FRED: I was annoyed with her.

LEE: What did you do with the annoyance?

FRED: Well, I teased her to some extent, or I needled her, not teased her. I needled her about—first I said that she didn't want to work, and then I think that there were a couple of comments. I don't remember what the content was, though I know the attitude was needling.

LEE: You needled her.

FRED: I needled her. That's right. That was sort of the attitude although some of the content of it was some confrontation about her not working.

LEE: You remember last week when she told you the dream—that she didn't remember? You made a fist and then you went "HUH!"

FRED: I remember something like a fist, but not—that was here, you mean.

[*Everyone talking at once*]

MADGE: [*To Lee*] Why didn't you say that Fred was angry?

LEE: I knew Fred was angry, but I didn't know *I* was angry. But seriously, Fred, were you aware of the fact that you were angry? "I had a dream, but I don't remember the dream. You know I don't remember anything."

FRED: I really, I remember being annoyed with her. I don't remember being very angry. I remember being very angry with her when she cut back one session. Then I was very angry. The last session I don't remember being very angry. I just remember being annoyed. If I was more angry, then I wasn't aware of it.

As I attempted to get Fred to focus, he became increasingly scattered. I found myself increasingly pressuring Fred, and his becoming evasive.

At this juncture, Madge interrupted us.

MADGE: I'm going to say something at this point. I have been feeling the last few minutes that you are doing with Fred what Fred does with his patient; and I'm sort of identifying with the patient and saying, "Stop! Slow down. Stop badgering. Let him say what he wants. It's moving in on him so much." I mean, not to protect you, 'cause you know . . .

LEE: I'm needling him; I'm pushing him.

MADGE: Yeah, and it's not like you.

I asked Fred if he was aware of the anger and irritability the patient evoked in him. He replied that he was somewhat aware of it during the session but much more so after it.

FRED: Now, if you're asking me what I do with those feelings, why don't I say, "Look, I'm feeling such and such," or find some other way of presenting it. [*Long pause*] Well, all I can think of is that, ah, it's hard for me to really be angry directly with any of my other patients. I tend not to become angry, I really don't share that very much with them. I might turn it around into a confrontation about something that if I understand what it means, I might—as I did that time—I think I confronted her about not working—and I was annoyed about it at the time. When she cut back one session, I was feeling very angry. I think I was afraid to confront her because I knew I felt that I would start yelling at her.

LEE: You were afraid that you'd become hysterical with her, and that you'd be too strong or too attacking.

FRED: Well, or hurt her feelings, push her away. I'd be very critical, and that—I'm not supposed to do that. You know, that was my problem, and I had to find a way to deal with what she was doing. But saying, "I'm furious with you," or "I'm very angry with you, and I feel you're pulling away"—I don't know. Maybe, also, I don't want to directly get into that kind of emotional entanglement with a patient, acknowledging how strongly I might feel one way or the other. That keeps me at a certain distance, I suppose, too.

LEE: Well, maybe it's a distortion on my part. I'd like to tell you what I experienced during the last session, and I think on the replay I heard it with greater impact. *I* felt irritable and that in some way, whenever I would try to make contact with you and get you to focus on what was going on between you and her, you would go back to Mel. I began to see the whole thing lacked directness, and there was a lack of contact. There was a quality of, I felt, elusiveness, which is not typical of you, and I felt frustrated and irritable, and trapped in some kind of way.

MADGE: I think there's something to that. Fred, were you aware that Lee felt that frustrated?

FRED: [*Sighs*] No. I felt I liked the session. I felt that I had left with what I thought were two valuable ideas. I felt the session, as I told Madge, was a little more formal because of the tape; but also I felt that it was more vigorous, and I didn't feel you were irritable or irritated particularly.

LEE: I wasn't aware of it at the time.

FRED: But *I* wasn't aware of it either.

LEE: [*To Madge*] What did you experience as we were discussing the session?

MADGE: Just now?

LEE: Before.

MADGE: Before was different from now.

LEE: How was it before?

MADGE: Before I thought that you were both angry at Helen, and I thought, "Yes, she's irritating." She doesn't remember. She's not working. And I thought what you are doing with Fred, and Fred was doing with her is what you obsessives would do. And she doesn't— she won't hear you. What I object to with this whole thing—with this hysterical patient, you know—and granted, it's my bias—is that you people act as if it is within her conscious power that she should recall a dream to work better, to talk about what's going on between the two of you. And experientially, she really can't do that at the moment. And I think when you make interpretations and you tie up genetic material, she thinks she's trying very hard. I don't think she would know what you meant. If you had suggested another way of dealing with her, which I thought was more effective, in terms of saying how you felt or telling her what you think she's doing, not feeling or thinking—I think she might be able to hear you. She can't do what you're asking her to do.

LEE: In retrospect, about the supervisory session, as with everything in life, when you hear it another time, you can hear it at a more profound level. And I think you're right, Madge, because what I heard was that when I tried to make contact with you, Fred, you were evasive in the way you report her being evasive with you. And I felt that I was responding with irritability to a situation where I couldn't make contact with someone and where there was evasion in some kind of way, wittingly or unwittingly, I don't understand why or how.

FRED: The question about why I have difficulty sometimes, maybe many times, confronting the patient or using the feelings—I can't solve that or excuse that question. I can't answer that right now exactly. The trouble with being angry with my patients in some ways, I think, goes against my conscience in certain ways. I have trouble sometimes believing that because I have a feeling, it's not necessarily induced by the patient; it might be my headache or hang-up about the patient. So to use that with them, to me, sometimes is this side of being omnipotent, which I think a lot of people do.

LEE: I agree wholeheartedly with you there. You have to be very careful to know what you're responding to. But one thing did come through, very clearly to me, was that had *I* listened more carefully, had I been— put it this way: I was only half aware of what was going on in some of the feelings between you and the patient, and I was only half aware of what was going on in *my* feelings in supervision with you.

See, for me, the key issue when I listened to that session again was, Why is it that I didn't say to you, "Hey, Fred, I'm feeling irritable." And then it dawned on me. That really is a key issue with Helen. You're not saying to her, "Hey, what are you doing to me?" Is it my imagination? I feel irritable and exasperated, and I can't make contact; and I feel defeated. What's going on between us? Something along that line.

MADGE: Because you're not blaming her.

LEE: That's interesting.

FRED: Say that again.

MADGE: The way Lee verbalized it just now is not blaming you. You do your thinking for yourself. He's saying, "*I* feel frustrated, *I* feel angry, *I* can't make contact. What's going on between the *two of us?*"

LEE: Do you feel I attacked you this session?

FRED: I don't usually feel that. No, I don't feel it was an attack. I feel like we were arguing. It doesn't feel like an attack on me. Uh, in fact, if you take a strong position on that, then that frees me to take a strong position back. I mean, I can feel myself being tempted to argue with you, some of it just to wrestle, for wrestling's sake. But I don't really— I can't say that I really mind that; in some ways I like it. I don't like hearing that I was evasive; it's not pleasant to hear that.

LEE: Is there a reason in your own background, without going into detail, why you should be that caretaking?
[*Long pause*]

FRED: Yes. I think my sister and I are like that with my mother, that we were very careful about her. We were very well behaved. We had occasional battles with her, but they were relatively rare; and I think— my understanding of our behavior wasn't so much that we were frightened of their not loving us or becoming furious with us. She got angry, but she wasn't really that frightening when she got angry, but that she was very nervous. She was very anxious. I don't think we really knew until later, certainly by high school. But before that I don't think we really knew how anxious she was. I had mentioned that my mother, when we moved to a new neighborhood, was phobic for quite a while, didn't go out very much. I didn't even know it. I never realized why my father was shopping on Saturday until many years later. So I never could understand why my sister and I were so good as kids. It didn't make sense to me that we were just afraid that they would get angry; that never seemed to be quite enough. But that in combination with my mother being very anxious and worried, the idea of feeling guilty and crummy because she would be upset, and some other areas where I think I did things to please her that I didn't even really want to do, because she would be hurt or something like that.

LEE: So without going into any details, in your own growing-up years there was limited opportunity to use yourself honestly or with authentic feelings, especially if they were strong feelings or negative feelings or separate feelings.

FRED: I think that it was with feeling negative feelings that it was true. The other kind, I don't know. I think that I don't know so much about my father, but I think my mother was kind of affectionate, mushy kind of stuff with the little kids but not once they got older, as far as I can see. She was very huggy, and that kind of stuff, with babies; but my recollection was after that she was really not that way any more; she was available but not very emotional. She reserved that kind of stronger expression of feeling much more for infants, for my sons. But I think it's much less with my nephews, who are now 6 and 10. She's much more reserved with them.

I think that I always felt, many times felt frustrated with women, the girls when I was in high school, because they always seemed like they were, the pie was being held out and I couldn't quite get to it. Very frustrating. It was all out there, and you can't quite, didn't know quite how to get to it, couldn't get through. I would find if I were in a situation where that was going on, I would prefer, I didn't realize this until later, but I would prefer to get out of it than to feel the frustration and the anger about it.

LEE: Well, just try to bring it back to the case material now. Because here is a woman who holds out the pie, and then it's not available; she's very frustrating. She starts off being very warm and needy, and that's the kootchy-coo stage. And now she's very remote and distant; she's holding you off. So there are elements of needing to protect, experiencing her distance. So this is material of your own that would somehow play into it. But we're not here to do that analytic job. That's your thing. But we are trying, we do try to understand what this woman could trigger off in you, and therefore your need to avoid contacts of a certain kind with her, which prevents you from using yourself in terms of what she needs in therapy.

[*Fred further notes the similarities between his patient and his mother and the similarities in the way he responds to both of them.*]

LEE: You know, something that happened between us might be of help, in keeping in mind. I found myself on the replay experiencing with greater consciousness my irritability. Right? And as it came out here, you picked up that I was coming on very strong in some kind of way, maybe angry; I was coming on strong.

MADGE: Pushy.

LEE: And I think that when I feel frustrated and impotent and irritable and manipulated—that when I finally do start to move, I move too strongly, perhaps. I think that's an all-too-human tendency.

FRED: Maybe that is something of the way I responded to her. Because I think what happened was that I would translate the feeling into speaking to her more vigorously, more confrontingly, and maybe some more needling, instead of saying I'm feeling irritated. So maybe that's very similar.

LEE: So what she succeeds in doing is provoking rage, rejection, distancing, finally disgust, and the other person walking away.

MADGE: The thing she wants least.

LEE: Whenever I tape a session, a supervisory session or an analytic hour, and play it back—even if it is a good hour—I realize how not so good it really is in some kind of way. How much better it could be with hindsight. Maybe that's the tragedy of our work. We're always writing first copy of our material. We never see the finished product. But on the replay, I certainly began to realize that I wasn't using me, and I felt trapped and irritable, and that was what you were reporting going on with this patient. That I wasn't experiencing my anger and/or my frustration with you, which is not in my usual style, as you know. I'm not very shy when it comes to that. And for whatever reasons, I was not using this part of me, with you; and that in retrospect, I think I was responding to Helen's vulnerability in you, which you had picked up, and were reporting and experiencing. So that something is going on; I can't make it clearer because I don't know enough about that process yet. This kind of induction where you and your patient merge in some kind of way. And then what happens is that I am responding to you and to her in the same kind of way. And I want to say that I, seeing you in supervision, know you were different with her, in discussing her, than you were, for example, in discussing an obsessive male patient. There is something about this girl's anxiety and your fear of moving in on her which is very anxiety laden to you.

And I think you are right, Madge. She does things which alienate people. She doesn't know what she does, she doesn't know how she does it, and Fred, if she could learn what and how with you, it would be of enormous help. And for her to learn that, you have to be authentic and to be able to share with her what you experience her impact to be. Not irritated, not enraged, as I started to overrespond to Fred, but without hostility. Then she's not being attacked, and that something is being examined, her self-defeating impact. That's a very difficult thing to do because I think we're talking of an analytic growing edge, and something which your patient needs from you, Fred, which is anxiety laden for you but which you cannot postpone in the service of her therapy.

[*There is further dialogue on this theme.*]

FRED: Well, I'm not leaving the session with more of a sense of Helen, but more reflecting on the difficulty that I may have in sharing some of these kinds of feelings. Not so much to apply it immediately to Helen, but even as I was sitting here, I was thinking about where else this happens with a patient. Last time the feeling was, I have something to work on with Helen. Now I have something specific to go on—an approach, and so on. So it's a different thing.

THE MODEL

At this juncture, I would like to state again the model for this clinical study. It includes two candidates working in cosupervision with a supervisor; a peer supervisory group of which the supervisor is a member;

and the replay and study of the supervisory tapes in the peer supervisory group. Obviously, the model permits the simultaneous study-teach-
ing of the overlapping processes of therapy and supervision.

Perhaps more important, the model also permits the study of the
overlapping and patternings of the relationships between patient and therapist, patient-therapist and supervisor, and patient-therapist-supervisor
and the supervisory peer study group. This permits the supervisor to
simultaneously be the observer and the observed, the expert and the
learner, empathic and cognitive, participant and observer.

Hopefully, the model permits the study of such basic but subtle
processes, in therapy and in supervision, as empathy and participant
observation, and most assuredly the ubiquitous, little understood, usually overlooked, but potent parallel and reciprocal processes.

SOME CLINICAL IMPLICATIONS OF THE PARALLEL PROCESS FOR SUPERVISION

I believe the parallel process in supervision is probably always
there. We in our peer supervisory study group were amazed at the
consistency with which the parallel process was present—either in the
foreground or background. It was usually clearly discerned by the peer
group, once we became alerted to look for it, but at best in the partial
awareness of the supervisor.

Members of one supervisory study group that met over two years
report that the parallel process always occurs, regardless of who presents, and that the supervisor is usually at least partially unaware and
startled by apparent oversights when they are pointed out to him.

When in the midst of the parallel process, the candidate and the
supervisor are each struggling through for themselves—each is at his
own growing edge. The implications: Obviously, in parallel processing,
the controlling variable is the supervisor. For the parallel process to be
truly usable in teaching-learning in supervision, the supervisor must be
aware of himself, what he experiences in the supervisory relationship. If
the supervisor is not "inside" and actively participating in the process
but rather functions cognitively and separate from the ongoing process—a didactic approach—the focus inevitably falls on the candidate's
countertransference to his patient, his "inability" or "negative attitude"
toward learning in supervision. The supervision becomes a morass.

Where there is parallel process, there is *always* transference and
countertransference operative for the patient, analyst candidate, and

probably for the supervisor as well. Each has to be clearly seen, weighed, and separated out.

The parallel process occurs more dramatically when the patient, therapist, and supervisor have a juncture or crossing of blind spots with resultant heightened dysjunctive anxiety and decline in empathy. Examples, in the case discussed are: the patient's transference to the therapist as father or lover; the therapist's countertransference to the patient as mother; and the supervisor's countertransference to his own family history of overprotecting the woman who is easily upset. I should like to underscore that these overlapping transferences and countertransferences are operative *without* awareness.

What makes the parallel process work? First, we have the overlapping transference and countertransference factors. Second is the therapist's confusion—of being caught in a bind he cannot leave or resolve—and therefore the need to preconsciously react to the problems in supervision with himself in the patient's role and the supervisor in the analyst's role. I believe part of this is in the service of emotional learning in supervision. But I must again emphasize that once *in* the process, what transpires is no longer in the service of cognition-growth-learning but rather in the service of a more primary process: The need to go beyond one's impasse that is authentically experienced, even though the source may be primarily evoked in the parallel process and only secondarily derive from the supervisor's own countertransference.

I should like to reiterate: Though the parallel process may at times be a small or a large part of the supervisory relationship, it is always there. When the supervisor and student analyst are not aware of it, a glorious learning opportunity is missed. When the parallel process is not recognized, there is the danger that what transpires will be understood solely in terms of transference and countertransference. The analyst–supervisor relationship may then deteriorate in the same way as did the patient–analyst relationship—an unaware parallel processing is going on with the therapist and the supervisor bending to the contours of the patient's pathology. When this occurs, the supervisor frequently shows the same behavior with the therapist that the therapist showed with the patient. Searles (1955), in discussing a group supervisory research seminar, reports the following:

> We have been impressed not only with the influence of the seminar upon the therapeutic relationship (an influence which came to be clearly beneficial), but also with the striking influence which the current mode of relatedness between patient and therapist exerted upon the mode of relatedness among the members of the seminar. The influence in this latter direction was effected, apparently, both by the therapist's verbal and nonverbal communica-

tions to us and, very importantly, by our hearing the patient's and therapist's own affect-laden voices from the recordings. Most impressive of all was the capacity of the schizophrenic patient, whose anxiety was generally so much more intense than our own, to influence the therapist's functioning and, in turn, our relatedness within the group. (p. 146)

It is my contention that good supervision cannot take place without awareness of the parallel process, without which pathological processes may win out. Or there may be some preconscious collusion between the supervisor and candidate; there may even be an ongoing love affair with minimal or no attendant anxiety or dysjunction between them, but also peripheral pseudolearning and pseudogrowth.

THEORETICAL DISCUSSION OF THE PARALLEL PROCESS

The Parallel Process and Empathy

What is this process where three different people (Jim, Philip, and Lee) or five (if we include Madge and Fred) are all evoked in the same receptive, plastic (moldable) way?—that we are all evoked to respond in the same uncritical manner?

Please note that we are *not* speaking of "acting out," which implies that each of us would respond countertransferentially to unique aspects of his dissociated self and that each would respond in his own style. To the contrary, we are speaking about an opposite phenomenon where unique and disparate persons are all evoked to respond in a similar and uncritical way.

This process is normal (normative) emotional learning and emotional communication and does not involve conscious mentation. This process of emotional learning and emotional communication can be identified as H. S. Sullivan's (1947) basic concept of *empathy*.

If the observations of our peer-group seminar are valid, we three, while hearing the first supervisory tape, were evoked to react in the same unthinking way. This was true when the evoked state was pleasant and not anxiety provoking. Responding in the same uncritical way was also true when the evoked state was noxious or anxiety provoking. Our similar responses were geared to voiding these unpleasant intrusions. Again and again we were struck by how much of our responses were uncritical and unaware.

All of this sounds like *repetition compulsion*, where the patient evokes or programs a certain response to fit the interpersonal integration he needs to gratify his repetition compulsion. Somehow, what is evoked has implicit within it a programmed or anticipated response. All this is communicated and received and responded to without awareness; that is, by empathy—the noncognitive process of emotional learning and emotional communication. For example, the tug of the evoked response was so strong that, upon hearing the replay of the first supervisory session, Jim and Philip were evoked to experience the same apathy, loss of focus, impotence, frustration, and irritability as I had during the supervision.

How much of one's behavior is due to cognition (conscious thinking); how much is due to empathic response in the interpersonal field where one is evoked to respond with a nonaware paralleling of the anticipated response; and how these two ways of learning, communicating, and responding—the empathic and the cognitive—how these resonate and ultimately determine behavior poses a most fascinating question. As we explored this further in detail in our study group, we became less and less certain that we were cognitively on top of it all.

The Parallel Process and Participation Observation

The study of the parallel process offers some implications for aspects of H. S. Sullivan's (1954) concept of participation observation.

In the participant part, the therapist enters into the patient's subjective interpersonal field. In the empathy part (emotional learning and emotional communication), the therapist experiences a tug (noncognitive) toward paralleling the interpersonal response needed and evoked in him to complete the patient's repetition compulsion or anticipated integration. For example, Fred responded to Helen, as did Mel, with the same evoked affects of irritability and avoidance that were programmed by Helen's need for this kind of interpersonal integration.

In the observer part of the participant observer, cognition dominates. There is *always* a lag between participation and observation—objectification comes later after the primary process data have been apprehended—evoked in the empathy.

We are speaking of *participant* as an empathic function and *observer* as a cognitive function. *The empathic tugs toward an uncritical merged parallel process response that is contoured to the patient's anticipated interpersonal integration.* In this sense, the attuned therapist as participant is constantly experiencing emotional learning and communication evoked by his patient—a parallel process contoured by the patient's interpersonal integration needs. The process is initiated by, evoked by, and centered in the patient's self. The therapist as observer experiences himself as cognitive (thinking), responding with a delayed reaction, autonomous and centered in his own need system.

THE RECIPROCAL PROCESS

By reciprocal process, I refer to the intrapersonal response evoked in the recipient in the parallel process.

What is this process where the supervisor (Lee) acts out with at most partial awareness the dissociated and unacceptable aspects of the supervisee (Fred)? The same question can be raised regarding Fred the therapist acting out dissociated and unacceptable aspects of Helen, the patient.

When we talk of parallel processes, we are in the realm of field theory; that is, all respondees who are unique are responding in similar nonunique ways to the conscious and preconscious cues of the evoker. In Sullivan's terms, "We are more simply human than otherwise."

However, parallel processing does not explain the *intrapersonal* process evoked within the recipient in the parallel process. This reciprocal process—the intrapersonal response of the recipient to the evoker in the interpersonal field—has fascinating implications clinically and theoretically. For example, the interface between the intrapersonal and interpersonal fields may help us in understanding the intrapersonal operations that make interpersonal integrations work, that make them predictable.

How does the reciprocal process work? Perhaps my subjective experience with Fred during the first supervisory session that surfaced during the first supervisory peer-group discussion can shed light on at least my reciprocal process—which, hopefully, may be typical.

> What was I being sucked into [in this parallel process]? Fred was relating to me as the patient had to him. I was experiencing Fred's anxieties, frustration, etc., not primarily my own. Why? It was *not* a logical process, nor was it consciously "in the service of learning." Rather, it felt toxic. I was taking over Fred's feelings, perceptions, and so on, or, rather, they were taking me over. I was experiencing his dilemma firsthand, his impasse that was—as he experienced it with his patient and I in supervision with him—beyond my control. During the peer supervisory group *replay* of the tape, I doodled and scribbled: "Why did I not see my rage??? I feel shut out . . . neglected . . . I feel irritable . . . I can't function, can't think . . . I can't get across to him . . . He won't listen to me" My BIG, BIG doodles: "Why did I *not* cope with his rage??? My irritability!"
>
> I was *stuck in the situation*, just as he was. There was no resolution, just this exasperating, anxiety laden, *not clear thinking process* going nowhere. I felt that I could not move or alter the situation to make cohesion out of *my*

The Third Ear

PHILIP M. BROMBERG

> One of the peculiarities of this third ear[1] is that it works in two ways. It can catch what other people do not say, but only feel and think; and it can also be turned inward. It can hear voices from within the self that are otherwise not audible because they are drowned out by the noise of our conscious thought processes. The student of psychoanalysis is advised to listen to those inner voices with more attention than to what "reason" tells about the unconscious.
>
> Theodor Reik

INTRODUCTION

Among Freud's (1912/1958) basic ground rules for establishing the psychoanalytic situation, he describes the appropriate stance for listening to the patient and refers to the proposed technique as "a very simple one" (p. 111).

> It consists simply in not directing one's notice to anything in particular and in maintaining the same "evenly-suspended attention" (as I have called it) in the face of all one hears. . . . Or to put it purely in terms of technique: "He should simply listen, and not bother about whether he is keeping anything in mind." (pp. 111–112)

---

[1]The expression *the third ear,* which I borrowed from Theodor Reik (1949), was, according to him (footnote, p. 144) originally borrowed from Nietzsche (*Beyond Good and Evil,* 1891/1967, Part VIII, p. 246). The influence of Reik's work in writing the present chapter is not intended to suggest any formal connection with the interpersonal approach to psychoanalysis, but rather an appreciation of the similar humanity in Reik's clinical thinking and the richness of its expression, particularly with regard to the experience of becoming an analyst.

PHILIP M. BROMBERG • Supervising Analyst, William Alanson White Institute of Psychiatry, Psychoanalysis and Psychology, New York, New York 10023, and Assistant Clinical Professor of Medical Psychology, College of Physicians and Surgeons, Columbia University, New York, New York 10027.

Few analysts today would agree that what Freud described is simple, and few psychoanalytic supervisors would consider it simple to teach. The Zen monk Takuin, when asked how long it took him to paint one of his portraits of the legendary Daruma, is said to have replied: "Ten minutes and 80 years." It is an answer that expresses a non-western view of both the nature of man and the nature of education. A Westerner who says it takes 10 minutes and 80 years to be able to do what Takuin did is usually talking of the years of study and practice necessary to develop the skill, compared to the brief time spent in rendering the particular piece of art. To the Japanese, the 80 years refer to the self-realization needed to become the person who can paint Daruma, while the 10 minutes signifies the study and practice of the necessary technical skill no matter how lengthy that "10 minutes" might be in measured time.

In the following pages I will outline my current clinical perspective on the process of psychoanalytic supervision. It is a process that, when it goes well, I see as bridging the boundary between the "10 minutes" and the "80 years" in the development of a psychoanalyst. But in order to be as clear as possible about how I see supervision of psychoanalysis, I feel it would be helpful to first clarify how I see psychoanalysis itself, and the interpersonal approach in particular.

In a paper attempting to compare the interpersonal paradigm with the classical Freudian model, Merton Gill (1982) stated tongue in cheek that "an analyzable patient is a patient with whom the analyst can maintain the illusion of neutrality." It is precisely because this remark from a classically trained analyst was made with humor, that it so beautifully underlines the weariness with which psychoanalysts continue to grapple with an unresolved philosophical dilemma that has its roots as far back as man has systematically thought about the nature of his own relationship to the universe.

Consider, for example, the two neo-Confucian schools of thought. The first postulates "the investigation of things leading to the extension of knowledge" and implies the objective study of things within the universe from the stance of an outside observer. The second holds that "the universe is the mind and the mind the universe." This position teaches the realization of what is already within oneself by allowing full confrontation between the self and the other so as to reveal the psychological realities behind appearances. Now consider a statement from the current psychoanalytic literature (Abrams & Shengold, 1978, p. 402). In discussing the differences between what they call "the *traditional* model and the *new* model of the psychoanalytic situation" and the fact that "some analysts have developed substantially different views of the psychoanalytic situation," Abrams and Shengold report that "in the new model . . . the psychoanalytic situation is seen primarily as an *encounter* between two people, rather than as a setting whose purpose is the examination of the intrapsychic processes of one of them." Then, as now, the truth is elusive, and the line between "neo-Confucian" and "neoconfusion" is not always clear. Fundamental differences in how far we can legitimately depart from Freud and still call what we do psychoanalysis have woven into the fabric of the psychoanalytic literature two threads whose colors have been historically difficult to bring into harmony. One emphasizes the primacy of interpretation and conscious insight, with transference being the chief source of data through which insight occurs. The other emphasizes the interpersonal experience of the patient–analyst relationship, with transference being the most vivid and immediate experiential element in the overall process, one aspect of which involves insight. To put it another way, the first perspective, which is most readily identified with Freud's structural theory (Freud, 1923/1961), is more *content*-oriented than the other. Its clinical structure has been well expressed by Arlow & Brenner (1966):

> Psychoanalysis aims at nothing less than a major realignment of the forces within a patient's mind, a realignment which is to be achieved by means of interpretation and insight. . . . Accordingly, in the psychoanalytic situation, a set of conditions is arranged in which the functioning of the patient's mind, the thoughts and images which emerge into consciousness, are as far as is humanly possible, endogenously determined. . . . This is what is uniquely psychoanalytic. Because the psychoanalytic situation is relatively uncontaminated by the intrusion of ordinary, interpersonal relationships, the interaction of the three components of the mind—the ego, id, and superego—may be studied in a more objective way. (pp. 30–32)

The ordinary interpersonal relationship between patient and analyst, to the degree it is not analyzed, is thus viewed as a contaminant of the analytic situation. The one value assigned to the nontransferential bond (the therapeutic alliance) is that of a necessary tool for the analysis to proceed. It is treated as a means to an end—a working collaboration between the observing function of the analyst and the mature portion of the patient's ego. The observing function of the analyst can thus be theoretically kept separate from the analyst as a participant in a relationship, and conceptualized as a tool with which to objectively gather and organize the patient's unconscious fantasy content as revealed by his unevoked, endogenous associations. Since the psychoanalytic situation has been divided theoretically into two components—how to listen and what to do (i.e., technique)—the traditional training of classical analysts has been similarly shaped around the teaching of a listening stance and the teaching of intervention (i.e., breaking into the flow of associations) as separate entities. This polarity is further reflected in the model for the supervisory process itself. At the 1974 conference of the committee on psychoanalytic education (COPE) of the American Psychoanalytic Association, it was stated (Goodman, 1977, p. 36) as follows:

> The dual requirements of precise content analysis and of nondefensive utilization of the material should be met in a flexible manner. *The constant attuning of the analyst to the ego state and the analytic process, to determine the appropriate dosage of interpretations, etc.,* may be looked upon as a process parallel to the teaching relationship of the supervisor and student analyst. (Italics added)

The problem with this perspective in unmodified form, as its critics as well as some adherents have pointed out, is that because it is cast in overly mechanistic and content-oriented imagery, it can too easily lead to a clinical approach that fails to reach the patient and fails to let the patient reach himself through reaching the analyst. The patient may simply talk about himself without ever *being* himself in the analysis. The old self-contained "truths" are simply replaced by a *new* egoistic image of "analytic self-awareness," which changes nothing because the current character structure remains impermeable. A supervisory process that is similarly patterned runs the same risk. The analytic enterprise or supervisory enterprise is led to a diagnosis of "unanalyzability" or "unsupervisability," or to a drawn-out process of self-indulgent rumination, with the fantasy, which is often shared by both participants, that change will somehow come later.

The interpersonal school of psychoanalysis—and Harry Stack Sullivan in particular—has modified this perspective in a central way by developing and teaching an approach that rebalances the original overemphasis on content—the approach of participant observation. It has helped shift the clinical perspective from content to process as the primary data base, and in so doing it has made the task of maintaining "evenly suspended attention" more complex for the analyst and more challenging for the supervisor to teach. The interpersonal approach does not view the analyst's participation as a contaminant of the field of observation. Rather, the analyst's participation is seen as an ongoing element in the field of observation and inseparable from it. Part of what the analyst must always be observing includes the immediate and residual effects of his own participation. This is, of course, equally true for the more classically trained analyst, but it is less built-in to his training. He is educated to rely upon the process of free association and the resistance to it as sufficient and to "simply listen and not bother about whether he is keeping anything in mind." As Freud (1912/1958, p. 112) put it:

What is achieved in this manner will be sufficient for all requirements during the treatment. Those elements of the material which already form a connected context will be at the doctor's conscious disposal; the rest, as yet unconnected and in chaotic disorder, seems at first to be submerged, but rises readily into recollection as soon as the patient brings up something new to which it can be related and by which it can be continued. (Italics added)

A major contribution of the interpersonal approach was to recognize that, despite Freud's genius, he was not accurate in this statement. What is achieved simply by listening in this manner is not sufficient for all requirements during treatment and certainly not for all patients treatable by analysis. Thus, the process of "detailed inquiry" (Sullivan, 1954) into what the patient means, as he is associating, found its place in the analytic situation, and it counterbalanced the earlier classical emphasis on working only with what the patient produced spontaneously as sufficient.

The benefit, however, is not without cost. The listening process becomes more complex as the analyst feels freer to use himself interactively. During an interactive inquiry, the analyst's attention becomes more concentrated and focused. Here, Freud's warning is both accurate and vital (Freud, 1912/1958, p. 112):

For as soon as anyone deliberately concentrates his attention to a certain degree, he begins to select from the material before him; one point will be fixed in his mind with particular clearness and some other will be correspondingly disregarded, and in making this selection he will be following his expectations or inclinations. This however is precisely what must not be done. In making the selection, if he follows his expectations he is in danger of never finding anything but what he already knows; and if he follows his inclinations he will certainly falsify what he may perceive.

The goal, then, albeit a difficult one, is for an analyst working from an interpersonal perspective to be a *skilled* participant observer, and to develop the facility of participating while still maintaining his perspective of the entire analytic field—including his own participation in it. It is the development of this facility that I have in mind when I discuss psychoanalytic supervision and *the third ear*.

There is nothing more disheartening to a student-analyst as the notion that analytic skill is derived not from what you do but from who you are. But he often feels equally disheartened to perceive that despite excellent technique, he feels he is somehow missing the point of it all and is doing what Levenson (1982, p. 5) refers to as "painting by the numbers." As supervisors, how do we facilitate the process that helps these two elements blend? In a recent paper (Bromberg, 1982) I discussed psychoanalytic supervision as an apparent paradox that attempts to teach a set of rules—one of them being spontaneity. What I mean by spontaneity approaches what Reik (1949, p. 20) conveyed when he compared the young analyst to an actor:

> The actor should, when he walks out upon the stage, forget what he has studied at the academy. He must brush it aside as if it had never been there. If he cannot neglect it now, in the moment of real performance—if it has not gone *deep enough* that he can afford to neglect it—then his training wasn't good enough. (Italics added)

For an actor, *deep enough* means being embedded in the role so that all ongoing experience is processed through it. The saying of the lines is an expression of what is experienced, not of what has been learned. For an analyst, *deep enough* means something similar but not identical—the ability to hear in such a way that he *does not have to* play a role. His interventions are an expression of what he hears, not what he has learned.

My specific goals as a supervisor are determined by the needs of the person I am supervising, but my fundamental goal that encompasses all of the others is always the same: to supervise in such a way that the "learning of the rules" is gradually blended into a natural and comfortable analytic stance within which appropriate technique is largely a spontaneous outcome of participant observation. Inasmuch as I am trying to help the analyst to look at his interventions as an expression of what he hears, it should come as no surprise that I structure much of the supervision around a method designed as much to improve his hearing as to teach him the principles of clinical psychoanalysis.

PSYCHOANALYTIC SUPERVISION

Reik (1949, pp. 428–429), in discussing his own struggle to integrate *being* and *doing* as an analyst, describes a crisis in the career of Bruno Walter as reported by the conductor in his memoirs. This description could well serve as a model for what I see as the integral relationship between analytic supervision and the "10 minutes and 80 years" in the Zen parable.

> He came to the conclusion that he did not know how to conduct, that . . . "excessive watchfulness of details interfered when I had to anticipate a longer phrase or tried to satisfy the demands of synthetic interpretation." *He increased this watchfulness and self-criticism at the rehearsals. "On the other hand, I vetoed every bit of self-observation during performances, forcing myself to concentrate exclusively upon the music as a whole . . ."* He tried successfully to regain his self-respect and his former firmness of strength. This double method bore fruit and led to a reinvigoration of his musical work. During his perfor-

mances he now felt he could use his growing technical accomplishments; *"that I was able to insert a certain amount of critical listening and observation without jeopardizing the flow and continuity of the music."* (Italics added)

In essence, he is describing a process of self-supervision. He came to the supervisory situation (rehearsal) already an accomplished professional, not a novice. But he came prepared to take apart and reexamine the basic ingredients of what was already the basis for his professional self-esteem in order to mature beyond that.[2] He then allowed the actual performance to play a synthesizing role by restructuring the old perspective with the new data as he was concentrating his full being upon the music *as a whole.* He relied upon the natural process inherent in ego growth to integrate what he learned during rehearsal as he fully and spontaneously invested his "evenly suspended attention" in the music.

Psychoanalytic supervision, in order to be successful, must, in my opinion, provide a set of conditions that facilitates this kind of growth. I have referred to it elsewhere (Bromberg, 1979) as "a change in the self-representation out of which behavior will organically and naturally reflect reorganization of the self at increasingly higher levels of interpersonal maturation" (p. 651).

In supervision the student must be able to scrutinize what he *already* does. He must have an opportunity to hear his sessions, to hear himself with his patient and his patient with himself, in a way that goes beyond what he heard during the sessions as they were in progress. What he hears must be more than that which fits comfortably into his current perspective; but he must also be able to take in what he hears as compatible *enough* with his current perspective so that his need to protect his self-esteem does not get in the way of his gradually integrating the new into the old as he works.

This does not require, in my experience, the need for a particularly supportive or nurturant supervisory atmosphere—at least in the more common usage of those words. Self-disclosure and self-scrutiny in the presence of another person does arouse some anxiety. The student is most often quite able to handle his own self-esteem needs provided that the setting encourages activity and give-and-take between the two participants. This includes questioning and disagreeing, comparing the supervisor's opinion and perspective with his own, freedom to comment in an ongoing way on the supervisory process itself and the supervisor's

---

[2]As in psychoanalytic supervision, the student is most often not a novice as a therapist, but is relatively experienced within his own frame of reference and does not start from "scratch." He instead has to accomodate how he already works as a therapist and grasp a new perspective that cannot simply be added on to the old.

impact, and in general, an atmosphere that encourages self-regulation rather than passive ingestion.

This principle is certainly nothing new to educational theory. Piaget (1936), for example, has emphasized that self-regulatory processes are the basis for all genuine learning. In order for new mental structures to develop from old ones, the person must *act* upon his environment. The passive reception of facts and concepts is unproductive for intellectual growth. Furthermore, in a setting such as analytic supervision, where the facts and concepts may pose a threat to the student's current foundation for his professional self-worth, his activity with the concepts becomes the *one* productive way that he can take care of who he is now while at the same time allowing it to change. If this process is interfered with, some students will retreat into passivity while others will struggle abortively and resentfully against supervisory strangulation.

With regard to students in training at analytic institutes, I have made a similar observation as a teacher—that seminars as opposed to lecture courses evoke a much lower level of hostile integration as a form of intellectual calisthenics. The students tend to listen to the instructor and to each other with greater interest and to be more involved in collaborating on the development of an idea than engaging in virtuoso performances. I have also had the impression that seminars tend to be evaluated by the students with more kindness, as if the seminar experience has an inherent value that makes it less important for the instructor to be brilliant, charismatic, and the like. It is perhaps for the same reason that the best supervisors are those who students do not remember as being particularly clever, because they experienced their own growing effectiveness as the heart of the process.

What do I do as a supervisor? To write about one's clinical approach to psychoanalytic supervision is a difficult task. In one way it includes a feeling often experienced by a supervisee when he is about to present a session to his supervisor. "I'll try to tell you what went on, but you had to have been there to really appreciate it." The mandate—if taken seriously—is much like that given to the supervisee himself: "Say what occurred; present what you do, but also share your conceptual perspective of what you are presenting; reveal all, including the experience of your own participation."

The fact is that a supervisor cannot reveal all, anymore so than can the patient to the analyst or the analyst to the supervisor. Indeed, anyone involved in an event and subsequently choosing to report the event to an observer cannot fully report the details of his own involvement. It is always in part a construction of selected perceptions that then becomes assimilated as though it was a memory of an observed event.

Most people have memories of themselves from childhood or dream of themselves as children—often quite vividly and in great detail—seeing themselves engaged in various activities, as for example, swimming. For the most part these visual images tend to be accepted by them as memories, or at least as derived from memories, unless it is called to their attention that the image is often seen from a perspective that only an outside observer could have had, and it could not have been their own visual percept—as for example, a view of one's back while swimming. We can only remember what we observe, but what we construct becomes our "truth" and our "reality." These are sometimes in jeopardy when we are suddenly required to observe from a different angle.

There is a phenomenon in our field that I have come to refer to as "case-conference cleverness"—the uncanny ability of the members of a case conference to discover what the presenting analyst "missed" and to hear what he did not hear. As in supervision, the presenting analyst's reaction varies. Sometimes he may feel he missed something he should have heard; sometimes he may state that even though he did not hear it he was aware of the issue but working on something else; sometimes he may be the only one in the room who insists he does not hear it. Most often, however, there does seem to be something approaching a core experience of hearing with the group—hearing what the group hears, and sometimes a bit painfully, hearing it for the first time even though he was there originally. He does not necessarily feel, however, that what he missed is what was "really" going on, as is sometimes implied by the group.

The phenomenon is so common and cuts across so many levels of expertise, experience, and character styles that it is clearly reflecting something ubiquitous in the human communication process that is not exclusive to psychoanalysis. At the moment of the original event, which the analyst is now hearing in a different way for the first time, what the analyst "missed" took place when he was functioning more as a participant than as a participant observer. In any aspect of life, when a person is involved in something that is commanding his full, or almost full, attention in a highly focused way, at that moment he relinquishes his broader perspective. He is more solely a participant and less likely to register the event in which he is participating, with a "third ear." As an analyst, during the course of a session there is normally constant freedom of movement from participant to participant observer—in both directions. This is as it should be, and it allows the process of analytic inquiry to blend with analytic regression and analytic observation.

An outside observer—a supervisor or a member of a case conference—will *always* be potentially capable of hearing what the analyst is "missing," because he is not participating in the event. He is only an observer. He can therefore see the analyst and the patient from a perspective not limited by his own focal involvement in the event. It is only when the analyst's participation becomes enmeshed with the patient's transference that we normally talk of countertransference and can, with any justification as supervisors, label what we hear as something that was being *missed* or that was *really* going on. It is not countertransference simply because the analyst does not hear it and we do, but because it reflects a theme that seems to remain *systematically* outside of the analyst's participant–observer function. He cannot hear it with the "third ear," and falls victim to what Freud (1912/1958) warned against as *perceptual falsification* and what Sullivan (1953) called *selective inattention*.[3]

As a supervisor, I am always functioning in this sense as the analyst's auxilliary "third ear" while attempting to help him to sensitize his own. Since the participation aspect of analysis involves a communication level that is difficult for the analyst to hear when it is occurring, I try to structure one aspect of the supervision to emphasize the level that permits almost pure *observation* of the original event. For this reason, I find the use of tape-recorded analytic sessions extremely valuable when integrated into the overall supervisory situation. The reason the supervisor hears differently than does the analyst includes the fact that he is listening to the event without participating in it. By using tapes of sessions, this channel is now also open to the supervisee. He has the opportunity to integrate new data from what the supervisor hears and communicates into what he, the analyst, hears as he listens without participating, and what he processes as he compares the current experience with his "memory" of the original event.

I am interested in what the supervisee hears, and primarily in that context, what he does. What he does, informs me of what he is hearing. What he is hearing informs me of a number of different things that can then be addressed individually depending upon their relevance for a given student; how he is listening, how he thinks, his ability to conceptualize as he hears, his depth of knowledge, his values, and his possible blind spots due to unresolved personality conflicts of his own. I will frequently make suggestions that relate to principles of technique, but I try not to comment often on "what he is doing" *per se*. I try to address

---

[3]The issue of a person's blind spots resulting from anxiety-induced selective inattention was central to Sullivan's (1953) work. He saw it as one outcome of the developmental achievement during early school years, of learning *to control focal awareness*. This achievement, as Sullivan pointed out, results in "a combination of the fortunate and unfortunate uses of selective inattention" (p. 233). One theme of this chapter has to do with enlisting one of its more "fortunate" uses in the supervisory process of psychoanalysis.

the relationship between his actions (including silences and voice tone) and what he hears and does not hear; what material he uses and does not use. I pay particular attention to how much of a discrepancy I perceive between the effect of patient and analyst upon each other during a particular session or period of time, and the effect of each upon me. If the discrepancy is great, I think about whether there may be something going on between them that is systematically being unacknowledged, or whether the discrepancy is more likely due to something in myself. I am also interested in helping the analyst to think about how he relates what he is hearing on the tape to how he conceptualizes that particular session, how he is viewing this particular patient, and to his developing overview of the psychoanalytic process as a whole.

As an analyst the student must become a sensitive observer. His fundamental commitment is to listen to the patient—not to the patient's words. By this I mean what Reik (1949, p. 136) meant when he quoted Socrates: "Speak, in order that I may see you." He should listen to his manner, posture, gestures, and voice. He should listen also to himself— to his own interior dialogue while listening to and interacting with the patient. Listening to his own tone of voice as spoken and unspoken responses pass between them; how does he sound to himself? Why is he at this moment sounding tender, irritable, indifferent? Why is he at this moment offering or thinking of offering the patient the "real" meaning of his behavior? Why does the "real" meaning feel so compelling to convey at that moment, and why the equally strong feeling that it will have no impact? When his patient drifts off into reverie, why then? Why that particular fantasy? What does the analyst imagine is the patient's fantasy about whether or not he will break into the reverie or let him go on?

An analyst in this stance is more than an observer; he is, in the fullest meaning of the term a *participant observer*. The concept of participant observer, in my view, has only indirectly to do with the analyst's *manifest* level of activity, whether he is interacting with his patient, whether he is speaking or remaining silent, whether he is inquiring about details and meaning or allowing the patient to pursue his own associations freely. The implication of participant observation is, from my perspective, not that the analyst is more interactional than in a classical stance, but that the "conditions which facilitate *regression* must be balanced with those that facilitate *inquiry* within the total analytic climate for any given patient" (Bromberg, 1979, p. 654). The participation that I hold to be central is the freedom of the analyst to use himself in such a way that his presence in the patient's inner world is analytically optimal: That the patient is freely able to utilize transference regression, that he is able to reveal himself maximally in the relationship and to integrate what he sees into his experience of self through his own efforts. The therapeutically optimal level of regression does not have to be induced. It is my belief, as I have expressed elsewhere, that it will eventually occur with most patients if not interfered with by over-clarification of meaning or by being systematically conversational (Bromberg, 1980, p. 234). By listening with what Reik calls the "third ear," the analyst is attempting to hold a constant perspective on the analytic process as such; to monitor where he stands in the patient's representational world and the effects of his own participation upon it. Part of my job, as I see it, is to help him increase his ability to do that while he is simultaneously working with the manifest details of the patient's life as they are being reported.

In other words, along with whatever else I may be doing, I am trying to help him experience several levels of "reality" simultaneously—to hear the transference level as an ongoing channel along with the "content" level.[4] Only within this context do I attempt to deal with psychodynamics, clinical theory, development, history taking, and technique as part of supervision. For each supervisee I first try to determine where he is along the "80-year" path; that is, his personal maturity and comfortableness with himself. I then try to assess what the supervisee knows, how he thinks, what his strong and weak points seem to be, and his conceptual rationale for the way he works. In other words, his position in the domain of the "10 minutes." Beyond that, I try to observe how the supervisee has structured the analytic situation and his facility for remaining within it without being either detached or swallowed up.

The supervisee is asked to present an overview of the week's sessions, trying to give the flavor of how he is thinking about the analysis as it is in progress. This sometimes stirs up a certain amount of anxiety in the supervisee during the early weeks of supervision that usually diminishes once he realizes he is not being tested, and that revealing both what he does and how he thinks about it, brings out a level of mastery the supervisee was not fully aware he possessed. The presentation of the overview is designed to get the supervisee accustomed to

---

[4]Edgar Levenson (1972) has dealt in great depth with the same issue, but he does not view it as a simultaneous occurrence of several levels of perception. He sees it as the analyst's "ability to be trapped, immersed, and participating in the system and then to work his way out" (p. 174). I believe that this is really a special case of the capacity to be fully immersed without loss of the analytic field, and that the more highly developed the capacity in an analyst, the more fully immersed or "trapped" he can safely be for potentially longer periods of time, without the danger of being unable to "work his way out."

thinking about his work conceptually as it is in progress and to keep the responsibility for providing meaning primarily in *his* hands. In other words, what comes across is that he is in charge not only of the analysis but of understanding it. The overview, therefore, is not designed to cover detailed process but rather to present a picture of process themes in the context of how the supervisee is viewing the development of the work and the development of the patient.

If the supervisee has agreed to work with tapes of sessions, these will also play a role in the supervisory process, but the role will vary, depending upon what seems most useful for each particular student and for the different points in supervision. I will not try to deal here with the differences of opinion among analysts as to the benefits and liabilities in using tapes both with regard to the analysis itself and to the supervision. I am aware that there is a certain trade-off, but in my experience it more than repays the investment. As far as the patient is concerned, he seems, more often than not, to "know" when the analyst is in supervision even when he is not told directly. Thus, the introduction of a "mechanical third ear," while it undeniably has an effect, eventually tends to blend into the overall context of the analytic situation and becomes grist for the mill as particular transference issues surface.

There is no implication in the use of tapes that the student is untrustworthy or incapable of reporting process verbally. By listening to portions of a tape together with me, he can, in addition to getting my input, hear as an observer what he heard as a participant observer and get a chance to hear what he did not hear at those moments when his focal attention was invested mainly in participating. Sometimes the supervisee will select a particular portion of a particular session he wishes to listen to; sometimes we will select a session and a portion at random; and sometimes I will ask to hear a particular portion of a session I feel might be illuminating. At the beginning of supervision I often find it helpful in getting to know the supervisee, to listen with him to the beginnings and ends of sessions for a while. It is sometimes surprising and extremely helpful to the supervisee to realize how much of what went on during a session can be heard during the first and last few brief minutes and to realize further that he has the capacity to hear it.

By listening with me, he can often see an issue being unconsciously played out between himself and his patient at the same time it is being consciously identified or even interpreted through external events or prior transferential material. The supervisee becomes more aware that there is no "time out" in the *process* while he is dealing with "content," whether he is asking a question, clarifying a point, formulating an interpretation, confronting a denial, or having an interchange. While his attention is focused upon that task he is less the observer; he does not have the same distance, the same perspective to hear as sensitively that the most vivid expression of the theme has shifted from that which is being said to the interpersonal context in which he is immediately immersed while saying it.

When a student allows me to share in his work with his patient on an ongoing basis, he permits me to know him in some depth, both through the relationship with the patient and through his relationship with me. Both contexts can serve an educational function. One aspect of his work that he allows me to know pertains to the problems or difficulties he is having with his patient. When this focus is the central frame of reference, it is what defines *consultation* and distinguishes it from *supervision*. In supervision it is but one element of a more complex process of learning, but it is most often the source of greatest anxiety for the supervisee. Because it is thereby something that becomes frequently excluded from awareness by the analyst and thus not consciously reportable to the supervisor, the supervisory relationship itself can become the data base for its disclosure.

Part of the supervisory relationship involves a channel of communication referred to in the literature as *the parallel process*. (See Bromberg, 1982; Caligor, 1981; Doehrman, 1976; Gediman & Wolkenfeld, 1980; Sachs & Shapiro, 1976.) It appears to be a phenomenon that most often occurs when the supervisee is unconsciously enmeshed in an unresolved treatment difficulty, resistance, or impasse with his patient, although it can and does sometimes develop out of the supervisory process itself. Most writers feel that because the supervisee wants to but is unable to verbalize the position in which he is stuck, the experience can only be communicated by his behavior—specifically by behavior that unconsciously appears to parallel that going on between the supervisee and his patient. The supervisee, with no apparent awareness, behaves with the supervisor in a manner strikingly similar to the way his patient is behaving with him. And the supervisor often plays the reciprocal role—equally unconsciously.

Used judiciously and selectively, this process can be a valuable source of data to broaden the analyst's perspective, but if it occurs routinely it may suggest the existence of a problem in the supervision itself that needs attention. In *both* instances it provides a fascinating opportunity for a shift in perspective to occur in a powerful and vivid way. It is also probably the one experience in supervision where there is a chance for the supervisor to at least come close to a participant observer stance vis-à-vis the patient, as distinct from his role as observer—that is, to know directly, albeit by analogy, what the analyst himself is experiencing.

In summary, my approach to analytic supervision is contextual and perspectivist. It is reflective of the movement away from a model of the human psyche as a piece of machinery whose faulty energy system can be observed and adjusted from a position outside of it. It recognizes the interpersonal field as the basic medium of mental growth, whether in normal personality maturation, therapeutic change, or psychoanalytic education. The "third ear" metaphor is borrowed here to highlight what I see as one of the most valuable contributions a supervisor can make— to help increase the analyst's sensitivity to the ongoing interpersonal context, so as to most effectively use the interplay between its constantly shifting perspectives in bringing about the deepest and most self-perpetuating analytic growth in the patient.

REFERENCES

Abrams, S., & Shengold, L. Some reflexions on the topic of the 30th Congress: "Affects and the psychoanalytic situation." *International Journal of Psychoanalysis*, 1978, *59*, 395–407.

Arlow, J. A., & Brenner, C. The psychoanalytic situation. In R. E. Litman (Ed.), *Psychoanalysis in the Americas*. New York: International Universities Press, 1966.

Bromberg, P. M. Interpersonal psychoanalysis and regression. *Contemporary Psychoanalysis*, 1979, *15*, 647–655.

Bromberg, P. M. Empathy, anxiety, and reality: A view from the bridge. *Contemporary Psychoanalysis*, 1980, *16*, 223–236.

Bromberg, P. M. The supervisory process and parallel process in psychoanalysis. *Contemporary Psychoanalysis*, 1982, *18*, 92–111.

Caligor, L. Parallel and reciprocal processes in psychoanalytic supervision. *Contemporary Psychoanalysis*, 1981, *17*, 1–27.

Doehrman, M. J. G. Parallel processes in supervision and psychotherapy. *Bulletin of the Menninger Clinic*, 1976, *40*, 3–104.

Freud, S. Recommendations to physicians practicing psychoanalysis. In J. Strachey (Ed. and trans.), *The complete psychological works: Standard edition* (Vol. 12). London: Hogarth Press, 1958. (Originally published, 1912.)

Freud, S. The ego and the id. In J. Strachey (Ed. and trans.), *The complete psychological works: Standard edition* (Vol. 19). London: Hogarth Press, 1961. (Originally published, 1923.)

Gediman, H. K., & Wolkenfeld, F. The parallelism phenomenon in psychoanalysis and supervision: Its reconsideration as a triadic system. *Psychoanalytic Quarterly*, 1980, *49*, 234–255.

Gill, M. *The distinction between the interpersonal paradigm and the nature of the interpersonal relationship*. Paper presented at a meeting of the William Alanson White Psychoanalytic Society, April 1982.

Goodman, S. (Ed.). *Psychoanalytic education and research: The current situation and future possibilities.* New York: International Universities Press, 1977.

Levenson, E. L. *The fallacy of understanding.* New York: Basic Books, 1972.

Levenson, E. L. Follow the fox. *Contemporary Psychoanalysis,* 1982, *18,* 1–15.

Nietzsche, F. W. *Beyond good and evil: Prelude to a philosophy of the future* (4th ed.). London: Allen & Unwin, 1967. (Originally published, 1891.)

Piaget, J. *The origins of intelligence in children.* New York: International Universities Press, 1936.

Reik, T. *Listening with the third ear.* New York: Farrar, Straus, 1949.

Sachs, D. M., & Shapiro, S. H. On parallel processes in therapy and teaching. *Psychoanalytic Quarterly,* 1976, *45,* 394–415.

Sullivan, H. S. *The interpersonal theory of psychiatry.* New York: Norton, 1953.

Sullivan, H. S. *The psychiatric interview.* New York: Norton, 1954.

Can Psychoanalysis Be Taught?

GERARD CHRZANOWSKI

I have been a teacher, seminar leader, and supervisor of psychoanalysis for the last three decades or longer. It may be argued successfully that a person who has done this kind of work and is doing it with some conviction would be an outright hypocrite if he taught something that basically cannot be taught. At the same time, I fully appreciate the fact that what I have been taught by some and what I have been teaching to others in the name of psychoanalysis will not find a consensus of opinion as to whether the content of my teaching fulfills the requirement of what one or the other would consider psychoanalysis to be.

THE MANY FACES OF PSYCHOANALYSIS

Today neither psychoanalysis nor psychotherapy can be viewed as uniform in theory or in practice. Almost every major construct of the analytic theory and practice has been challenged from within and outside the profession as well as from followers or descendants of a given school of thought. It means, in its present form, that psychoanalysis can no longer be taught, learned, or practiced as a homogeneous theory of therapy. The present-day fragmentation of psychoanalysis complicates the process of supervision but, as I hope to document in this chapter, it does not preclude the teaching of generally valid principles in undertaking intensive analytic work with patients. There are political, territorial, economic, and ideational differences between the increasing number of

GERARD CHRZANOWSKI • Training and Supervising Analyst, William Alanson White Institute of Psychiatry, Psychoanalysis and Psychology, New York, New York 10023 and Associate Clinical Professor of Psychiatry, Psychoanalytic Division, New York Medical College, New York, New York 10028.

different schools of thought that make communication difficult and complicate the task of teaching the field. It is my firm conviction that all schools of thought must deal with the same underlying predicaments, the same human difficulties, and the same psychiatric complexities. What we observe, then, is a number of heterogeneous approaches that look at similar clinical manifestations from very different vantage points. The situation is comparable to what we are shown in the brilliant Japanese movie *Rashomon* in which the self-same event is witnessed by four different people. Each person experiences the event from a different vantage point and accordingly sees something that is in contrast or seemingly contradicts what the others had seen at the same time in the same situation.

There are certain approaches that undoubtedly are more applicable to some patients than they are to others (Havens, 1973). Much of our present dilemma can be dealt with if we are addressing ourselves to genuine differences based on the position of the observers and the particular areas that they are observing. This point of view is in contradiction to the dogmatization, concretization, politicization, and religionization of a particular school of thought. Similar considerations apply to the great debate over the DSM-III and other nosological symptom complexes. The fact remains that we cannot treat a psychiatric disease as such: We can only treat a person, that is, an individual with psychological or psychiatric difficulties. Nevertheless, it is essential that we have meaningful, traditional constellations so that we have the capability of interprofessional communication to gauge change, progress, or deterioration lest we subscribe to a free-for-all.

In this chapter I wish to focus my attention on common territory that permits an analytic supervisor to deal with disciples of different schools of thought. For instance, we find Kernberg and Kohut as spokesmen of different points of view within the overall setting of classical Freudian psychoanalysis. We find supervisees who lean toward Melanie Klein or Ludwig Binswanger, Fairbairn, Winnicott—to mention just a few of the present-day heroes. It is my opinion that some basic principles of intensive analytic work with patients can be taught in the supervisory process that transcends the particular adherence to the point of view within the quarreling branches of psychoanalysis.

THE SUPERVISORY PROCESS

Psychoanalysis is basically a dyadic or two-way phenomenon. For all practical purposes, two people are engaged in a reciprocal process of interaction with due respect to the uninvited presence of introjects and similar undesired phenomena.

By contrast, psychoanalytic supervision centers on the interplay of at least three actual people in which two people usually address themselves to a third party who is not present (Eckstein & Wallerstein, 1958; Fleming & Benedek, 1966). Some of the other presences are the supervisee's analyst and the supervisee's psychoanalytic institute. In practice, the focus of supervisory attention is on the therapeutic relationship between the supervisee and his or her patient. An important additional component in the supervisory setting is the mutual awareness of what transpires between supervisor and therapist on a didactic, personal, and often institutional level.

As I see it, psychoanalytic supervision serves a dual role. One aspect of the process is of a basically didactic nature. The supervisor transmits fundamental technical procedures to the supervisee and offers clinically useful recommendations. The nature of the particular didactic process and supervision will be discussed in some detail later on. The other aspect of supervision focuses on the particular therapeutic instrumentality that is embedded in the supervisee's personality structure. Much supervisory effort is expended in encouraging the supervisee to develop his personality as a technically competent and humanly sensitive therapeutic instrument. It is my firm conviction that all supervisory difficulties must be settled within the framework of the supervision, and they cannot and should not be referred back to the analyst. It is unrealistic to expect the patient to wait until the analyst has worked through whatever remaining difficulties he may have in dealing with the patient. There are some technical, clinical ways in which he needs to deal with the situation even if the analyst is not basically quite ready for it.

It should be stated that supervision is a particular form of teaching that cannot be compared to a conventional teacher–pupil situation. As supervisors, we do not merely show a less experienced colleague how to do or how not to do it. This consideration is of great importance. Our primary aim as supervisors is not to create disciples or impose our particular therapeutic style on others. What we do as supervisors is to set examples, to suggest ways and means of dealing with the situation—all with the purpose of developing the supervisee's personality in dealing with a particular situation that he or she encounters with that particular patient. Much has been written in recent years about the *parallel processes* (Bromberg, 1981; Caligor, 1981; Searles, 1955). In my opinion, there are limitations involved if we focus excessively on the supervisee as a reliable mirror of his or her analytic patient in the supervision.

The supervisory process is basically different from an apprenticeship except in the initial phase of setting up the analytic situation. Otherwise, there is less of a master–pupil relationship and more emphasis on the supervisee's capability of psychoanalytic listening. In the final analysis, a clarification of the person-to-person contact between supervisee and patient becomes a key area of supervisory inquiry. I will discuss these points and others in some detail after presenting a checklist of points that I consider to be central in the supervisory process. Among the categories to be covered in supervision are roughly the following: A clarification of the analytic process as it is viewed by supervisee and supervisor, respectively; overlapping and diverging aspects of psychotherapy compared to psychoanalysis; a reciprocal role definition of supervisee and the supervisee's patient; and a mutual expectation of what can and cannot be accomplished in the analysis.

Also necessary is discussion of the patient's presenting problem and the particular life situation in which it occurs, including the network of the present personal environment as well as its historical roots. A diagnostic consideration of differential diagnosis and the suitability of the patient for analytic work are all factors of significance. Then we need a checklist of the basic rules and agreements pertaining to fee, number of hours, cancellations, vacations, changes in hours, and sundry mundane policies that are to be worked out.

A key issue centers on an elaboration of the basic principles of psychoanalytic listening, the need to focus on the contextual nature of the process, and the impact of the listener on what is and what is not communicated by the patient. We also have the task as supervisors of enlarging the supervisee's observational acumen in regard to conception, thought, intervention, and the capacity to hear and pick up differentiations in the patient's moods, attitudes, and what have you (Chrzanowski, 1977).

Another important area deals with the encouragement of the supervisee to use his own personality as a therapeutic instrument in tuning in to the patient's verbal and nonverbal communication. This process is in the broad sense of the word the constructive use of countertransference. Next comes an awareness of transferential manifestations and a vigilance to countertransference that indicates personal involvement on the part of the analyst in response to certain difficulties of the patient.

Another field significant in supervision is the use of dream work of unconscious processes, of interpretations, confrontations, and specific communications to the patient. Particular reference is also required to elicit unconscious material in the patient. When such material emerges, the analyst needs to share his conception of the material with the supervisor and discuss different approaches of how to deal with it clinically.

A discussion of motivational, cognitive, volitional, and effective phenomena and their potential interrelatedness are explored by supervisor and supervisee along with the recognition of anger, anxiety, and acting out when they appear on either side of the dyad in the therapeutic situation.

Last but not least is the appreciation of the nontechnical, actual relationship between supervisee and patient—in particular, the impact of their respective personalities on each other. Included here are reciprocal role commitments, collusive aspects, hostile integrations as well as constructive alliances.

Now I wish to elaborate on some of the points that have been sketched in an almost abbreviated way.

THE ANALYTIC PROCESS

The clarification of the analytic process is among the more difficult tasks in teaching psychoanalysis. It tends to evoke either a dogmatic approach or a free-for-all. In a similar vein, there is no easy way to make a clear-cut distinction between where intensive psychotherapy ends and where analysis begins.

Some of this difficulty may be eased when we define psychoanalysis in more general terms without being unduly parochial about it. For instance, we can speak of the process as a long-term commitment by both patient and analyst to work together on the patient's problems and conflicts in a long-haul therapeutic setting. In such a setting there needs to be some openness about the frequency of weekly hours. Again, it becomes somewhat arbitrary as to where we draw the line. In most instances three hours or more a week are required in order to call the process *analysis*. The purpose is to have an assurance of an intensification of contact between the participating parties in the therapeutic process. We also have the so-called basic rule of saying everything that comes to mind without censorship. That rule still applies in most situations. Also, the process calls for eliciting unconscious material as well as for the recognition of some aspects of transference and countertransference.

Now, every practitioner in the field will be aware of the fact that there are many exceptions to the basic rule, and the question is what can be taught about the core issues involved in the psychoanalytic process. Some of those core issues have to do with what comes from within the patient and what comes from outside. Where is the sickness actually located or anchored? Are we able to find any cause-and-effect relation between early life experiences, hereditary, environmental, social, cultural, and other factors? In this connection, we easily become caught between the Scylla and Charybdis of dogmatism versus excessive ecclecticism. The introduction of certainty tends to ease the minds of supervisors and supervisees alike. There is something to be said for the assumption that one knows the answers and knows exactly what to do. At the same time, if one just acts helpless and does not know how to proceed, one encourages an attitude of nihilism and therapeutic incompetence.

It seems to me more and more that it is not terribly important which underlying theory of therapy we accept or adhere to as long as we have a basic belief, a basic assumption, and, I believe, a basic ideology with enough flexibility not to become unduly rigid about it. In every supervisory and in every analytic situation we are dealing with a number of phenomena that must be included in our overall considerations. There are cognitive distortions that invariably need to be dealt with and call for corrective experiences of one kind or another. Some of them occur with a supervisee, some of them with a patient, and some of them with the supervisor. The correction can take place in many different ways. I doubt that there is one specific way that is necessarily best. However, the capacity to talk to the patient in a way that the patient understands and that actually makes sense to the analyst seems to be a great advantage. The avoidance of slogans, the avoidance of stereotypes and cliches rather than the reliance of personally experienced and felt impressions and expressions are of a recurrent nature. The result is a pattern that deserves to be used for checking and verification and confrontation when indicated. For instance, it is important that both patient and analyst have an awareness of a patient's seeking situations repetitively that represent the core of the patient's difficulties in a good many areas. The selection of one's personal environment can be a good indicator of the particular difficulties a person has. Then we need to learn to what degree the patient's attitude structures the interpersonal situation into a hostile integration or something that has a better working basis. In other words, the patient is rarely a total victim of his environment; he is always an active director in molding the environment to suit his or her neurosis.

In a similar vein, within the scope of the transference certain early repetitive phenomena can be observed as well as the here-and-now contribution of the actual people and their respective personalities as they meet under the circumstances that prevail. In my opinion, the observable pattern always underlies the here and now, while the here and now has an impact of its own that is not merely a clear-cut repetition of what has been done to a person that is being relived exactly as it used to be. The emphasis on exclusively intrapsychic or exclusively intraper-sonal or cultural phenomena strikes me as being one-sided, and only by considering both sides of the coin are we in a position to have a larger perspective of the situation that always includes the analyst in terms of his or her own contribution to the situation.

In discussing the patient's presenting problem and arriving at a diagnostic consideration, we need to keep in mind that we cannot ever treat a disease as such but must deal with the person who has whatever difficulties they have. It becomes a matter of utmost significance to have a working diagnosis as the total orienting point in every long-range and even short-range type of therapy. The idea that we can treat every condition exactly the same way and every patient the same way is not acceptable. In this connection, we also need to have clarity in discussing the situation with the supervisee as to whether the patient is suitable for analytic work that means more intensive work and/or is better suited for a psychotherapeutic approach. We need not quibble about the specific line of demarcation where one ends and the other one begins.

There is no doubt that from a certain point on, the intensity of contact brings out different aspects of the respective personalities of patient and analyst. Similar events may happen to a lesser degree in a less concentrated, less intensive and less frequent get-together. In this connection, special emphasis needs to be placed on the degree to which the supervisee, analyst, or both may be taken in by the patient's ra-tionalizations. Many collusive experiences can be documented where both parties avoid coming to terms with the particular conflict of the patient and have an unwitting unconscious pact to stay clear of it. This particular dilemma can occur at any phase of the psychoanalytic treat-ment. It may enter into the situation from the very beginning. It may come to the fore in the early or middle phases, and very often it can become a special problem when it comes to actually concluding the analysis, or as it is unfortunately called, terminating it.

The question of who is and who is not responsive to psychoanalytic work is also a complex issue. Much has to do with the capacity of the analyst to be responsive to the particular security system or symp-tomatology of the patient without becoming unduly defensive, involved with it, and what have you. In other words, some analysts have the personalities and capacities to do analytic work with narcissistic pa-tients, with borderline patients, and with outright psychotic patients. At such a point one need not quibble unduly about what specifically is being done that is helpful. What matters is that something of a rapport has been established forming a workable situation in which both parties can engage. The term *workable* here is used by me as being capable of

problem solving in terms of human interactions between the two participants along certain lines.

There are certain ground rules that have been connected with psychoanalysis. Some of these have been eased over a period of years. It is
not important to explore carefully what is and is not in vogue today.
There is a certain element of ritualistic practice involved as well as a
certain mystique. Here, I only want to address myself to those aspects
that require a clear understanding as to what agreements need to be
made between the two parties in a long-haul psychoanalytic situation.
What one needs to discuss is an understanding and clarity about setting
the fee, the number of hours to see each other, policies about cancellations, vacations, changes in hours, and other mundane aspects. Clearly
spelled-out details must be worked out sooner or later lest something
goes seriously wrong.

Aside from contractual aspects of the analytic situation, each analyst and each analysand has some personal requirements depending on
their respective life situations. It ordinarily suffices to spell out with
clarity what individual arrangements are compatible with the factual
needs of both parties. Appropriate modifications can be agreed upon as
long as they do not obscure power struggles, faulty communication,
resistance, or similar obstacles to the flow of the therapeutic process. In
this connection, transferential-countertransferential as well as actual relational barriers need to be explored when and where they interfere with
basic arrangements. Here are two abbreviated illustrations of potential
complications of this kind.

A patient has a seriously ill husband who requires emergency hos-
pitalization at frequent intervals. This leads to last-minute cancellations
on a basically legitimate foundation. Over time, a clear pattern emerges
in spite of the husband's grave illness, since it blends with the patient's
controlling personality and her constant need to "call the shots." An
element of righteousness and entitlement comes to the fore and needs to
be dealt with forthrightly. A major barrier in this respect turns out to be
the analyst's guilt feelings about appearing somewhat less than human
in the face of a tragic illness. The situation is further aggravated by the
patient's expressed ambivalence toward her husband and her repetitive
avoidance of discussing her intense feelings with the analyst.

In another case, a patient in intensive analysis requests a change of
the analytic hour by a period of 10 minutes, which is no hardship for the
analyst. The patient has a severe obsessive-compulsive disorder and is
excessively preoccupied with getting his way. It turns out that the analyst unwittingly retaliates by his insistence upon keeping the issue of the
10-minute change alive for a prolonged period of time without either

complying with the patient's wish or moving on to another aspect of their interpersonal conflict. In my opinion the analyst would not have aggravated the patient's neurosis by giving him a 10-minute goodwill present instead of being afraid of placating the patient's need. The obvious requirement in this case is to transcend the relational impasse that manifests itself in the way analyst and patient unproductively lock horns.

One of the key areas of the analytic process in my experience is an area that can be taught. What I am addressing myself to is the elaboration of the basic principles involved in psychoanalytic listening that is the need to focus on the contextual nature of the process. The impact of the listener has to be stressed on what is and what is not communicated in many situations by the patient. The emphasis is on the fact that patients never talk to a wall; they always read into the situation a potential *yes* or *no* as to what is and is not encouraged. There is a conscious as well as an unconscious element involved in what the analyst nods or shakes his head to, often before it is said and before it reaches the communicative level.

In my professional experience, patients often want to know what they are supposed to talk about in the analytic situation. There is not a satisfactory answer to such a question, since we need to make it clear to all patients that they need to talk about whatever they want to talk about. It must be understood that this does not stop many patients from trying to read the analyst's mind and talk about things that they are expected to talk about. The analyst may not catch on to this particular phenomenon, and it may lead to a certain deadlock. There needs to be a challenging quality in comments to the effect that there is a problem when the material becomes unduly monotonous or repetitive, obscure, or uncommunicative. One needs to explore such a deadlock along general lines or based on interactions in the analysis. The other side of the coin is a statement made by Bion whereby the analyst has to clear his mind of previous perceptions and start every session with a clean slate. This particular aspect can be further complicated by certain topics that may make the analyst uncomfortable and get him into an anxious or tense mood of listening. The result is either a distortion or a failure to pick up a specific personal communication. There may be certain shifts in the analytic role relationship that brings a particular difficulty to the fore. For instance, an analyst–patient relationship may have a parent–child model or a teacher–pupil relationship, and at a given point it may change to a more egalitarian atmosphere. At that point the analyst may have difficulty in shifting gear and still listen "to the more child-like or the more structured communication of the patient rather than to the dialogue that now exists between two potential fellow adults." I believe that self-monitoring of one's listening capacity in the analytic process is one of the basic requirements of every analyst. There are many other nuances to the psychoanalytic listening process in its contextual nature that I have described elsewhere in more detail (Chrzanowski, 1980, p. 146).

The supervisor's clinical experience permits him to be aware of a large number of seemingly peripheral phenomena that often assume a center position. The idea is not to point it out in every single situation, but after a pattern has formed and it is clear that the supervisee repetitively has difficulty in seeing something that can be documented. When this happens, it is the supervisor's task to point it out to the supervisee in a matter-of-fact fashion. This is particularly true when the patient sends an obvious message to the analyst that calls for a response in one form or the other. There are certain critical situations that require intervention or recognition for the commitment on the part of the patient. There are times of decision making in which the analyst needs to be sensitive to the dilemma the patient is in and must approach the process of problem solving in a fashion that gives the patient a clearer notion of the options at his or her disposal, and then be in a better position to do something about it. It is not always easy to distinguish between a false alarm on the patient's part and something that actually calls for an intervention or clarification and decision making on the part of the patient.

The supervisor needs to call the analyst's attention to the total impact that the patient has on the analyst and the range of his emotions, reactions, and responses, both in terms of positive, negative, and seemingly detached reactions. This use of countertransference in psychoanalysis has been elaborated on in many publications and books from John Klauber (1981) to Margaret Little (1981), to Epstein and Feiner (1979) and Winnicott (1958), and many others who have expressed their points of view on this topic.

WORKING WITH DREAMS, REVERIES, AND FANTASIES

Dream work is an essential part of every psychoanalytic practice. The discussion of unconscious processes, of dreams, of fantasies, and thoughts that take place "while the person is not looking" constitutes a key part of what transpires in every psychoanalytic situation. It is understood that the analyst's response to all the unconscious manifestations and partially conscious ones is to elicit the patient's thoughts and ideas as much as possible about what the material presented by the patient means to the patient. The analyst's response, then, is simply a way of looking at it from the outside without necessarily changing the frame of reference. It is not in the nature of a *right* or *wrong*. It deals with the sensitivity and clarification of certain means of communication at the patient's disposal that are not fully appreciated and that often require some encouragement and elaboration. There are some patients who use dreams excessively—to the point of being an outright resistance. I saw one patient who always brought more dreams into every hour than possibly could be discussed and then sent an additional batch of dreams at the end of the week to be reviewed by me over the weekend. This made any spontaneous discussion that had not been structured by the patient practically impossible. Then there are many patients who need to be asked about their dreams and be clearly encouraged to recall what goes on in that respect and to tune in to the fact that the dreams have taken place and to find out what they have been about. In a small number of instances, an analyst may have dreams about the patient that can tell the analyst much about perceptions and observations that he or she had not been clearly aware of. A discussion of such material with the supervisor is helpful, and once in a while a discussion of some of the material with the patient can also be clinically useful.

The recognition of anger, anxiety, lethargy, withdrawal, and similar forms of interference with the analytic process needs to be focused on. It calls for a confrontation of the analyst with his own reactions as well as a confrontation of the patient to see whether they are in touch with the kind of manifestations of feelings that have come to the fore. The next point addresses itself to the patient's capacity to see with clarity the options available to him or her at a given point. These are the choices that have to be made in problem solving and decision making. In this connection, the element of volition and commitment play a part here. Volition is seen as the implementation of choices, depending on the situation that prevails at a given time, while commitment—similar to motivation—is an element that indicates the patient's desire to stick to a particular course of action (Chrzanowski, 1982).

My supervisory approach is based on the firm conviction that psychoanalytic theories, as essential as they are, cannot cure mental disorders or cope with human malintegrations. Psychoanalytic theories are not scientific tools capable of cutting the Gordian knot that liberates people from their conflicts. Every successful supervision, similar to every successful psychoanalysis, requires a dynamic quality, a mutually challenging teamwork that inspires both parties to listen to themselves more carefully and thus be able to listen to the partner in a more understanding way.

Psychoanalytic listening, as I have pointed out elsewhere, is a contextual phenomenon that can have a number of consequences. It may encourage a novel point of view in looking at familiar and repetitive thoughts. A new facet or dimension may be added. An element of excitement may be evoked in sensing a reverberating response on the analyst's part. If all goes well, a creative and mutually satisfactory accommodation between the participating parties may take place. The patient often discovers new options and different ways of coping and of dealing with existing problems that may appear in a new light. The feeling of commitment to the pursuit of one's exploratory journey, which is shared with the attentive ear of the concerned analytic listener, is an experience that needs to be brought to the fore in the supervisory process. New discoveries of the supervisee about the interplay with his or her patient enliven the supervisory teamwork.

Transference may originate with either party with due respect to the usually greater intensity on the patient's part. My point is that every analyst is entitled to some degree of transference to the patient that is not invariably a countertransference, that is, something that originates predominantly with the patient. I have observed the emergence of a transference psychosis in some severely disturbed patients where the analyst played a distinct part in the exacerbation of the phenomenon.

Supervision, in order to be successful, benefits greatly from an initial structure along points previously outlined. Next comes the mutual process between supervisor and supervisee to get some spark going that adds a vitality to the process. It permits a certain loosening of theoretical and technical guidelines, while emphasizing the vitality of the patient's working issues through with the supervisee. At the same time, the supervisor enlarges the intensity, the scope, and the quality of listening on the part of each of the involved people.

Patient, supervisee, and supervisor need to keep their respective identities intact, which means a basic absence of placating all around. The capacity for genuine empathy often lies in the freedom to retain one's own stance by adhering to the particular difference of one's personality, rather than to look for real or imagined similarities between the patient, supervisee, and analyst. This is not to question the validity of Sullivan's well-known dictum that, as humans, we are all more basically similar than different. When it comes to empathy, however, it often pays dividends to be more different than similar to the patient. It brings to mind Lyman Wynne's well-known term *pseudomutuality*. Wynne's concept refers to a playacting family unit that he considers to be tributory to certain schizophrenic disorders. My comment obviously refers to a pseudofamiliarity in the supervisory triad that is based on preconceived assumptions rather than on prevailing circumstances.

As a final point, I wish to say something about my own experience as a supervisee. For the most part, I had it pretty good. There is no doubt in my mind, however, that my most enjoyable and profitable supervision took place after my graduation when I had fulfilled my quota requirements. My postsupervisory experience was very special to me. Some candidates who worked with me under similar circumstances went beyond the boundaries of my experience. They confessed that they actually had falsified material or censored data in supervision. They felt that they did not feel free to present some material as candidates, out of fear that it could hold them back in the way they would have been evaluated by their supervisors. There have been a number of reports in the literature on the transference connected with the candidate's training institute (Brazil, 1975; Chrzanowski, 1975a,b; Dannevig, 1975). In a similar vein, the roles of analytic supervisors as elite groups of judges has been a topic of some controversy. In many cases the institutional aura and the potential power of the supervisor's hierarchy are not major obstacles in the supervisory process. Nevertheless, they are factors to be considered and dealt with when they arise.

REFERENCES

Brazil, H. V. On the complexities of teaching and learning psychotherapy: III. The dilemma of training analysis. *Contemporary Psychoanalysis*, 1975, *11*(2), 243–245.

Bromberg, P. The supervisory process and parallel process. *Contemporary Psychoanalysis*, 1981, *18*, 92–111.

Caligor, L. Parallel and reciprocal processes in psychoanalytic supervision. *Contemporary Psychoanalysis*, 1981, *17*, 1–27.

Chrzanowski, G. On the complexities of teaching and learning psychotherapy: I. Introduction. *Contemporary Psychoanalysis*, 1975, *11*(2), 1. (a)

Chrzanowski, G. On the complexities of teaching and learning psychotherapy: IV. In-group dangers. *Contemporary Psychoanalysis*, 1975, *11*(2), 246–250. (b)

Chrzanowski, G. *Interpersonal approach to psychoanalysis: Contemporary view of Harry Stack Sullivan.* New York: Gardner Press, 1977.

Chrzanowski, G. Reciprocal aspects of psychoanalytic listening. *Contemporary Psychoanalysis*, 1980, *16*(2), 145–156.

Chrzanowski, G. *Volition and change: An interpersonal perspective.* Paper presented at the Harvard University Symposium on the Process of Change in Psychotherapy, Cambridge, Mass., June 1982.

Dannevig, E. T. On the complexities of teaching and learning psychotherapy: II. Changes in social structure. *Contemporary Psychoanalysis*, 1975, *11*(2), 241–242.

Eckstein, R., & Wallerstein, R. S. *The teaching and learning of psychotherapy*. New York: International Universities Press, 1958.

Epstein, L., & Feiner, A. *Countertransference*. New York: Jason Aronson, 1979.

Fleming, J., & Benedek, T. *Psychoanalytic supervision*. New York: Grune & Stratton, 1966.

Havens, L. L. *Approaches to the mind*. Boston: Little, Brown & Co., 1973.

Klauber, J. *Difficulties in the analytic encounter*. New York and London: Jason Aronson, 1981.

Little, M. I. *Transference neurosis and transference psychosis*. New York and London: Jason Aronson, 1981.

Searles, H. F. The informational value of the supervisor's emotional experiences. *Psychiatry*, 1955, *18*, 135–146.

Winnicott, D. W. *Collected papers*. New York: Basic Books, 1958.

4

Stimulation of Curiosity in the Supervisory Process

ALLAN COOPER AND EARL G. WITENBERG

Our purpose in supervision is to teach students that the practice requires the creative use of oneself as well as a sound knowledge of theoretical and technical principles. Mastery of all these aspects of the process is essential to helping the patient toward change—which is, after all, the goal of treatment. The accumulation of knowledge alone is thus not enough. Nor is it enough for the analyst to understand the patient only in theoretical terms. Rather, the analyst must be able to communicate to the patient himself that he is being understood, or the analysis will become a static exercise in intellectual dynamics instead of a vibrant, meaningful experience. We teach students that such empathy (i.e., an understanding of the patient) can only be achieved if the analyst is able to observe his own responses to what the patient tells him in the session, and to use these observations as a sounding board while he listens. Then, and only then, can the subtleties and nuances of the patient's communications be really understood and utilized to expand his awareness.

Although in his own practice with patients, the senior analyst has comfortably mastered these skills—knowledge of theory, the use of techniques related to the theoretical premise, and the creative use of his own responses—in his role as supervisor, he has a more complex task.

This chapter first appeared as *Stimulation of Curiosity in the Supervisory Process of Psychoanalysis,* in *Contemporary Psychoanalysis,* 1983, *19*(2), 248–264. It is reprinted with the permission of the William Alanson White Institute.

ALLAN COOPER • Director of Curriculum, Fellow, Training and Supervising Analyst, William Alanson White Institute of Psychiatry, Psychoanalysis and Psychology, New York, New York 10023. EARL G. WITENBERG • Director, Fellow, Training and Supervising Analyst, William Alanson White Institute of Psychiatry, Psychoanalysis and Psychology, New York, New York 10023 and Past President, American Academy of Psychoanalysis, New York, New York.

Whereas in practice it is up to the analyst to "see" his patient as clearly as possible, in supervision the supervisor must develop a picture of the patient indirectly from what the student tells him; he must develop a picture of the student, and he must be clear about the relationship between the student and the patient. Finally, he needs also to be aware of how his own relationship with the student affects the student's relationship with the patient. It is here that the true skill in supervision becomes apparent. The supervisor cannot simply tell the student what to do. He must be able to lead the student to discover for himself the answers to the problems he is having. Is it lack of theoretical understanding? Is the student misinformed about technique? Is the student not using himself when he listens to his patient? Or is it that crucial information is missing or is not being heeded? How is the supervisor to determine where the difficulty lies? Using himself creatively as he listens to his student, the supervisor often becomes aware of significant differences between his reaction and his student's to what the patient is saying. He becomes aware that his own approach toward the patient would have been different from the student's. All this requires inquiry and clarification to determine in what area to focus in order to enable the student to use himself more effectively when listening to the patient.

When the issue involves theory or technique, the supervisor should make clear the principles that guide his own work with patients. Our practical and philosophic orientation is *interpersonal*. The term comes from Sullivan (1970) who specifically stated: "In every case, whether you know it or not, if you are to correctly understand your patient's problems, you must understand him in the major characteristics of his dealing with people" (p. 13). We have also been influenced by Fromm, Thompson, Fromm-Reichmann, and many others at the White Institute. We also feel that it is important not to be exclusive, and we encourage students to read widely in *all* psychoanalytic literature. Ultimately, however, every analyst must think for himself and find the way of working with patients that best suits his own personality and outlook on life. He must compare his own clinical experience with what he reads in books. No theory has final answers or the ultimate truths about people. At its best, all that theory can do is to provide a way of organizing one's thinking about people, the nature of their problems, and a way of helping them.

Experience in supervising analytic candidates indicates that the first and often most difficult problem they encounter is gaining a coherent picture of who the patient is. Students usually can see symptoms, various dynamics, bits of transference, and some historical data, but they generally have no overview of the patient. Some students continue to listen in the hope that things will become clear eventually, but even when they present a case they have been working on for a year, they still cannot present a clear overview. It is not from the emergence of more data that the picture becomes clearer. Clarity comes from the analyst's ability to organize, formulate and structure the information he receives. The way he does this will depend upon his theoretical orientation, and how he uses himself when listening to the patient. Clarity also comes from knowing where to inquire in order to obtain a clearer perception of event, and to expand the awareness of the patient.

How do we develop an overview of the patient? The most effective way is to observe and understand the patient's characteristic ways of relating to others. This should tell us what the patient wants from people, how he interferes with reaching his own goals, and his habitual ways of warding off anxiety in interpersonal situations. We can often begin the process with a simple observation. What follows is an example: A candidate began presenting a patient whom he described as a transvestite. This symptom preoccupied the patient with worry and shame. The patient hated himself for dressing in women's clothing but was often compulsively drawn to do so. The student had many relevant details about the symptom, such as when the patient first began wearing these clothes, the types of clothing, and the various fantasies associated with this symptom. Dreams, free-associational material, and transference reactions had been examined to understand the dynamics of the symptom. There was ample additional material about the patient, such as current life experiences, historical material, and data about work. However, the data appeared like a collection of interesting facts with no unifying thread. Listening to the material from an interpersonal perspective, an obvious pattern emerged in the patient's life. He seemed to be very lonely and craved closeness. Moreover, as soon as he began to develop relationships, he suddenly inhibited his own reactions of friendliness and managed to stay distant from the people he wanted to be close to. This pattern was repeated in what he described about his male friends, potential girlfriends, and in his relationship with the analyst. The pattern is also apparent in the historical material he presented. Once this was pointed out, the student analyst recognized it immediately. Probably he had not formulated the material this way because he was not looking at the patient's life from that perspective. The candidate was encouraged to point out this pattern to the patient and to ask him what he made of it. It was further suggested that he ask the patient if he had always related to people this way in the past, and when had there been exceptions?

Presenting such a simple observation to a patient has several advantages. The patient can recognize this pattern in himself once it is formulated, and can see for himself that it causes difficulties in living. The patient can then become curious about himself apart from his symptom and begin to look into his paradoxical approach to people. Organizing the material in this way, along with the suggested follow-up inquiries, represents theoretical and technical supervision of the candidate. It does not yet deal with the creative use of the candidate as an analyst. Before going into that aspect of supervision, there is another aspect of technical supervision that we must discuss.

Very often candidates do not understand the principles underlying different techniques. They usually learned techniques in training from various supervisors in the form of *rules of thumb*. They usually believe that they should not say too much and should not reveal their reactions or their opinions. At the same time, they have learned that their neutrality should not lead to lifelessness and therefore they often struggle in a confused way to remain neutral while being lively. The best way to approach this situation is to ask the student if he understands the principles underlying some particular point of technique. If the student's explanation seems vague or confused, the supervisor must clarify the underlying rationale for a particular approach to treatment. If student and supervisor differ in their approaches, it is important to discuss these differences in terms of theoretical orientation and to show how differences in technique complement the different theories. Different techniques are used to reach different goals.

For instance, when a student is not obtaining enough information from the patient to understand him, or when he does not comment enough on what he hears, the basis for his silence is open to question. The student's silence might be caused by several different factors. It could be that his idea of correct technique is to remain silent. It could reflect a fear of countertransference, or it could indicate a passive character structure. Although it may be true that countertransference reactions are responsible for many of the student's problems, ignorance should not be confused with countertransference as is too often the case. When the problem is lack of knowledge, the supervisor must act as a teacher—not an analyst.

The idea that everything is countertransference is probably a corollary of the old Freudian notion that the patient really "knows it all" but has simply repressed this knowledge. Even if this were always true with patients, it cannot be true with a student who has large gaps in his knowledge of theory and/or technique. In fact, it often seems that many students would rather discuss their countertransference reactions than admit ignorance.

For instance, when a student says that he has not obtained certain information because he did not want to interfere with the neutrality of the analytic situation, it is important to ask the student what he means by neutrality. Why is it so important in psychoanalysis? If the explanation seems vague or incomplete, it is appropriate for the supervisor to offer a brief lecture to explain that in *Freudian* and *object relations* approaches, neutrality is designed to allow the transference to develop in an uncontaminated situation where it is not distorted by the intrusion of the analyst's personality. Ultimately, this will lead to the final goal of recalling the infantile fantasies that are the expressions of forbidden wishes. In those theories, it is predicted that when these wishes are recalled and worked through, the neurosis will be cured. It is through the medium of the transference that the patient reveals to the analyst the nature of the repressed impulses. Through the analyst's interpretations, the patient eventually recalls his repressed impulses in the form of fantasies. In that system, it is believed that the more the transference comes solely from the patient's reactions and is not distorted by the real personality of the analyst, the more accurately and faithfully the transference reflects the patient's impulses. In these systems of thought, *neutrality* means not revealing oneself in order to keep the transference pure.

In the *interpersonal* approach, the transference concept is used in somewhat different form. While it is extremely important, it is used in a different way. Although Sullivan's term *parataxic distortion* is not popular even with interpersonalists, it reflects more accurately what he meant than does *transference*. Basically, it means that the patient treats the analyst as if he were someone from the patient's past. However, this way of relating to the analyst does not necessarily reflect libidinal desires. Moreover, the reaction to the analyst is rarely only a simple carryover of early feelings toward a parent. The way the patient relates to the analyst may, or may not, be the way he relates to other important people in his life. This is because while a person's character has consistency, it also has complexity. One's way of relating to others is very much determined by who the other person actually is and in what context the two people are together. From the interpersonal perspective, it is most important to clarify communication, to learn what distortions exist in the patient's perceptions of others, and what purposes these distortions serve. Ultimately, the patient must learn what interferes with his gaining new experiences that would make his life more rewarding. He must then engage in this new experience and learn from it. He should know what satisfactions he seeks with others, find the people who will share in these experiences, and not let his antianxiety defense interfere with developing better ways of relating to others.

In the interpersonal approach, free association alone is not expected to help the patient become clearer about himself and others. In fact, attempts at free association often are used defensively and lead away from clarity. The *transference neurosis* and its resolution is also not expected to cure the patient. Clarification of the distortion inherent in transference can be very interesting, but it does not provide the new experiences that are needed to live a life that is both satisfying and secure.

In order for the analyst to understand the patient, the patient must be helped to feel free to speak openly in his sessions. This requires trust. Trust and respect are developed only as the patient comes to experience the analyst's goodwill and the validity of his interventions. The patient develops confidence in the analyst's ability to clarify his fears and desires and to identify his antianxiety techniques that got him into trouble. The analyst listens carefully, knowing what to ask about and when. The inquiry may range from simple clarification to questions about why the patient thinks he organizes his life in a certain way. Or, the analyst may inquire into areas that the patient would never have brought up spontaneously because he had not attended to these issues. In short, the analyst tries to learn as much as possible about the patient—often by direct questioning. This, then, helps the patient inquire into himself about matters that he was previously unaware of.

In this model of doing therapy, being totally neutral is a practical impossibility. It would not be considered desirable even if it could be attained. Pertinent, focused inquiry—especially when it brings the patient's attention to areas he usually overlooks—is considered the more valuable approach. If one was to use the term *neutral* in this system, it would have to mean that the analyst tries to see the patient as clearly as possible while maintaining a high level of objectivity and concern. From the interpersonal perspective, it would be incorrect *not* to interrupt the patient when it is necessary to gain clarification. Obviously this needs to be done with tact and good clinical judgment, but the analyst should not expect that continued free association will bring clarification on its own.

This type of teaching is a very important aspect of supervision. The student must be helped to realize that the interpersonal orientation requires active, collaborative inquiry and often the presentation of tactful but direct formulations to the patient. Thus, at such times when there may be confrontation with the patient about his patterns of relating to people, collaboration and thoughtful reflection are encouraged, while regression to an infantile state is not considered useful. Recall of significant life events takes place without the artificial induction of a regressive state.

Some students become concerned that the analytic relationship is not sufficiently warm and understanding. They often appeal to the concept of *creating a good holding environment,* and they worry that confrontation, direct formulations about character, and pointed questioning will not create the warm environment that some of the more fragile patients need. At this point we look at the essential ingredients of a good analytic relationship. The analyst must have basic respect for the patient and be able to present his interventions in a direct and nonthreatening manner. Students often confuse being empathic with being warm and totally accepting. However, the analyst's empathy for the patient will become evident only when he can follow the patient's phenomenological experience and can make this comprehension clear to the patient. Then the patient will know that he is with a person who understands him. Nonetheless, while the analyst must understand the patient's experience, he should still be able to maintain his own point of view about what he hears. If there are differences between his point of view and the patient's, the analyst should inquire about them in order to clarify his own understanding of the patient and/or the patient's awareness of himself.

On one occasion a student made a presentation indicating that his patient was panicky in new situations because he felt like a phony and was afraid of being exposed by people he was meeting for the first time. The patient seemed to be competent, but usually he exaggerated his abilities and accomplishments so that he was never really what he pretended to be. However, when it was suggested that the student analyst share these observations with the patient, he objected strongly. The student felt that the patient needed a warm and accepting environment, and he was afraid that the patient might react as if he was being criticized by the analyst. The supervisor then pointed out that the formulation about the patient's experience had been developed from information that the patient himself had given the analyst and that much reflection back to the patient might serve to heighten the patient's self-awareness. What is most important is that the patient feel that his experience of other people is understood by his analyst. Acceptance without the patient feeling that he is known by the analyst offers little comfort. The patient then feels he is accepted only because the analyst does *not* realize who he is as a person. In this instance, the student and the supervisor reached a compromise. The student did not present the hypothesis directly to the patient, but he did ask some questions pertinent to the patient's experience in panicky situations. Much to the student's surprise, the patient announced that he often felt he was a phony and that he was terrified that he would be exposed. The patient was obviously relieved to express this feeling, and now direct exploration of a central problem in relating to people could be pursued.

In discussing historical material one can outline, as Sullivan did in *The Psychiatric Interview*, areas that are useful to inquire into. However, after suggesting the areas of inquiry, the analyst must rely on his ability to use his own reactions while listening to the patient. For example, in a lengthy, rather dull recital of factual data about a patient's early life, a student reported a vignette that the patient said had been told to him many times by his mother. The mother had said that when the patient was 6 years old, he was a great nuisance to the neighbors. His mother told him that she had stopped letting him visit the neighbors because he would visit at dinner time and prevent the family from eating their dinner. When the student was asked what he made of this little story, he replied that he did not make very much of it at all, except that the patient's mother must have regarded him as a nuisance. The student was then asked to picture what he had been told as if it was a movie. When he tried to do this, he realized that there were many gaps that he could not fill in. He could not picture how the little boy had prevented the family from eating. He could not picture the mother's attitude when she had told the patient that he could not visit the neighbors.

This vignette that the patient told was hard to picture. The lack of clarity about the incident raised questions that could be asked of the patient. And even if he could not answer them, at least he would become curious about this piece of family mythology that he had heard so many times in his life. He might become curious about what his mother was really trying to tell him. This kind of lively exchange—in which the analyst pictures what he is being told, becomes curious, and asks questions to extend the investigation of some aspect of the patient's interaction and feelings about other people—should take place continuously during analysis. The analyst might be quiet for periods of time, but the process should be taking place as he listens. When the student learns to picture for himself what the patient tells him, and learns to make pertinent inquiries, the collection of historical material becomes a lively evocative interaction in which the patient learns to collaborate and to become curious about himself.

The student was then encouraged to use his own imagination to try to see what implications there might be in the story of the 6-year-old boy. What questions did he have? How could a 6-year-old boy keep a family from eating? Were they unusually polite to the little guest in their house? Did the mother consider her son to be very powerful even at age 6? Could the mother have been jealous and wanted to keep her son at home where she could enjoy him? As the supervisor and student continued speculating like this, various possibilities became evident. The student's curiosity was thus aroused in the same way that we hoped to arouse the patient's curiosity. In this experience in supervision, the student thus had a firsthand understanding of how his patient would feel if he was able to develop a similar interaction in the course of analysis.

We have also found that paying attention to a minor detail in the patient's history can sometimes open up a theme that is significant and runs counter to the main thrust of the patient's account of his life. A student analyst described the history of a young woman that was bleak and dreary. There was maternal deprivation, the absence of a father, and a harsh mother. Life was lonely and frightening. The mother remarried, but to a man who was immature and dictatorial. The patient reported one occasion when she went fishing with her stepfather and accidently brushed against his fishing pole that was leaning against a tree. When it fell and broke he became very angry with her. The point of this incident seemed to her to be the same as the rest of her life. Namely, that nothing ever worked out. Something always went wrong between her and the significant people in her life.

As the student repeated this story, he was asked to picture the last episode for himself. At first he said he could picture the story, but when asked if he could picture the fishing poles breaking when it fell to the ground, he agreed that that was hard to imagine. He then suggested that perhaps the incident never happened and that the recollection was a screen memory. This hypothesis would lead us to speculate about the symbolic meaning of the story—along the lines that perhaps her father felt castrated by her or that she secretly wanted to castrate him.

The problem with this type of hypothesis is that it does not usually lend itself to direct inquiry, and while the speculation may be interesting for the analyst, it does not make things more alive for the patient. Then we started to speculate about how the pole got broken. The student thought that the patient might have been fooling around with the pole and doing something with it that was mischievous. This hypothesis was particularly important to the student analyst because it was the only clue to indicate that the patient may have been lively as a child and that this might be an aspect of herself that had been dissociated. In this instance, the student went on to tell the patient about his speculation about her mischievousness, and this led her to recall some important details connected with the incident. Further recollections of her being mischievous and lively emerged and helped the patient expand her sense of self.

The process of using one's self does *not* mean that the unconscious of the therapist will necessarily understand the unconscious of the patient. In fact, many speculations will *not* be confirmed, but what is more important is that the patient and analyst are engaged in a collaborative effort that is lively for both of them. When the analyst uses himself creatively, the probability of developing useful hypotheses increases. Communication becomes clearer and more meaningful. This process will be especially helpful to the patient by focusing on aspects of his experience with other people that he does not usually attend to. The analyst's imagination, feelings, thoughts, and knowledge are all brought into play when he listens to the patient in this way. This is not a *countertransference reaction* even when that term is used in its broadest sense. It may contain countertransference, but it is a much more extensive reaction, including, perhaps, the analyst's transferences, countertransferences, and both the neurotic and productive elements of his character structure. Thus, the extent to which the analyst can use his own reactions with minimal distortions, determines whether he can listen responsively and appropriately—for if the analyst is afraid to use himself, the entire analysis will be deadened.

It is important to remember, however, that the use of one's self must always be integrated with one's theories about motivation, the healthy development of the person, and the factors that lead to a successful analysis. In terms of interpersonal theory, the analyst must focus on the way the patient relates to and interacts with other people. He is interested in discovering what the patient has learned about living with other people and in those reactions outside of awareness that prevent the patient from finding new and better experiences in living. The analyst focuses on experience, both his own and the patient's, rather than on hypothetical structures of the mind. The analyst does not concern himself with such concepts as ego splits, ego–superego conflicts, or introjected figures from the past. Because of this, the analyst can communicate his observations, speculations, and hypotheses directly to the patient, and together they can explore issues in a collaborative way. Finally, the very process of this collaboration itself can become the subject of their study—as a model of how the patient approaches other interpersonal situations in his life.

Although we know that there are very few assumptions about the nature of people or what is "contained" in the unconscious that can be definitively substantiated, we do know that there is a model of how patterns of interpersonal relationships evolve from infancy and throughout life. In infancy, the child cries when it needs something. The mothering person responds to the *clear* communication of the cry and wants to help the child. As a result of this cooperation, they both feel satisfied. As the child grows older, his capacity to cooperate in the integration rapidly increases. If his development continues in a healthy way, he begins to care about some other people in much the same way as he cares about himself. Although eventually the child becomes capable of *real* cooperation with others, life experiences unfortunately often lead to anxieties in interpersonal situations that frequently cause people to develop inappropriate techniques for maintaining feelings of security and self-esteem. Many of these techniques are learned as self-protective measures in the early family environment, and they function outside of awareness, seriously impairing their capacity for developing satisfactory relationships.

For example, misleading and distorted speech is often used to protect self-esteem rather than to serve the real purpose of speech, which is to communicate clearly and to bring people closer together. Satisfactions that may be seen as threatening or forbidden are often avoided in order to maintain self-esteem, and in some cases even the desires for these satisfactions are dissociated and removed from awareness. Fear of other people and of their abilities to reduce one's sense of self-worth often makes genuine relating difficult, and it can become almost impossible to care about another person or to be engaged in a fulfilling relationship because of one's own sense of vulnerability. All this can be reflected in the partnership between the patient and analyst so that full collaboration is hard to arrive at. What may look like cooperation may only be a pattern of submission that is designed to avoid interpersonal anxieties.

The goal of analysis is for the patient to become clear about who he is, what he feels and what he wants from others. He must be able to perceive accurately how he protects himself from anxiety and with whom he is likely to obtain satisfaction while maintaining his sense of security. It is especially important for the patient to distinguish between real and imagined loss of self-esteem in his interactions with other people. Becoming aware is not solely a matter of lifting repressions. It will require developing a new attention to aspects of interactions with other people that the patient has historically avoided looking at. The analyst can help the patient to formulate new patterns of interaction that will help him bring the old ones into focus. In order to do this, the analyst must be able to see the world through the eyes of the patient, and yet simultaneously be aware of his own reactions and perceptions of the events he is hearing about. The analyst's reactions may be similar to the patient's—or they may differ—but either way, the awareness of these differences and/or similarities will allow the analyst to understand the patient and to bring to the patient's attention aspects of a situation that the patient has not previously attended to.

A student analyst describes a particularly dramatic interaction between a patient and his father. In high school the patient had been a soccer star. The father attended all the games and afterward would critique his son's performance. The father was himself not much of an athlete. The patient received a soccer scholarship to college, but because he was smaller than most of his teammates, he rarely played in the games. He hated the daily practices where he was often physically roughed up by the bigger players. He suffered from headaches and took aspirin and other medications that the trainers gave him. In his senior year, when he was expected to play in the games on a regular basis, the headaches became more frequent and more intense. The team doctor sent him to the university hospital where he was told that the headaches were a result of continuous concussions that were probably suffered while playing body-contact sports, and that he could not continue to play on the team because further blows to his head could result in very serious injury. The patient said that when he told all this to his father, he was treated as if he was a malingerer. The father told his son that if he did not play he would be very disappointed and would never forgive him.

The patient is a man who does not express much feeling, and he has a rather stiff-upper-lip attitude. He did not elaborate on the incident nor on his feelings about what happened, proceeding to talk about other matters. The student analyst continued reporting the events of the session following the patient's associations, but he did not give any indications of his own internal responses. After this jarring account of the patient's father's sending him back to play for the father's glory and the potential for death or serious physical damage that could occur, is the student analyst wondering how the patient will express his rage, his profound disillusionment, or his despair about his father's treatment of him? Does the analyst wonder if there is more to this story, such as the father's realizing the brutality of his immediate reaction and becoming remorseful and trying to make amends? The patient himself had not touched on any of these issues, but he had gone on to discuss other topics. He did not give evidence of any powerful or profound reaction. Has the patient lived so long with this type of callous treatment that he has come to believe that he can expect nothing from others except mistreatment? And where is the student's curiosity?

In terms of our simple model about interactions between people, this man's experience is far from ideal. Does the patient realize this? Does he avoid people in his current life who are likely to mistreat him? Or is he unable to differentiate? Without the analyst using his own reaction to what he is hearing, there is little basis for his understanding the patient or of focusing the patient's attention to aspects of his own reactions that he has not attended to.

In this case, when first questioned about his own reactions to his patient's story, the student had little to report. However, when the story was played back to him by the supervisor, and he was able to visualize the scene accurately, his own reactions were intense and vivid. He was able to see the implications of the father's behavior and the patient's apparent passivity that raised many questions that he wanted to ask the patient about. The student analyst now seemed more alive, responsive, and curious about the patient.

At a technical level one does not listen to every verbalization from the patient as if it was free association. The analyst must *evaluate* the flow of what the patient is talking about, especially if there is a shift in topic when he—the analyst—would not expect it. And he must always bear in mind that obsessive patients are particularly prone to use what could appear as free association to avoid issues and feelings that are anxiety provoking. Now how was it that in this instance the student was able to listen to the patient's dramatic story without having more of a reaction? Was it a matter of countertransference or elements of his own neurosis that got in the way of a spontaneous reaction? In any case, one technique that can improve a student's ability to use himself and to open himself up to his own reactions, is to try to picture in his own mind what his patient tells him as if he were watching a movie. If he cannot picture clearly what he is being told, he should know that he has to ask some questions. As with watching a movie or a play, he will have many reactions, and he should try to use them. If his reactions are different from that of the patient, he should inquire about the differences and in this way focus the patient's attention on something very valuable.

In all situations, it is helpful to ask the student frequently what he makes of what he is describing, what other reactions he has to the material he is reporting, what implications he sees, what inferences he draws, and what questions he would like to ask the patient. Sometimes the student's lack of responsiveness is because he does not want to do or say anything wrong and does not want to make any mistakes. This attitude needs to be confronted by the supervisor and discussed with the student. It can help the student for the supervisor to share his own reactions to the material and to try to develop a lively interaction with the student about different thoughts, feelings, speculations, and perceptions.

Another problem is that students often use plausible constructions derived from theory in the absence of their own reactions to what is being said by their patients. For example, a student analyst is treating a young woman who came to treatment with complaints of depression and concerns about working out a relationship with a man. The student felt that the most prominent features in her history were a separation from her parents at ages 2 to 3, and that the patient's younger sister was beautiful and preferred by her father. The woman had recently begun a relationship with a young man, but she was already worried that he would grow tired of her and abandon her. The student analyst felt that, having been traumatized by the early separation, she was always afraid of abandonment and that having been displaced by a younger sister added to her fear. Finally, since her father preferred her sister, the patient was always afraid that she would lose her man to another woman. These constructions were quite plausible, but the student found it difficult to use them in the analysis. The analyst had offered some interpretations along these lines, and although the patient agreed that they might be true, they did not have much impact on her. She had no further observations dealing with the issue, no recall of incidents from the past, no dreams, and no transference reactions related to the interpretations. The student analyst suggested that the patient might be very defensive and that she was resistant to letting the transference develop. The supervisor suggested that although this might be true, it would be worthwhile to look more closely at the relationship that was developing with the new boyfriend, and to pay more attention to, and to inquire about, the details of any interactions that the patient described.

A few sessions later, the patient complained that while making love, her boyfriend was holding off having his orgasm to give her time to have her orgasm. She was very upset about this. She did not elaborate, but went on to talk about other aspects of the relationship. When the student was asked if he had noticed what the patient had said and what his reaction was, he stated that he had had little reaction to this story at first. However, as we talked about it he became more curious. The supervisor then suggested that the two of them—the patient and her boyfriend—were in a situation together where their own and each other's satisfaction was the goal. The boyfriend at least appeared to be concerned about the patient, and he appeared to be offering her something. It was curious that she could not simply accept it and feel good. Were there other ways in which the couple gave to each other? As he reviewed what he knew about their interaction, the student then found that the data seemed to indicate that the patient had difficulty with simple give-and-take, cooperation, and working together. In later sessions, this pattern was also revealed on the job, with her parents, and with her analyst. The patient wanted people to give to her, but she was ashamed of wanting this and feared that the other person would become resentful. She was willing to give something to the other person as long as it gave her a sense of power in the relationship. If she felt that the other person was expecting too much, she became resentful, but she did not address the issue lest she offend the person and lose the relationship. From a technical point of view, the student was helped to make a formulation about how the patient related to other people characteristically. He was also being encouraged to use his reactions to understand her, to raise hypotheses, and to inquire into these hypotheses with the patient.

A few sessions later, the same student reported that the patient spent two sessions wondering if she should be in analysis. She said she was confused about how analysis worked—confused about the efficacy of the procedure. The student finally interpreted the confusion as a resistance and suggested that she was avoiding talking about something else that was important. In discussion with the supervisor, the student analyst was able to recognize that this current wonderment about analysis followed an interplay with the patient's sister in which the sister told her that she should not rely on and depend on analysis. The sister said she should stand on her own feet. Her sister also told her that she was simply afraid to do things that needed to be done and that instead of talking to an analyst about it, she should just pull herself together and do what had to be done. The supervisor then asked the student what he thought the patient felt during this exchange with her sister. He said he thought that, under the impact of the aggressive persuasion of the sister's arguments, the patient had become confused, and that she was using the confusion as a resistance. The student remained vague about how the patient had been feeling during the discussion with her sister. It was then suggested that he try to present the interaction between the two sisters to the supervisor as if it was a movie. The student began by acting the part of the sister, making a face of disgust as he launched into a lecture on why she should stand on her own feet. In playing the part of the patient, he was tentative, apologetic, and almost pleading for understanding—acting very embarrassed. Thus, once he was willing to put himself into the situation, the student had many more reactions than he originally had when he had not pictured what he was being told. He now had material from his own reaction to use in trying to understand the patient, to speculate about, and to inquire into with the patient. His speculations about the patient were no longer simply constructions based on theory. They also came from projecting himself into the situation he was hearing about, visualizing it, and using his own responsiveness. Now he would have the opportunity to ask the patient about his hypotheses and to see how she would respond—perhaps creating also in her, as in himself, a new awareness of self.

SUMMARY

Here we see that the process of supervision—like analysis—is very complex, and that the supervisor must act both as educator and analyst. Throughout the course of supervision, the supervisor must stimulate the student's curiosity about his own responses as he listens to patients and enlarge the student's capacity to use himself as a sounding board—always bearing in mind the theoretical premises upon which the goals of treatment were based.

REFERENCES

Crowley, R. M. Human reactions of analysts. *Samiksa*, 1952, *6*, 212–219.

Ekstein, R. & Wallerstein, R. S. *The teaching and learning of psychotherapy* (2nd ed.). New York: International Universities Press, 1972.

Fromm, E. *The forgotten language*. New York: Grove Press, 1951.

Saul, L. *Teaching and practice of psychoanalysis*. Philadelphia: Lippincott, 1958.

Sullivan, H. S. *The psychiatric interview*. New York: Norton, 1954.

Tauber, E. S. Observations on countertransference phenomena. *Samiksa*, 1952, *6*, 220–228.

Thompson, C. Counter-transference. *Samiksa*, 1952, *6*, 205–211.

5

Being and Doing in Continuous Consultation for Psychoanalytic Education

RALPH M. CROWLEY

Continuous Consultation means what is currently referred to as supervision of psychoanalysis—formerly known as controls or as controlled cases. I borrow the new term from Levenson (1982), who rightly criticizes the term *supervision* as a misleading misnomer. It encourages the consultee to think of his consultant as having superhuman vision, which, in order to be a psychoanalyst, he must acquire somehow. The truth is that none of us has it. None of us, including the patient, can have more vision than our humanness allows us. Yes, we can all learn to expand our visions and use them more skillfully. Doing so, however, is inhibited, discouraged, and perhaps even prevented by the view of the consultant as superhuman. So I shall be using the term *consultation, consultant,* and *consultee* instead of supervision, supervisor, and supervisee because the connotations of the former terms emphasize and corroborate, rather than contradict, what I mean to say.

I have long inveighed against the term *psychoanalytic training,* opting for *psychoanalytic education* instead. We are not dumb animals who get trained, nor do we train dumb animals. We educate human beings who have voices, voices in what they perceive, hear, understand, feel, and do. The process called *psychoanalytic* can be described as a mingling of voices, out of which come new voices in both analyst and patient[1] and in

---

[1]Although the terms *analyst* and *patient* are not ideal, it would be too confusing to substitute others for them.

RALPH M. CROWLEY • Fellow Emeritus and Training and Supervising Analyst, William Alanson White Institute of Psychiatry, Psychoanalysis and Psychology, New York, New York 10023 and Past President, American Academy of Psychoanalysis, New York, New York.

consultant and consultee. This does not mean that I regard psychoanalysis and psychoanalytic consultation as the same process. On the contrary, while they are both dialogues and educational in nature, they have different purposes and goals and, consequently, different methods for meeting these goals.

This chapter was written not only to honor Lewis Browne Hill, but it was stimulated by his paper "On Being Rather Than Doing in Psychotherapy" (1958). My orientation is that psychoanalysis is one kind of psychotherapy, and that they overlap, so that there is no sharp distinction between them (Paolino, 1981). Therefore, what I write applies to psychoanalysis as well as to psychotherapy. Both differ from any other kind of bipersonal relationship and from each other only in terms of their purposes (Sullivan, 1962). A psychoanalyst needs to be a good psychotherapist. Psychotherapy generally has the more limited goal of helping patients learn enough about themselves and other people so that they become better able and freer to cope with certain of their problems with living with people. Psychoanalysis also has this as a goal, but in addition it has the goal of the patients' growth and development as real persons and improved integration of the conflicted and fragmented elements within themselves. However, some of the latter may occur even with psychotherapy, although it is not oriented to the more ambitious goal of psychoanalysis.

If being a person is essential for good psychotherapy, it is all the more necessary in practicing psychoanalysis. The candidate in psychoanalytic consultation needs to have a consultant who serves as a model. Needless to point out, the candidate needs even more of a model in his personal psychoanalysis and also in his teachers of didactic courses. Discussions of supervision in the past have tended to concentrate on what the supervisor does. They have dealt with the supervisee's learning techniques (S. Kaiser, 1955). They tend to stress and overstress the role of countertransferences on the part of the supervisee. I believe that the consultee needs rather to learn to use the optimum of his native endowment and education and to learn to use his own person in his work with patients. Learning this in consultation depends on how the consultant uses himself in helping the consultee. So much for my orientation to this topic.

In my title I use the term *being*, but I also include in being, *being-in-becoming*—a term I borrow from Florence Kluckhohn by way of John Spiegel (1981). Spiegel has analyzed various psychoanalytic and psychotherapeutic schools in terms of the same cultural values that Kluckhohn used in analyzing whole cultures. One value pertains to the kind of personal activity most valued by the culture or therapeutic school—

namely, doing or being or being-in-becoming. Applying this to the consultative process, it refers to the consultant's emphasis on doing or being or being-in-becoming in his own activity and in that of the consultee with his patient. I believe that being-in-becoming is implicit in Hill's (1958) discussion of being and doing. He regards them as inextricably interwoven. As he says, "A therapist is what he does. Conversely put, what the therapist does is an expression of what he is" (Hill, 1958, p. 2). I am certain that, like Sullivan, Hill would also say that consultant, consultee, and his patient are continually changing, not just being and doing but also being-in-becoming. Although I regard these three as inseparable, for purposes of thinking and writing it is possible to focus only on one of these at a time. In other words, they are all equally important, therefore inseparable. Because our culture and many discussions of psychoanalysis and psychoanalytic consultation have emphasized what one does in terms of the technical rules, which are purported to follow the "true" theory, both Hill and I emphasize more the role of being. This means emphasizing more the role of the psychoanalyst both as consultant and therapist, as a person who is real to himself and to his consultee or patient, and emphasizing the psychoanalytic dialogue as a real human communicative transaction. This of course includes consideration of all aspects of being human—the imaginative, the cognitive, the affective, the conative, and the active doing. Conceptualizing psychoanalysis in this way is admittedly more abstract, nonspecific, and vague than are many other ways—whether classical or some variant. Its advantage lies in its being a higher level of abstraction that is capable of resolving many of the currently argued and controversial aspects of the consultative process.

The key theme in all this is the person or personality, if you will, of the people involved in these dyadic relationships of psychoanalytic consultation and psychoanalytic therapy. Although alluded to in various tangential ways from Freud on (his emphasis was on eliminating the personal), it is only recently that the analyst as a person has been singled out for the positive attention such a concept deserves. One of the first to do so wrote on transference and countertransference in the light of field theory (Colm, 1955). She wrote that

> in field theory there is no place for this approach of first, accepted and utilized transference, and, second, controlled and interdicted countertransference. In field experience there can only be spontaneous acting and reacting to the situation and countertransference becomes merely one facet of the common humanity of patient and analyst. (p. 339)

Thompson (1956), discussing the role of the analyst's personality in therapy, opts for positive gains from including consideration—in both theory and technique—of the analyst's personality, rather than attempting to exclude it or minimize its influence. Such consideration opens new fields for investigation, and it obviates the need for feeling defensive about being natural and spontaneous. It thereby facilitates more genuine reactions on the part of the psychoanalyst. In supervision, it makes available new data for observation, such as uncovering unconscious emotional involvement. It allows for becoming aware of the effects of current problems in the life of analysts, and it facilitates additions to the analysts' experience, when merely inexperience or lack of knowledge is the only difficulty. As Schimel (1981) has pointed out, lack of information or knowledge is not countertransference—a distinction that is often overlooked. In considering the personality of the psychoanalyst, Thompson and others make the obvious point that a therapist relates to a patient with more than intellect. There are always two total personalities engaged in reciprocal reactions. Applying this to supervision enables us, according to Thompson, to include as data for understanding the supervisory process the values held by both supervisor and supervisee.

The question of whether there is one type of personality that produces optimum therapeutic results, Thompson (1956, p. 358) answers in the negative. She does mention some personal qualities that she finds tend to produce optimum results, but such qualities can be manifested by many quite different types of persons. Qualities that she stresses include the ability to keep a flexible and open mind about oneself, thus facilitating freedom from blind spots; the ability to interact sensitively with others, while at the same time continuing to learn about oneself; and the ability to have and convey genuine respect for others. We need, she writes, a great variety of personality types for the varying needs of patients. Since patients often come because of conflicts between conforming and not conforming to cultural expectations and the expectations of others, it is good also for the psychoanalyst—both as therapist and consultant—to have had problems in nonconforming himself, and to have worked them out in a way that allows him to have empathy for the nonconforming aspects of his patients.

Thompson is most sympathetic to Colm's (1955) approach to the analytic situation in terms of a mutual human relation. Taking her cue from field theory, she sees the total personalities of any therapeutic dyad as two different fields interacting with one another. These total personalities include, of course, countertransference and transference attitudes, or, if you prefer, parataxic distortions, but they are not limited to them. In her application of field theory, Colm includes not only the person's present being but his potential—his being-in-becoming. She states (Colm, 1955, p. 340) that "not only the person's conscious *here and now* but his potential, his *becoming*, is carried into the field and is experienced in the encounter by the other person. . . . the analyst must be acutely aware of the becoming part of the patient." Also, the consultant must be acutely aware of the "becoming" part of the consultee.

Another outstanding paper dealing with the psychoanalyst as a person was written by Klauber (1968). Other papers that consider this theme in relation to the consultative process have come largely from psychoanalysts associated with the William Alanson White Institute in New York. These include papers by Tauber (1952), Caligor (1981), Issacharoff (1981), Bromberg (1981), and Levenson (1982). Other important contributions include those of Searles (1955), Eckstein and Wallerstein (1958), Doerhman (1976), and Sachs and Shapiro (1976).

In considering what a consultant does, we must include who and what he is. This means his being aware of who and what he is, his feelings and anxieties, and how his way of expressing them are perceived and felt by the consultee. In addition, the consultant must be aware of the anxieties of the consultee, both in doing a good job with the patient and in becoming a good psychoanalyst. There are also anxieties about being recognized as a good analyst by the consultants and by the institute's educational committee—the candidate's evaluators. Few non-institute candidates or institute graduates come for consultation with patients who come three to five times a week. With those who do come, the consultant and consultee are freed from the complications inherent in making evaluatory reports. However, evaluating and being evaluated is always present in any situation involving a teacher–student relation. In fact, making reports has a positive aspect in the consultant's having to confront the consultee's overall talent or lack of it and the consultee's having to face this issue. In our profession, this issue may be bypassed too often. A writing or music teacher who fails to let a student know whether he has the artistic ability required for adequate performance of his art is not only failing his responsibility as a teacher but also his social responsibility of encouraging only those who can serve adequately.

So I return to the usual less demanding situation in which the consultant shares responsibility for evaluation with another evaluatory body—usually an educational committee (perish the term *training committee*) of a psychoanalytic institute. It is impossible to exaggerate the anxieties of a consultee in reaction to his consultant's evaluation. The more the anxieties are out in the open, the better. Some consultants feel easier with these valuation anxieties than others—just as some consultees do—so that in many consultation sessions, evaluation is explicit rather than implicit. With those relationships in which it tends to be implicit, institute requirements of a periodic evaluation report shared with the consultee guarantees open discussion of the candidate's ability. No matter how evaluation is dealt with, it is never easy for the consultant to be both evaluator for the consultee and for the institute while also serving as a source of learning the art of psychoanalysis.

Usually a psychoanalytic candidate has a minimum of three consultants on continuing analyses. This fact tends to balance the personal biases of any one consultant for both consultee and consultant. Just as a psychoanalyst cannot be all things to any one patient, so a consultant cannot be all things or teach all things to any one consultee. The more minds the better, although the consultee may at the time find varied opinions—even contradictory ones—confusing. Fromm-Reichmann pointed out to me one day when I complained of what to do in face of the fact of contradictory advice that the essence of the learning process in an art such as psychoanalysis is in the ability of the student to synthesize such opinions in his own way and in terms of himself and with what works best with his own personality. He learns to absorb and integrate what is valuable and useful to him and to discard that which is not useful at any one moment in his education. What is discarded and what is valued and kept is subject to change throughout psychoanalytic education and throughout life.

Other chapters in this volume discuss specific aspects of the consultative process. I will discuss these only insofar as they relate to the overall framework of the importance of the person and the integration of his being and doing. By *being*, I refer to what and how he thinks, perceives, and feels—what goes on within himself. Any separation of thinking, perception, and feeling is, of course, contrived for purposes of writing and discussion. Every idea or thought or concept has some particular percept and some feeling or emotion connected with it, just as there is some thought behind every feeling. What the consultant does depends on his inner being, just as his inner being is expressed in what he does. Included in *doing* is not only gross muscular or body action but also speaking—how and what one expresses in words as well as in nonverbal postural and other bodily ways.

How does all this relate to the concrete experience of consultation and to currently debated issues in what is known still as supervision? Of great importance is the issue of whom consultation is primarily for—the consultee and his education or the consultee's patient and his therapy. Just as there are limits and structures in the psychoanalytic relationship and process, as Levenson (1982) has so ably discussed, there are limits and structures in the consultative relationship, the violation of which risks failure in achieving its purpose. What is its purpose? Primarily, I believe, it is to educate the consultee, which is distinct from the therapy of the consultee, and from vicarious therapy for his patient. To become an alter therapist or for the consultee to use his consultant as an alter therapist violates the structure of the consultee's being his patient's therapist and his being solely responsible for that therapy (H. Kaiser, 1965). To regard his relationship with his patient otherwise would in turn minimize or obviate the consultation's being primarily education for the consultee. Otherwise, the consultee becomes, as some have phrased it, merely a conduit for the consultant's therapy of his patient, thus destroying both the consultative relation with the consultee and the therapeutic relation with the patient. *Being* implies being wholly in one place at one time for one person, not being in two places at once for two people at the same time.

Another issue is, however, whether education of the psychoanalyst involves his therapy, and if so, how. I have no doubt that one's education—analytic or not and whether by a consultant teacher or a course teacher—will perforce involve the student's personal psychoanalysis. What he learns and how the learning process impinges on his personal problems, these are the materials for his psychoanalysis. That is not the issue. The issue is whether personal problems arising in the consultation, either those brought out by the consultant or those expressed by the consultee, need referral by the consultant to the consultee's analysis. For the consultant to make such referral is, to my mind, an infringement on the responsibility, the autonomy, and the being of the consultee. It is the consultee who has the responsibility for his psychoanalysis, not the consultant. Moreover, it is probably futile advice, and it furthermore interferes with the principle of free, or responsible, association. Whether advised or not, the student will or will not bring the material into the psychoanalytic purview.

One of the trickiest issues is the one that involves the consultant's becoming therapist for the consultee when personal problems, which are often regarded solely as countertransference, obstruct the consultative process. (It is not relevant here to discuss whether the student's analyst should ever presume to give consultative opinions, but I surmise that the answer to that does not have to be identical with that for the consultant's "doing therapy.")

If we believe that the purpose of the consultation is that of the student's education—that is, learning the processes and the art involved in treating people—it is then apparent that the consultee's voicing personal problems needs handling by the consultant, not by commenting on or interpreting them, but by educational methods. By those I mean comments on inquiries about what goes on between the patient and consultee in regard to the consultee's job as therapist.

For example, the consultee asks such questions of his consultant as

"What should I do when the patient says this or that?" or "What do you think is going on with my patient?" As Hill (1958) and Levenson (1982) have pointed out in different ways: Why such questions? Why is the consultee not clear about the answers? What is blocking him?

Sometimes, the consultee is playing a game, knowingly or unknowingly. He has some ideas on what is happening, but asks as if he has none in order to see what the consultant will say, hoping of course, that he will be confirmed in what he is thinking or sometimes hoping to hear something he has not thought of. It is useful when one suspects this sort of game, or even if one does not, to ask for the consultee's thoughts and feelings about what is going on and what he should do about it—whether or not he should intervene in some way. If, then, nothing of importance is said, it is useful, as Hill (1958) has described, to explore with the consultee what feelings he has in reaction to his patient and to what is being communicated. Most important in this are feelings of anxiety that tend to inhibit the consultee's being able to think about or respond to his patient. Oftentimes, bringing his anxiety to the level of communicated awareness results in the consultee's perceiving what is going on, what could be said, or what other sort of intervention might be helpful in furthering a psychoanalytic process.

For example, a consultee asks the consultant, after presenting material from a series of sessions, "What's going on with the patient?" Since the consultant may be quite clear about some problem or other that has been presented, such as how the patient tends to become a victim in one after another of personal encounters, the consultant might well wonder, if it is so clear, then why does the consultee ask him (Levenson, 1982). So one asks the consultee what he thinks is going on—in case the consultee is pulling his leg. In the event that this seems not to be so and that the consultee does not have a notion of what is going on, the consultant needs to ask questions like the following: What were you feeling this session? What was making you anxious? What were your perceptions of the patient that tended to make you anxious? Who does he remind you of?

Such questions inevitably stimulate personal associations and the consultee may be all too willing to reveal and confess personal information that belongs in his personal psychoanalysis, thus diluting it. The trick is to sidestep being involved in such problems and information and to bring the discussion back to being aware that he experiences anxiety. The consultee needs to consider how his anxiety is related to his being distracted from who his patient is, where he is, where he is coming from, what might be really relevant to his patient. This type of consideration often results in the consultee's being able to use himself more with respect to his patient.

What I have been describing is an example of the pre-parallel process, and it lessens the necessity for that more indirect approach. As an example of the parallel process, which was well documented by Caligor (1981) the consultant reacts to the consultee's questions of what should he do or think with anxiety or irritation or some other feeling. Following that lead, the consultant discovers that the patient has been pressuring the consultee to give advice or do his thinking for him. Therefore the consultant concludes that the patient has stimulated the same feelings in the consultee that the consultee has stimulated in him. The consultant then confesses his feelings and suggests the presence of similar feelings in the consultee, with the idea that he might well inform his patient of what effect the patient is having on him, as a way of clarifying what is going on.

In my view the use of the parallel process or reciprocal emotions in this fashion becomes necessary only if the consultant has not been doing his job of educating the consultee in the psychoanalytic process. This will be reflected in the consultee's work with his patient without having to rely upon, or without the occurrence of, parallel processes. The parallel process is a useful paradigm to keep in mind, but it is not the only one.

A way in which the consultant's memory of his experience as a consultee can be useful is as follows. Klauber (1968) has rightly shown, as Waelder (1960) did before him, the fact that all psychological phenomena are multiply determined. The psychoanalyst, at any given moment of intervening, selects for comment, interpretation, or what have you, one of the many aspects of what is presented. In so doing, he is influenced not only by the guiding principles of psychoanalysis but also by his personal values, preferences, and perceptions of how to apply psychoanalytic principles. In brief, what he does and says expresses who and what he is.

Returning to the experience of consultation, Bromberg (1982, p. 99) has noted that comments or instruction in consultations concern past material that will never again be repeated. Therefore, when the consultee next sees his patient, he will not be dealing with the same material nor even with the same patient as in the session before. One cannot step into the same brook twice. And one is reminded of one of Sullivan's (1940) presuppositions underlying the therapeutic interview, namely, "that nothing is static, everything changes in velocity and organization . . . all will undergo insidious change as the interview goes on" (p. 13). In regard to consultations, this fact can be frustrating to the consultee.

Many therapists have confirmed my own experience that a given consultation was helpful with all of my patients except the one on which the consultation was based and supposed to help. This again supports the position that consultation is for the education of the consultee—not primarily for the therapy of the patient being presented. Realization of all this can be helpful to the consultee in that it tends to disabuse him of the myth that the consultant can tell him what to do and that he can learn from the consultant how to do psychoanalytic therapy. It helps also in allowing the consultee to be the therapist, while at the same time learning the art.

Psychoanalytic theory, as Klauber (1968) has discerned, mainly fails to include the role of the person and personality of the psychoanalyst. This has meant that students of psychoanalysis often find little help from theory insofar as actual practice is concerned. It is common knowledge that theoretical papers on psychoanalysis fail to reflect what the author does in practice. Experienced psychoanalysts, even of quite different schools, tend to be more alike in their practices than not. In our present state of knowledge, we have no adequate theory about the human personality. Hill taught that if a patient did not fit the book, we would have to write a new book. Freud developed his theories by intense self-observation and observation of the productions of his patients. We must do the same as Freud did all over again with each patient. This means we need to use our own eyes, ears, and powers of thinking, evaluating, and judging in what we do as psychoanalysts. As consultants, this is the most important aspect of being a person who can be a role model for our consultees—that of being and changing, that is, becoming. We can do this in words and in how we behave. By so doing, we obviate the false dichotomy between theory and practice. This dichotomy arises out of the tendency to say one thing and to do another. By integrating what we are with what we do, this problem is eliminated. We no longer need to carry out theory into practice, only ourselves, of which our theories are only a part, although a necessary part. Theories and hypotheses satisfy our needs to reason and explain what goes on in our lives and in the lives of other human beings, who are like ourselves also. Theories are never facts, but we need more than facts; we need to understand relationships among facts and the meaning of facts. Theories are always changing, and we choose from theories what is useful in our lives and practices, but we need not substitute theories for ourselves or our lives.

Psychoanalytic theory has tended to deal mainly with contents of consciousness and their meanings—usually unconscious meanings. Left out of much psychoanalytic theorizing is what those contents are being used for; what are their purposes and functions. The meaning of content or subject matter is found in what it is being used for, what it is expressing or expected to accomplish, and what it is meant to effect in the person with whom one is communicating. If the consultant can bring his consultee's attention to the meaning of the communications of his patient in terms of their function, the consultee will be much less at sea, while listening with his third ear to his patient.

Consultee's attempts to understand communications without their inducing their patients to clarify what they mean or to what they refer leads to miscommunication, misinterpretation, and eventually to stasis in an analysis. For example, a consultee reports the following series of statements from his patient: "I think about myself and things." "I guess my parents drilled notions in me that I can't shake off." "Money is not personal for me." "I like to go out with Susie because she is easy to communicate with."

These all occurred in one hour, with talking about other things in between, but with no additional information about any one of them. The therapist let them pass without further inquiry, but he wanted his consultant to tell him what was going on. How could a consultant know without the consultee's knowing? How could the consultee know unless he asked the patient to clarify what he was talking about? He needed to ask the following: What was his patient referring to when he thought about himself? What were his thoughts? What notions did his parents drill in him? What does he mean by *drill*? What does he have in mind when he makes such an astounding statement that money is not personal to him? And who is Susie, and what is there about their relationship that makes communication with her "easy." What does he communicate with her that he finds hard to communicate to other people or to his analyst?

This example glaringly portrays how the consultee leaves himself out of the psychoanalytic dialogue. The consultee fails to manifest his own natural curiosity about what the patient is talking about, his curiosity to know his patient. The consultee fails to be aware of and to act on feelings of frustration with the patient's vague, unrevealing, and incomplete communications. Sullivan (1940) insisted that "one has information only to the extent that one tended to communicate about one's self or one's experience." What the consultee has to do here is to facilitate communication by satisfying his own personal needs in the situation. If he uses himself creatively, he will know where his patient is, and "how to do" psychoanalysis will proceed to a different level.

Psychoanalytic theory has worked on the basis that the only function of the psychoanalyst is interpretation. By this is generally meant interpretation of content, not the function of what was being communicated. Little attention was given formerly in psychoanalytic supervision, which was known then as "controls," to whether or not there was interpretable material, either of content or function. Still less attention is paid to how to interpret or communicate with a patient (S. Kaiser, 1965). In order for interpretation to take place, ways must be found to elicit analyzable communication. Most important in the analyst's repertoire is asking the right questions. This means looking in the right places, clarifying what is being said, asking for more information, as in the preceding example. To do this means development of oneself as a person, becoming a person who has access to and can use as much of his human potentiality as possible.

Facilitation of this process is one of the consultant's main tasks. Accomplishing it depends on how much of a real person the consultant has become.

REFERENCES

Bromberg, P. The supervisory process and parallel process. *Contemporary Psycho-analysis*, 1982, *18*, 92–111.
Caligor, L. Parallel and reciprocal processes in psychoanalytic supervision. *Contemporary Psychoanalysis*, 1981, *17*, 1–27.
Colm, H. A field-theory approach to transference and its particular application to children. *Psychiatry*, 1955, *18*, 339–352.
Crowley, R. Human reactions to patients. *Samiksa*, 1952, *6*, 212–219.
Doerhman, M. Parallel processes in supervisors and psychotherapy. *Bulletin of the Menninger Clinic*, 1976, *40*, 3–104.
Eckstein, R., & Wallerstein, R. *The teaching and learning of psychotherapy*. New York: International Universities Press, 1958.
Fromm-Reichmann, F. *Principles of intensive psychotherapy*. Chicago: University of Chicago Press, 1950.
Hill, L. On being rather than doing in psychotherapy. *International Journal of Group Psychotherapy*, 1958, *8*, 1–9.
Issacharoff, A. Countertransference in supervision: Therapeutic consequences for the supervisee, *Contemporary Psychoanalysis*, 1982, *18*, 455–472.
Kaiser, H. *Effective psychotherapy*. New York: The Free Press, 1965.
Kaiser, S. The technique of supervised analysis. Report of a panel. Introduction by E. Windholz. *Journal of the American Psychoanalytic Association*, 1955, *4*, 539–549.
Klauber, J. The psychoanalyst as a person. *British Journal of Medical Psychology*, 1968, *41*, 315–322.
Klauber, J. *The vicissitudes of relationship*. New York: Jason Aronson, 1981.
Leavy, S. *The psychoanalytic dialogue*. New Haven: Yale University Press, 1980.
Levenson, E. Follow the fox. *Contemporary Psychoanalysis*, 1982, *18*, 1–15.
Loewald, H. Reflection on the psychoanalytic process and its therapeutic potentials. *Psychoanalytic Study of the Child*. New York: International Universities Press, 1979.

Paolino, T. Some similarities and differences between psychoanalysis and psychoanalytic psychotherapy: An unsettled controversy. *Journal of Operational Psychiatry*, 1981, *12*, 105–114.

Paolino, T. *Psychoanalytic psychotherapy: Theory, technique, therapeutic relationship and treatability*. New York: Brunner/Mazel, 1982.

Sachs, D., & Shapiro, S. On parallel processes in therapy and teaching. *Psychoanalytic Quarterly*, 1976, *45*, 394–415.

Schimel, J. In discussion of Issacharoff, A., 1981.

Searles, H. The informational value of the supervisor's emotional experiences. *Psychiatry*, 1955, *18*, 135–146.

Spiegel, J. *Psychoanalysis, varied therapeutic interventions and personality change.* Keynote address. American Academy of Psychoanalysis, December 1981.

Sullivan, H. *Therapeutic aspects of the psychiatric consultation with special references to obsessional and schizophrenic states.* Unpublished address to the Neuropsychiatric Society of Baltimore, February 8, 1940.

Sullivan, H. *Schizophrenia as a human process.* New York: Norton, 1962.

Tauber, E. Observations on counter-transference phenomena: The supervisor–therapist relationship. *Samiksa*, 1952, *6*, 220–228.

Thompson, C. The role of the analyst's personality. *American Journal of Psychotherapy*, 1956, *10*, 347–359.

Waelder, R. *Basic theory of psychoanalysis.* New York: International Universities Press, 1960.

6

Countertransference in Supervision
Therapeutic Consequences for the Supervisee

AMNON ISSACHAROFF

Education, as Professor Whitehead (1929, p. 6) wrote, is the acquisition of the art of utilizing knowledge. He added that this is an art that is very difficult to impart. Most psychoanalysts are engaged in some educational pursuit, whether in classrooms, hospitals, or liaison work with other professionals. Most of us also educate through supervision—that is, teaching the art of utilizing technical knowledge and the utilization of the self as an "analytic instrument," as defined by Isakower (Balter, Lothane, & Spencer, 1980).

The psychotherapeutic aim of supervision is to improve the quality of the analyzing instrument—that is, the student's therapeutic personality. The psychotherapeutic consequences for the supervisee derive from the supervisory experience itself and from its influence on the supervisee's concurrent analysis, if he is a candidate in training.

This chapter is an attempt to pull loose ends together. Interweaving supervision and psychoanalysis is not firmly anchored in traditional paths of psychoanalytic education. On the contrary, as Daryl DeBell (1981) writes:

> Perhaps one of the earliest and most persistent questions about appropriate supervisory activity is how much one should treat the analyst versus how much one should simply teach him. This is a peculiar question and becomes more strange the more it is discussed. For one thing, it is difficult to find

This chapter was first published in *Contemporary Psychoanalysis*, 1982, *18*(4), 1–15, and is reprinted by permission of the William Alanson White Institute.

AMNON ISSACHAROFF • Fellow, Training and Supervising Analyst, William Alanson White Institute of Psychiatry, Psychoanalysis and Psychology, New York, New York 10023 and Attending Psychiatrist, New York Hospital-Cornell Medical Center, New York, New York 10021.

proponents of the explicit "treatment" of candidates during supervision, certainly no one in the group[1] advocates analyzing the supervisee. Still, every member of the group agrees that it is sometimes necessary to point out to the analyst certain obstructive patterns, and even on occasion to comment about and even inquire into their possible meaning and motivation. Such interventions by the supervisor are not necessarily thought to be unacceptably intrusive, i.e., "therapeutic." There is rather a tacit acceptance that such actions are often both useful and salutary. . . . The supervisor is demonstrating the existence of faulty technique, and is then permitted to pursue the matter by illustrating the possible origins of the error. To state the matter in extreme terms, everybody appears to oppose "treatment" of the supervisee, and yet everybody does it. Some do it with misgivings, and some without. (pp. 41–42)

The examples I choose to illustrate the interweaving of supervision and psychoanalysis are based on my experience in the conduct of both of these roles. At the William A. White Institute a candidate in the course of training is required to conduct several analyses under the guidance of several senior analysts. Different triads are thus formed, and each triad offers a different learning opportunity. The aggregate of these experiences enables the student to form the basis of his professional identity. As these experimental triads evolve, the student applies his learning effort to two simultaneous tasks: first, acquiring psychoanalytic technique, and second, understanding his emotional reactions to his patient—that is, countertransference. The emphasis on either one of these two tasks depends on the particular student, the particular supervisor, and the combination of the two. Personally, I discuss countertransference extensively with my students. Since candidates know about me through word of mouth and what I have written, those who are interested in countertransference request my supervision. There is a self-selection. It is, therefore, explicit in our initial contract that we will explore this.

In discussions of supervision in the 1930s and 1940s, the two learning tasks were seen as different areas of competence, which were to be handled by different teachers. The Hungarian system described by Balint (1948), recommending that both training and control analyses be carried out by the same person, was never approved by training conferences. In fact, the difference between the two tasks was emphasized. Teaching the student how to analyze a patient that presented problems different from the student's was termed *analysis Kontrol*. Analysis of the

---

[1]Study group on supervision of the committee on psychoanalytic education (COPE) of the American Psychoanalytic Association.

candidate's countertransference to his patient was labeled *Kontrol analysis.* (More recently, authors like Fleming and Benedek, 1964, have referred to analysis of the countertransference as supervisory analysis.)

In spite of the often-stated rule that supervision should not have therapeutic aims, it remains a fact that supervision touches upon unresolved conflicts of the supervisee. After all, as Tauber has observed (1952), we as psychoanalysts do not encounter all the facets of our analysand's personality. It is a fact of life that everyone is different, according to different roles, situations, and people with whom we interact. The supervisee brings to the supervisory situation transferential attitudes for both his patient and the supervisor. In that context, supervision is not only a didactic experience, but also it is one that includes the emotions that are brought into play both in treatment and in the supervisory process. In that sense, supervision is a kind of analysis. It provides an opportunity for further psychotherapeutic change as well as the study of technique. When the supervisory psychoanalyst deals with such a complex task, he may be able to help the student in his handling of the therapeutic situation as well as contribute to the development of the analyzing instrument—that is, to the further integration of the student's psychotherapeutic personality.

For example, a student described a situation that took place during the initial phase of the analysis of a male homosexual patient. During one session both had paid much attention to nonverbal communication: whether knees were overlapped (feminine fashion) or one leg made a *T* over the other (masculine fashion). The supervisee said that the demeanor of the patient—a psychology student—made him uncomfortable. In that same session, the patient described in great detail some sadomasochistic sexual encounters to which the student reacted with repulsion. The rest of the session was devoted to a description of the patient's only, older brother, a Vietnam veteran, who was so violence-prone that his application to the police had been rejected after psychological tests. The brother appeared confused and disoriented, and the patient's mother was constantly concerned with him. The patient added bitterly that this concern for his brother represented a shift from his mother's exclusive attention to the patient in earlier years. The student made no intervention during that hour.

In this first supervisory meeting the student assertively announced his intention of focusing primarily on the interaction in the here and now and letting the patient's historical background fall into place as it emerged. I was conscious of his paying attention to how I crossed my legs, and I wondered if this student, who had limited psychoanalytic experience, had considered what my contribution might be to his train-

ing. Upon reflection, I felt that this student experienced a reactive assert-
iveness toward me and had reenacted the patient's aggressive control as
an initial gambit. I assumed my initial irritation and temptation to set
him straight and to be a mirror of his own repressed hostility toward his
patient. The focus on the here and now and the watchful sitting face-to-
face and legs-to-legs were all part of a rationalized technique for defensive purposes. The student was under the impact of aggressive impulses
that emanated from the patient.

This initial assessment is an example of an approach to supervision
that attempts to resolve resistance to the learning situation as well as to
the patient's own resistance. The student was caught between his own
counterresistance to the controlling tactics of his patient and his reenactment of that situation with the supervisor. When this occurs, the supervisory situation is in a *jam,* as Emch (1955) calls it, and the supervisor has
to make a choice between addressing didactic and technical issues or
paying attention to the ways in which the student responds by identifying with the patient. The activity of the supervisor, if he chooses the
latter, is similar to what a psychoanalyst would do with his patient. He
is concerned with bringing into the student's awareness what has been
dissociated in the response to the patient. The supervisor has to take
into account matters of transference and countertransference between
himself and the student as well as between the student and the patient.
And finally, there are similar problems of strategy, timing, and phrasing
of what amounts to an interpretation.

This kind of supervisory work is quite different from the usual
didactic atmosphere of the regular supervisory hour where the two participants are engaged in enriching the understanding of the psychoanalytic process. In that situation, there are often "happy hours" that
enhance feelings of competence. But when supervision is in a jam and
the bells go off, so to speak, the supervisory reaction described before is
motivated by a therapeutic concern. When things work well, the
therapeutic aim is ultimately manifested in the student's work with his
patient.

In the situation I described, I chose to emphasize the empathic
nature of the student's identification with his patient. Noting how
quickly this process had been established allowed for direct access to the
understanding of a fundamental psychodynamic issue that was probably central in that patient's life: To control aggressively the abandoning
object. When the reenactment of this dynamic interplay in the supervisory situation was understood, the student's ability to tolerate his
empathic identification with his patient was reflected in a lessened resistance to the learning situation.

The immediate result of this approach was a noticeable decrease of tension both in the supervisory and psychoanalytic situations. The neurotic aspect of the countertransference was not predominant, and the student soon began to take a more active role in getting to know his patient. The stiffening of the facial and spinal musculature that often followed my comments gave way to a more relaxed posture. We began the slow journey to where occasional and productive collaboration was possible.

The perennial controversy between those who will teach and those who will treat (in DeBell's terms) in order to achieve the goal of optimal psychoanalytic competence was particularly highlighted in the supervisory problem presented by this student. Although we did not have an established learning alliance, I felt it was important to confront the parallel process at the outset of our work, just as a negative transference requires direct confrontation in the ordinary psychotherapeutic situation, even at its very beginning. Otherwise the repetitive elements of this process in the supervisory relationship might have led to equally intractable learning difficulties.

There is no doubt that there is an element of supervisory countertransference in this situation. Bromberg (1982) emphasized this point of confluence between supervisory countertransference and the parallel process, and he also referred to the difficulty of remaining neutral as a supervisor because of the supervisor's responsibility to respond to crisis, stalemates, and other problems in the treatment he is supervising.

In making the revolutionary discovery that transference was not an obstacle but rather a facilitating and necessary condition to the solution of the conflicts brought into therapy, Freud also made it possible to utilize the emotional conflicts brought into supervision by the student— to the benefit of the learning task. The supervisory task is complicated, however, by the fact that the student brings into the supervisory process his emotional attitudes toward both his patient and his supervisor.

In the current literature, *countertransference* is defined either classically—that is, as the unconscious, unresolved conflicts in the psychoanalyst that are expressed in mistakes in technique—or totalistically, as encompassing every conscious and unconscious reaction of the psychoanalyst toward his patient. I would place under the heading of *countertransference* any reaction on the part of the psychoanalyst that reflects a partial or complete blind spot or "dumb" spot (Jacob, 1981) in regard to his patient. This blind spot may be a cultural attitude, an aspect of character structure, a conflict from any developmental epoch or its related defense, a dissociated displacement or parataxic distortion, an empathic counteridentification, a patient-induced complementary reaction, and so on.

From the point of view of countertransference as a working instrument, it is important to assess its impact on the psychoanalyst. When the countertransference is overwhelmingly empathic in nature, it reduces the objectivity of the analyst's thought processes. On the other hand, when countertransferential information suggests a discrepancy between the psychoanalyst's feelings and the content of the patient's communication, as Paula Heimann (1977) describes it, this alerts the psychoanalyst to understand the content of the patient's expression to account for the affective disparity.

The student I described before was under the impact of the type of countertransference that is overwhelmingly empathic. This induced regressive phenomena leading to the parallel process. His identification with his patient was also a good example of what Arlow (1963) calls *transient identifications* that are unconscious in nature but not deeply rooted. This type of empathic undercurrent between the patient and psychotherapist that results in transient identifications is particularly important to understanding the patient. The shift from experiencing these identifications to self-observation grows smoother as the student gains experience and is more able to tolerate and accept them as a necessary and useful (albeit often disturbing) part of the psychoanalytic process.

If that shift from experiencing to self-observation does not take place, the supervisor can be alerted by the discrepancy between what the student reports and the affective climate in the supervisory session. The student's countertransference, resulting in a transitory identification with his patient, goes unreported, but it is reenacted in such a way that the affective disparity is accounted for. The student is no longer interested in learning, and the supervisor becomes preoccupied with what has gone wrong in supervision rather than in understanding the psychoanalytic process between the student and his patient. In that situation, it is the supervisor's task to make the shift from experiencing to self-observation by clarifying the way the student's identification with the patient has been extrapolated to the supervisory process.

Searles (1955) calls this parallel phenomenon a reflective process by which a student, in Hora's account (1957), "unconsciously identifies with the patient and involuntarily behaves in such a manner as to elicit in the supervisor those very emotions which the student, himself, experienced while working with the patient, but was unable to convey verbally." This is more likely to happen when the patient makes a powerful impact on the student, who may react with a temporary identification based on similarly repressed wishes or defensive needs. The emotional bombardment coming from the patient creates the necessary condition under which the identification synapsis clicks into place and closes at the same time the student's access to verbal memory.

The regressive quality of this process has been noted by several writers. Gediman and Wolkenfeld (1980) describe it as "transmitting in action what fails to be reported in words." This transient regression has a quality that is opposite to recollecting and repeating in words. But because of its transient nature, it is more readily accessible to interpretive activity in the supervisory situation. This is particularly true if the learning alliance has a positive quality and the supervisee has advanced sufficiently in his own analysis. The more advanced candidates are less defensive about their temporary identifications with their patients and can explore these reactions to learn more about themselves and about their patients.[2]

The following are some thoughts on the mutual impact of supervision and the student's own analysis. It has been my experience that most students tend to present their work in such a way that it describes the behavior of the patient and whatever historical antecedents help to

---

[2]In teaching a clinical seminar on borderline and schizoid pathology, the students were instructed to present an interactional difficulty with a patient who filled the requirements of the course. In a second go-round, the students presented the same patient, focusing this time on a detailed account of the last session prior to the presentation. The class was instructed to respond to the presentation with their appraisal of the treatment situation. Similarly to what Sacks and Shapiro (1976) found in their study, the presenters often reenacted the roles of their patients and elicited responses from the class similar to their own vis-à-vis the patient. This parallelism between what transpired in the seminar and in the treatment situation derived its driving force from the focus on the difficulties aroused in the treatment by the severe pathology of the patients discussed in the seminar.

What is "normal and essential process in reporting" (Arlow, 1963)—namely, the oscillation between transient identification of the student with his or her patient and objective reporting—was also accentuated by the inevitable reaction to the group situation. Although the climate that evolved in the seminar was one of openness and trust, it was difficult—for some students more than others—to describe impasses and stalemates that necessarily aroused feelings of inadequacy. I noted an atmosphere in the group that was complementary to the attitude of the presenter that suggested the enactment of a parallel process. My role was to point out that parallel process, when it was clearly discernible, and to interpret it as a problem emanating from the dynamics of the patient presented. Almost consistently, the class members reported in the follow-up presentation a sometimes dramatic resolution of the problem presented, following the discovery of the parallel occurrence. The experiencing of their identification with the patient in the peer-group situation facilitated its reversibility with the attendant relief afforded by regaining the objectivity of the observing role. The recurring consistency of this phenomenon suggests that a nonjudgmental supervision in the format of a clinical seminar may bypass some of the complexities introjected by transferential issues in the one-to-one supervisory situation.

elucidate it, but most students tend to omit their own participation and reactions. Thus, they maintain an emotional distance from themselves and from the material. But if the student's behavior and reactions become an issue because of some unresolved conflict on his part, the supervisory effort may be to recognize that such a situation exists and then to deal with it in terms of the student's problems in facing that particular situation.

Here the old problem of not transforming the supervisory process into a treatment process becomes an issue. If the supervisory relationship is a positive one and if there is enough trust to permit the airing of the problematic material, the issues at hand may conceivably be contained within the supervisory hour. Sometimes, however, these are not that easy to approach in this direct way, and then comes the famous recommendation, *Take it up in your own analysis.*

This recommendation is futile most of the time. The psychoanalytic process does not necessarily allow for the intrusion of an issue—on command—because it would be convenient in the training process. An issue that comes up in a supervisory hour may not be indicated at that time in the process of the student's own analysis. Therefore, the fact that the student may not bring the issue up in analysis does not necessarily indicate a resistance on his part, but merely the fact that he is engaged in other issues of his own analysis. However, at times it may be an indication of resistance, particularly when the issue reflects an ego-syntonic personality problem, in which case there may be reluctance on the part of the student to overcome the resistance to issues that he does not consider important in himself. If this situation becomes entrenched in the supervisory situation, we have a problem that may require other measures in order to overcome the resistance of the student, facilitate further growth, and most important, to tackle a situation that—if permitted to remain untouched—might hinder further growth in the student's capacity to analyze the patient as well as to grow as a person.

Martin Grotjahn (1955, p. 11) is emphatic about the role of supervision as an extention of analysis. He says that "the supervisor should take an active part in the interpretation of the countertransference of the student." Grotjahn avoids telling the candidate that "this is a blind spot of yours; this you have to take up in your own analysis." He finds that ineffective. It is warded off because of the candidate's resistance and reinforced by the training analyst's corresponding resistance. On the other hand, a candidate may sometimes accept interpretations given in relation to his behavior toward the patient that have been given to him many times without any result in his own analysis. The different structuring of transference resistance in the supervisory situation may enable the student to integrate this insight and then take the further step of resolving it in his own analysis.

Should the supervisor communicate with the student's psychoanalyst? To take advantage of this possibility may require a review of certain attitudes that have become traditional in the training system of schools such as the William Alanson White Institute. There is a wide consensus in the literature that indicates that there should be a clearly drawn line between supervisory intent and psychotherapeutic intent on the part of the supervisor. In their 1953 publication "What Is a Supervisory Analysis?" Blicksten and Fleming favored a collaborative conference between the supervisory analyst and the training analyst. This, I believe, can be especially useful when there is a positive, collaborative atmosphere among all the participants.

Emch (1955), commenting on the Blicksten–Fleming point of view about direct communication between the supervisory and training psychoanalyst, objected to that practice when the student is still in analysis. She doubted whether most training psychoanalysts would agree with the assumption that the supervisor becomes a kind of superanalyst because he knows of some more important resistance in the student of which the personal psychoanalyst has little or no knowledge. Emch went on to state that it was more probable that resistance noted by the supervisor relates to areas extremely important to the student's own analysis that will require repeated careful attention before clear and relatively constant awareness of their meanings can be manifested in conscious behavior and functioning. Emch also objected to this particular kind of interauthority communication, or supervisory collaboration, on the grounds that it might interfere with the use of free association.

However relevant some of Emch's points may be in terms of the psychoanalytic process and the fundamental resolution of conflicts in that setting, it seems to me that she overlooks the role of the transference resistance in the resolution of these problems and the fact that outside events—such as supervisory events—may act as active precipitants that crystallize issues at crucial moments. *Supervisory jam,* as Emch calls it, may acquire more importance than other conscious current events because it may represent an active split in the candidate's transference. The inclusion of this information in his own analysis can be a powerful integrative tool. To maintain an encapsulated relationship with the analyst is reminiscent of a more infantile type of relationship. At the White Institute, the training analyst receives feedback from the supervisory analyst in training-committee meetings. However, the kind of collaboration I am speaking of goes beyond that passive listening to the reports of the supervisor. It is a more personalized discussion, particularly around the problems that may arise in supervision and that have to do with character resistances—or particularly countertransferences—that may indicate resurgence of emergence of personal conflict in the candidate. He may have some resistance to dealing with this in supervision and possibly in his own analysis as well, if it is not actively encouraged by a collaborative relationship between the supervisor and the training analyst. Of course, this collaborative relationship between the supervisory analyst and the training analyst presupposes the existence of a harmonious "psychoanalyst family." The institutional setting may facilitate these collaborative relationships or increase the possibility of the sibling rivalry that is inevitable in even the most harmonious families. The tendency to protect the one-to-one relationships parallels to some extent the relationship that exists between a child and mother in the earlier stages of a child's development, as Fleming and Benedek (1964) note. This does not necessarily help the maturation process of the student, and that could be reflected in the student's attitude toward his own patient. This collaboration between the supervisory and the training analysts can take place only if the supervisor takes an active interest in the emotional attitude of the student toward his patient, that is, if he pays special attention to countertransference issues.

The following are examples in which the psychoanalyst was in a position to facilitate the resolution of a supervisory jam. Due to his knowledge of genetic components, the psychoanalyst could intervene and help the student acquire a perspective on the bottleneck where a disassociated conflict on his part was contributing to a stalemate with the patient and supervisor.

A young and attractive student started a psychoanalytic session by describing strong feelings about a recent supervisory session. Her supervisor, a mild-mannered and benevolent figure, had commented about the candidate's difficulty in confronting aggression and her emphasis (*overemphasis* as heard by the student) on sexual matters. The candidate's patient—also a young woman—had made sexual advances during the therapy hours and now had embarked on a persistent and vociferous devaluation of the whole treatment, which was about to end because of circumstances beyond the control of both participants. The candidate also reported that during the psychoanalytic hour her supervisor, who had made her feel she was his favorite in classes and seminars, had just announced an impending move to a distant city. At the time, the student was exploring in her own psychotherapy self-derogatory feelings that emanated from sex play in her childhood—admonitions by her mother not to engage in genital exploration with her female cousin. With these converging forces, the patient experienced acute self-depreciation and intense guilt about her sexuality. The transferential split between the supervisor and the patient's analyst was reinforced by the analyst's identification with her patient. That is, the analyst avoided the exploration in her own therapy of similar transferential wishes as expressed by her patient by focusing on her guilt in the supervisory situation.

The point emphasized is the triangle formed by the student, the supervisor, and the psychoanalyst. The student denies her identification with her own patient to avoid the experience of loss of the supervisory relationship and the impending termination of the therapy. She accepts her patient's negative feelings about the whole therapeutic experience. The devaluation is seen as the better alternative to the symbiotic tendency by means of sexual exploration. Sexual fusion induces excessive guilt that is reinforced in the supervisory experience. The supervisor's comments about her excessive sexual curiosity and the impending termination of his supervision point to defensiveness about painful loss in both participants. The reenactment of her mother's injunction against sexual exploration in the supervisory situation introduces an inhibitory element in her function as a therapist as well as a safety barrier between her and the supervisor. We could speculate on the possibility of the supervisor's contertransference and even of the possibly defensive nature of his comments on his supervisee's concern with sexual matters. But this is not necessary for our purposes. The fact is that, regardless of the supervisor's unconscious intention, the student experienced an acute crisis in role appropriateness.

The confluence of her sexual conflicts in different role levels (daughter, patient, supervisee) was finally brought to a boiling point by the supervisor's creating a crisis of therapeutic potential. With the transferential forces fully invested by the student in the triangle with her patient and her supervisor, my role was to sort out and bring perspective to facilitate learning in the supervisory process. The supervisee, having understood in her own therapy the dynamic roots of her reactions to both her patient and her supervisor, could regain the role and her objectivity in both situations. Only the supervisee's therapist could have been in a strategic position to reestablish the role equilibrium of all the participants.

Another candidate in psychoanalysis worked on understanding her tendency to become increasingly critical of any man with whom she tried to develop a serious relationship. One of her supervisors remarked on her recurrent difficulty in selecting the right patient, who was supposed to be a man, for her training requirements. This difficulty was not brought up as a psychoanalytic issue by the student, and I felt that their contract did not allow its inclusion in the work. However, when agreed on as part and parcel of the training system, a judicious use of collaborative consultation between supervisory and training analyst around specific issues can facilitate the exploration of recurrent neurotic patterns that overlap the professional and private aspects of the candidate's behavior as well as help overcome unconscious resistance on the part of the candidate to bringing such patterns to analysis. The argument is that the resolution of the underlying conflict in the analysis would be facilitated by the vicissitudes of the supervisory and training experiences without specifically focusing on such issues as brought to the psychoanalyst's attention by the supervising analytic colleague.

In the tradition of the White Institute, the training psychoanalyst would be able to use the information provided by the supervisory analyst only when it was appropriate to the process of the analytic situation and then only to clarify his own thinking and interpretation of the material. At present, however, a kind of informal collaboration does take place between the supervisory and training analysts when they are in communication about other matters. In these situations, a casual comment by the supervisory psychoanalyst may point to a problem area and alert the training psychoanalyst.

Issues that come up in the supervisory situation that are grist for the mill of the student's own psychoanalysis include the candidate's reaction to his patient's transference—that is, his countertransference reactions. When these issues are explored in a supervisory situation, they may provide opportunities to clarify what otherwise might remain as lacunae in the candidate's analysis because these issues may not become apparent in the transference in the analysis. In other words, when the emotional reactions of the student toward the patient are of such a nature as to actively and adversely affect the treatment, supervision may offer the possibility to explore the conflict in a manner that will bypass the transference resistances that the student may experience in his own analysis.

Interpretations in the context of the supervisory situation are different from the classical interpretations given in the analytic situation. In the latter, interpretations, when they encompass elements from the past as well as from the present in the transference situation, have a rounded quality of completeness. This—almost by definition—cannot be attained in supervision. The complete interpretation is neither desirable nor attainable in the supervisory situation. At most, the supervisor can comment on the emotional reactions of the supervisee toward the patient and some transferential reaction toward himself. Links to genetic aspects remain outside the supervisory situation, although at times a student may bring them up in spontaneous association. I do not encourage these associations to develop but accept them as corroboration of the issue at hand. The aim is always the resolution of the conflict between the supervisee and the patient, with the dual aim of improving the analytic instrument—that is, the capacity of the candidate to be free of internal conflicts and to analyze his patient, as well as an opening for further self-analysis or analytic work in the student's own analysis.

It is true, as Arlow (1963) states, that the genetic aspects of the conflict that the candidate may experience and its unconscious determinants are properly the realm of the personal psychoanalysis. He emphasizes that the supervisory situation is a part of reality and must be treated as such. Therefore, an attempt to make interpretations in the supervisory context may be compared to giving an interpretation to a patient without any knowledge of the unconscious genetic factors of the disturbance. Although we often do just that in the ordinary therapeutic situation, we abstain as supervisors because of the different contractual agreement with the supervisee. However, as Arlow also recognizes, the supervisory situation may sharply expose those aspects of interaction between the patient and therapist and thus provide an opportunity to observe the neurotic reactions that the psychotherapist may experience, which can then be studied phenomenologically. The difficulty in separating the two learning goals—the analysis of the student's countertransference, which is an extention of his own analysis, and the imparting of technical skills—is at the root of the difficulties that the supervisory psychoanalyst may experience, with a resulting overprotection of the candidate in the supervisory situation.

Benedek (1954) equates supervisory overprotection to parental overprotection and finds that the most significant problem is that of insecurity with respect to the child—"the fear of one's inability to handle the child and treat and educate him to his best advantage." This type of transference in the supervisor often leads to either the overprotectiveness I have mentioned or to an overly critical attitude—that the candidate may be a disappointing child. The supervisor may feel like a narcissistic parent whose offspring have to achieve perfection.

Another problem is discussed by Lucia A. Tower (Sloane, 1951), who suggests that students who are eager to report and analyze their own reactions in supervision may be suffering from unresolved exhibitionist masochism. She goes on to say that preoccupation with the student's countertransference can be detrimental to the conduct of the supervision for a variety of reasons:

1. It may shift attention from the patient to the student.
2. By threatening the student, it may cause increased defensiveness and hostility toward both the patient and the supervisor and create a greater confusion.

3. It may be an expression of the supervisor's countertransference toward the candidate or the training psychoanalyst, in which case the supervisor would be using the situation for personal reasons.

Tower affirms that the person who is best qualified to deal with countertransference reactions is the student's own psychoanalyst. Sloane (1951), quoting Aaron Karush, also reports a case in which analyzing countertransference seemed to have become a fad. The candidate spoke freely about his countertransference toward the patient, confessing his hostility in telling about his difficulty in grasping certain psychodynamic formulations. Since the candidate kept repeating the same thing, however, the supervisor began to suspect that he really did not know much about the psychodynamics of the patient. The supervisor also thought that the candidate was attempting to seduce him by discussing a pseudocountertransference with him. In this respect, a supervisory experience comes to mind that seems to corroborate Karush's view.

The student in question was all too eager to examine his countertransference, and he volunteered data from his own analysis to understand his patient. He was convinced that by not displaying curiosity over any aspect of the material presented by the patient, he could maintain an optimum level of neutrality. However, his sporadic interventions had a strong moralistic overtone, and when that was pointed out he was ready again to examine his countertransference. This apparently compliant attitude might be seen as a worthwhile goal in supervision, but in reality it covered an omnipotent fantasy of an ideal psychoanalyst engaged in the ideal psychoanalysis that would be made more perfect by pursuing the task of examining the psychotherapist's emotions in supervision.

In fact, the psychotherapist's aim was to create a system in which the patient would bring about reactions in him that would provide the material for his own treatment, both in his own analysis and in his supervision. His lack of curiosity about his patient's history and background was, in reality, a reflection of his need to avoid an interruption to the continuous stimulation of his own internal processes. There was therefore no need for a more complete picture of the patient's psychodynamic roots. Allowing the pieces to fall into place gradually is, of course, a tenable analytic posture. But in this situation there was an interesting and revealing dichotomy in the supervisory material. The student paid little attention to transference issues, but he was continually receptive to the patient's impact on the setting and on himself.

He insisted that by learning more about himself and his reactions to his patient he would become a better psychoanalytic instrument and eventually benefit his patient. In fact, he paid little attention to the unconscious meaning of his patient's words and behavior. In this situation, I felt that the supervisory situation required more attention to basics.

Edgar Levenson (1981) has described a supervisory mode that he termed the *algorithmic method*. This is a three-step approach that first establishes the setting, then a detailed history, and finally careful attention to the transference. The student described previously needed the discipline of a rigorous application of a learning approach that would redirect his attention from himself to the patient. Levenson's basic method well describes the changes required in this case—with good results culminating in a substantial improvement in the learning climate.

In conclusion, I have emphasized the value of an approach in supervision that constantly evaluates the student's talent in the area of self-knowledge and the constructive use of his countertransference reactions. There are always difficulties in this area. Sometimes these may be the result of anxiety attributable to inexperience, or the supervisor may have some questions about the student's sensitivity, ability to work with transference, capacity for self-analysis, and so on. But these problems may prove to be temporary. They should be kept in mind as the student continues in training, but to share them prematurely may not be helpful and could indeed be discouraging.

Sullivan (1947, p. 246) remarked that when people are adequately and appropriately motivated, they tend to understand each other and to collaborate to mutual advantage. He stated further, in his unique dry style, that "everyone, at least occasionally, understands and collaborates with another. Everyone, all too frequently, fails for a variety of reasons." This state of collaboration facilitates communication, which Sullivan (1947, p. 246) defined as an "exquisite triumph of trial and profit from shrewdly observed errors." He considered the chances for collaboration vastly improved when all those concerned know that (and he quoted Bridgeman) "a term is defined, when the conditions are stated under which I may use the term and when I may infer from the use of the term by my neighbor that the same condition prevail" (pp. 246–247). Assuming that this state of collaboration is reached, the conditions may be laid for an enjoyable and creative learning experience for both participants. In such situations there is a much increased tolerance of ambiguity and a temporary lack of understanding. Both participants can suspend their critical faculties and find new meanings in the material presented. If the stage of trial and profit is successfully dealt with, the collaborative state allows the supervisor to pay attention to the student as a psychoanalyzing instrument. The supervisory instrument in this task is the supervisor's own analyzing instrument, and therefore, the patient becomes a *mutually shared* patient. The questions the supervisor asks at this stage and his or her therapeutic suggestions derive from his or her own way of experiencing the psychoanalytic situation.

I have discussed a mode of supervision that emphasizes the exploration of the student's countertransference when the learning-about-the-patient aspect of the supervisory experience runs into problems. This may be caused by the inclusion of transference and countertransference issues both in the supervisory and the psychoanalytic situations. This approach to supervision requires a clear understanding and the collaboration of the student. I have indicated that this type of supervision is a kind of analysis that uses the same technical considerations as regular psychoanalysis, and its usefulness is apparent in situations where the student reenacts nonverbally in supervision his countertransference toward his patient.

I have commented on the interplay between supervision as an analytic process and the student's own training analysis, emphasizing the potential usefulness of a collaborative conference between the supervisory analyst and the training analyst, particularly during supervisory jams that may suggest a transferential split in the student—leaving out of his own psychoanalysis certain conflicts that appear only in the supervisory work.

Finally, I have reflected on possible misuses of countertransferential issues in supervision and the occasional bliss of the collaborative state.

REFERENCES

Arlow, J. A. The supervisory situation. *Journal of the American Psychoanalytic Association*, 1963, *11*, 576–594.

Balint, M. On the psychoanalytic training system. *International Journal of Psychoanalysis*, 1948, *29*, 163–173.

Balter, L., Lothane, Z., & Spencer, J. On the analyzing instrument, *Psychoanalytic Quarterly*, 1980, *49*, 474–504.

Benedek, T. Countertransference in the training analyst. *Bulletin of the Menninger Clinic*, 1954, *18*, 12–16.

Blicksten, N. L., & Fleming, J. What is a supervisory analysis? *Bulletin of the Menninger Clinic*, 1953, *17*, 117–129.

Bromberg, P. M. The supervisory process and parallel process in psychoanalysis. *Contemporary Psychoanalysis*, 1982, *18*, 92–111.

DeBell, D. E. A critical digest of the literature on psychoanalytic supervision. *Journal of the American Psychoanalytic Association*, 1963, *11*, 540–575.

DeBell, D. E. Supervisory styles and positions. In R. S. Wallerstein (Ed.), *Becoming a psychoanalyst*. New York: International Universities Press, 1981.

Emch, M. The social context of supervision. *International Journal of Psychoanalysis*, 1955, *36*, 298–306.

Fleming, J., & Benedek, T. Supervision: A method of teaching psychoanalysis: Preliminary report. *Psychoanalytic Quarterly*, 1964, *33*, 71–96.

Gediman, H. K., & Wolkenfeld, F. The parallelism phenomenon in psychoanalysis and supervision: Its reconsideration as a triadic system. *Psychoanalytic Quarterly*, 1980, *49*, 234–255.

Grotjahn, M. Problems and techniques of supervision. *Psychiatry*, 1955, *18*, 9–15.

Heimann, P. Further observations on the analyst's cognition process. *Journal of the American Psychoanalytic Association*, 1977, *25*, 313–333.

Hora, T. Contribution to the phenomenology of the supervisory process. *American Journal of Psychotherapy*, 1957, *11*, 769–773.

Jacob, P. The San Francisco project. In R. S. Wallerstein (Ed.), *Becoming a psychoanalyst*. New York: International Universities Press, 1981.

Levenson, E. Follow the fox: An inquiry into the vicissitudes of psychoanalytic supervision. *Contemporary Psychoanalysis*, 1982, *18*(4), 1–15.

Sachs, O. M., & Shapiro, J. H. On parallel processes in therapy and teaching. *Psychoanalytic Quarterly*, 1976, *45*, 394–415.

Searles, H. F. The informational value of the supervisor's emotional experience. *Psychiatry*, 1955, *18*, 135–146.

Sloane, P. Panel report: The technique of supervised analysis. *Journal of the American Psychoanalytic Association*, 1951, *5*, 539–547.

Sullivan, H. S. Remobilization for enduring peace and social progress. *Psychiatry*, 1947, *10*, 239–252.

Tauber, E. S. Observations on counter-transference phenomena: The supervisor–therapist relationship. *Samiksa*, 1952, *6*, 220–228.

Whitehead, A. N. *The aims of education and other essays*. New York: Macmillan, 1929.

7

Supervisory Crises and Dreams from Supervisees

Robert Langs

In recent years, psychoanalysts have begun to examine the specific structure of the supervisory situation and its techniques. The present chapter is an attempt to explore a particular dimension of supervision that is seldom examined in a specific fashion—the supervisory crisis. Because of the wide scope of this important topic, the present contribution will focus on a single aspect of this situation: The use of dreams spontaneously reported by supervisees to their supervisors as a means of conceptualizing and dealing with supervisory crisis situations.

I stress at the outset that the present study does not imply that supervisors should request from their supervisees the report of dreams or other personal communications. On the contrary, the model of supervision that provides the framework for the present study is focused on process note presentations from supervisees and the unconscious supervisory effort of his or her patients. Also, this presentation is based on a supervisory finding that on rare occasions supervisees spontaneously report dreams to their supervisors. Quite often, this occurs at a time of supervisory crisis when a supervisee is under severe stress from one or all of the following factors: (1) a personal crisis in his or her therapeutic work and more rarely in his or her outside life; (2) an especially troublesome and highly specialized problem with the patient under supervision; and (3) a special and highly disturbing difficulty with the supervisor to whom the dream is reported.

This chapter was first published in *Contemporary Psychoanalysis*, 1982, *18*(4), and is reprinted by permission of the William Alanson White Institute.

Robert Langs • Program Director, Lenox Hill Hospital Psychotherapy Program, New York, New York 10021.

The main hypothesis to be developed in this chapter is that all such dreams contain the supervisee's direct and encoded (derivative) unconscious perceptions and reactive fantasies of the supervisor, his or her work with the supervisee, and the underlying nature of the therapeutic technique in use. This particular thesis is, of course, in keeping with the principle developed by Freud (1900/1958) and reiterated by Kanzer (1955) that any dream reported to another individual must on some level deal with the relationship between the dreamer and that particular person.

In addition, it will be proposed that a supervisor can in some general fashion make use of such dreams in a highly tentative, though effective manner to formulate unrecognized factors in a particular supervisory crisis and as a basis for definitive responses to the supervisee. Nonetheless, the limitations inherent to such efforts must be recognized due to the fact that the supervisory situation is not structured as a treatment experience, and it especially cannot and should not provide an opportunity for the supervisee to express the full range of his associations to the issues at hand.

Because of these limitations, the present study is proposed not as a carefully controlled psychoanalytic investigation derived from the psychoanalytic situation, but, instead, it is proposed as a form of extraanalytic investigation that falls best into the realm of applied psychoanalysis. However, it has been carried out under highly favorable conditions—that is, circumstances where some measure of validating information is available to the supervisor based on the supervisee's ongoing therapeutic work and direct (though limited) responses in supervision.

Finally, it will be proposed that a supervisee's report of a dream is a signal to the supervisor to undertake a period of self-analysis regarding his relationship with the supervisee and the nature of his supervisory interventions. Dreams of this kind may reflect some incapacity within the supervisor to hold and contain appropriately the supervisee's inevitable stresses and learning difficulties as reflected in his therapeutic work with the patient under supervision. While such failures are always an interactional product with vectors from both the supervisee (and his or her patient) and supervisor, it is critical to consider first possible countertransference problems in the supervisor before taking into account other sources of difficulty.

The material for this study will be drawn from the literature (Freud 1900/1958; Spotnitz & Meadow, 1976), a personal report, and from four of my own supervisory experiences. Since the conditions of supervision greatly influence the frequency with which dreams of this kind are reported as well as their meanings and functions, I will first define a model of psychoanalytic and psychotherapeutic supervision before presenting specific clinical data.

A MODEL OF SUPERVISION

Elsewhere (Langs 1978, 1979a), I have proposed a model of supervision based on an extension of the classical psychoanalytic position that has been termed the *adaptational-interactional* or *communicative* approach (Langs, 1982). This position is founded on a listening process that takes into account three levels at which therapists may formulate the material from patients:

1. Manifest contents and self-evident expressions
2. Latent contents in the form of encoded derivatives that are understood in terms of evident encoded (usually intellectualized) inferences that may be derived from the surface of the patient's communications or that may be developed in terms of isolated intrapsychic responses—usually in the form of unconscious fantasy formations; these are termed *type 1 derivative formulations*
3. The consideration of latent contents as encoded derivatives that are constituted as responses to the manifest and latent implications of the therapist's interventions (adaptation-evoking contexts), for which specific meanings and functions are assigned in light of these interventions and the ongoing therapeutic interaction; these are called *type 2 derivative formulations*

It is proposed that the expressions of a patient's *neurosis* (a term used here in its broadest sense to refer to all forms of psychopathology) are mobilized within the therapeutic situation mainly as responses to the manifest and latent meanings of the therapist's interventions. As a result, it is only type 2 derivative formulations that can represent realizations that pertain to the true and dynamically active meanings of the patient's associations and behaviors. To state this proposition in general terms, the communicative approach places the spiraling conscious and especially unconscious communicative interaction between patient and analyst at the center (though not the totality) of all meaningful formulations.

It has been found empirically that patients tend to represent in derivative form highly perceptive unconscious perceptions of their therapists and the implications of their interventions. They provide extremely meaningful guidelines to their therapists as well. Patients appear to have an uncanny unconscious awareness and recognition of the ideal conditions for treatment (the ground rules and boundaries) as well as a proper holding and containing relationship and the use of sound (eventually validated) interpretations.

Unconsciously, virtually all patients engage in active supervisory and curative efforts directed toward the therapist when he or she has made a technical or human error. Such work occurs in its most valid form on an encoded or derivative (unconscious) level and can be recognized only with type 2 derivative formulations. This is in keeping with the finding that patients react essentially to the realities of their therapists' efforts and their implications—the here and now (Gill, 1979)—representing these actualities and their unconscious meanings and functions in encoded form. Anticipations of the future as well as genetic repercussions fan out from this central nodal point. It is this set of findings that are extremely condensed here that forms the basis for the supervisory model used by the communicative therapist supervisor in both psychoanalysis and psychotherapy.

Specifically, the supervisory situation is constituted by a set of ground rules and boundaries that include a set hour, length of session, fee, teaching context, and professional relationship. In contrast to the psychotherapeutic situation where the ideal ground rules and boundaries are relatively unvarying and maintained at an optimal level to the greatest extent feasible, there is in supervision some flexibility in the application of each of these tenets—though a general sense of structure is consistently conveyed. Within this framework, the supervisee presents *sequential process note material* of the sessions that have taken place prior to the first supervisory consultation or between each supervisory hour.

The supervisor adopts a type 2 derivative listening stance, and makes use of a basic listening and intervening paradigm that includes the recognition of the following:

1. *Patient indicators* or *therapeutic contexts*—signs of neurotic disturbance in the patient including symptoms, resistances, and breaks in the ground rules or framework of treatment
2. *Adaptation-evoking contexts* as constituted by the therapist's interventions, including the identification of the most active adaptive context for a given session, the best *representation* of these contexts in the patient's material, and a study of their main implications
3. *The derivative complex*—constituted by the patient's encoded perceptions of the implications of the therapist's interventions and reactions to these perceptions (Langs, 1982)

In essence, then, the basic means by which a supervisor comprehends the transactions of the therapeutic experience involves an interplay between expressions of the patient's (and/or analyst's) neuroses as they are manifested in a particular hour and as they are illuminated in terms of unconscious meanings and functions by the stimuli for these neurotic expressions (and virtually always, these involve the therapist's interventions) and the derivative communications from the patient that reveal the unconscious meanings of both the stimuli involved and the neurotic response itself.

To this basic schema, a 7-part informational or observational schema is added as a means of further organizing the analyst's listening efforts (Langs, 1982). Included here are, for both patient and analyst, the following:

1. The state of the ground rules or frame
2. The mode of relatedness (healthy and pathological autism and symbiosis and pathological parasiticism)
3. The mode of cure (action-discharge-merger as compared to genuine insight)
4. The mode and nature of the communicative relationship
5. The presence of dynamics and genetics and to whom these primarily apply—the therapist (in the presence of deviations and errors the patient's representations involve primarily valid and elaborated unconscious perceptions) or patient (in the presence of a secure frame and sound interpretive work the patient tends to respond with distortion and transference)
6. The realms of self, narcissism, and identity
7. Issues of madness and sanity

As a participant in the therapeutic interaction and as an individual with an enormous measure of unconscious perceptiveness and sensitivity, the patient in both psychotherapy and psychoanalysis has been found to have an unconscious but strong sense of the ideal therapeutic hold (ground rules, boundaries, and frame) as well as the ideal interventional approach (the judicious use of silence and the restriction of interventions to management of the ground rules and interpretation-reconstructions). Sound interventions obtain indirect, derivative validation (type 2 derivative validation, Langs, 1982), that includes both cognitive confirmation and derivative representations of inevitable and unconscious introjective identifications with the well-functioning analyst. Erroneous interventions, while they may elicit some form of flat, surface agreement, do not obtain type 2 derivative validation, and they generate negative and destructive introjective identifications with the poorly functioning analyst.

However, in addition to the patient's unconscious validating response or its lack, at times of error analysands virtually always adopt a curative and supervisory attitude toward the errant analyst. At such times, the *designated* analyst has become the *functional* patient, and typically the *designated* patient becomes the *functional* therapist (Langs, 1982). In general, these shifts occur outside the awareness of both participants to analysis. On the patient's part they involve intense unconscious supervisory and curative endeavors designed to call to the attention of the analyst the existence and nature of his or her error and the patient's speculations as to the unconscious basis (Langs, 1978; Little, 1951; Searles, 1975). These efforts are, of course, limited by the amount of conscious and unconscious information available to the patient, and they tend to be undertaken in rather general terms. Nonetheless, they are highly perceptive and usually quite sound.

If a therapist is aware of the adaptation-evoking context of a specific intervention that has evoked these encoded curative endeavors, he or she is in a position to decode their specific meanings and functions. On that basis, it is possible for the analyst to rectify his or her error, to engage in a period of self-analysis guided by the patient's unconscious confronting and interpretive efforts, and to interpret those aspects of the material that lend themselves to intervening based on sound principles of intervention. In all instances, such interpretations must be organized around adaptive contexts that are represented in the patient's direct and derivative material. There is no justification for self-confession and noninterpretive interventions even under these circumstances.

Based on this particular conceptualization of the therapeutic interaction, the overriding focus of a supervisor's teaching efforts is founded on the patient's own unconscious supervision of the treating analyst. It is the supervisor's responsibility to be aware consciously of the direct and encoded implications of the supervisee's interventions (the adaptive contexts), to anticipate (predict) the patient's derivative responses (perceptions and fantasies), and to identify those derivative reactions that were not previously formulated. In addition, the supervisor's recommendations regarding technique and responsive measures is founded entirely upon the patient's own derivative recommendations, to which the supervisor adds comments regarding the basis for such work in general psychoanalytic theory and in the specific theory of the therapeutic process.

Thus, a supervisor offers few extraneous remarks, though he or she may engage in occasional supportive comments, personal but illuminating remarks, efforts to cite the literature, empathic responses to the plight of the supervisee, and a variety of similarly supportive and constructive ancillary measures. However, at the heart of the supervisory process is the utilization of the patient's own supervisory responses to the therapist.

This particular approach safeguards against the influence of countertransferences in the supervisor to the greatest extent possible. It also offers a set of ground rules that tend to lessen the number of inadvertent and inappropriate responses from the supervisor, especially those that are highly idiosyncratic and that are bound to disturb the supervisee and supervisory relationship. The approach also helps to minimize the arbitrary qualities of many supervisory experiences, providing both supervisor and supervisee with a basic validating methodology through which all supervisory interventions can be measured. Thus, all formulations and technical recommendations offered by a supervisor are examined in the light of the patient's subsequent material for validation, or its lack. A sound supervisory formulation should indeed find type 2 derivative validation in the subsequent material from the patient and should therefore constitute a form of prediction. Failure to obtain such derivative validation should, in all instances, lead to a rejection of the supervisory recommendation and to efforts at reevaluation.

SUPERVISORY CRISES

With this brief and incomplete resumé of a fundamental supervisory approach, we may now turn to the issue of supervisory crises. As is true of all interpersonal relationships and interactions, major disturbances in supervision are indeed interactional products with major vectors from the supervisor, supervisee, and the patient under presentation. Because of natural tendencies toward defense, under such conditions it is critical that the supervisor engage in self-analytic efforts in the light of the nature of his or her supervisory work in order to determine his or her own contribution to these incidents, before taking into account the responsibilities of the supervisee and patient.

It is all too easy to project and identify projectively into the supervisee (and patient) through accusations, implied condemnations, and the like the supervisor's own contribution to such a crisis. The supervisee is seen as resistant, oppositional, competitive, having difficulty in learning and the like, while the patient is seen as too sick, resistant, prone to negative therapeutic reactions, and so forth. The opportunity for a supervisor's use of these mechanisms and for supplementary rationalization is enormous, especially in the light of the power of the supervisor over the supervisee. (Often, he or she is in a position to evaluate the supervisee and to help to determine the course of his or her career.) The possibility of an intense sadomasochistic misalliance between supervisor and supervisee or for open hostility on both sides is considerable. Nonetheless, a well-reasoned evaluation of contributions on all sides by the supervisor can do much to preclude such unfortunate responses to moments of emergency issue.

In principle, a supervisory crisis will always include some contribution from the supervisor. In order to determine this aspect, it is essential that the supervisor review his or her relationship with the supervisee as well as his or her responses to the material being presented and to the patient involved. As is true of psychoanalysis itself, supervisory presentations are frought with opportunities for unresolved countertransference-based responses, and these must be identified as part of the effort to resolve this type of crisis situation. Often, a period of definitive self-analysis is required of the supervisor. The use of his or her own dreams for free association and then integrated understanding tends to be a useful tool for these purposes.

A supervisory crisis may arise when the patient under supervision is doing poorly, and especially in the presence of an acute regression, suicidal or homicidal episode, or a threat to terminate treatment prematurely. It may involve as well direct criticisms and attacks on the student analyst, especially when there has been a high rate of error including breaks in the ideal therapeutic frame (Langs, 1979b).

Supervisory crises also take the form of direct opposition by the supervisee toward the supervisor. This may involve thoughts of leaving supervision, direct challenges to the supervisor's work, open complaints, and an expressed sense of dissatisfaction with the supervisory experience. All such problems are indeed interactional products and, as noted, their resolution requires the self-analytic understanding of the supervisor, the rectification of countertransference-based inputs on his or her part, and a candid discussion with the supervisee (within limits) in which the supervisor's role in the crisis is acknowledged.

It is here, of course, that both the limitations of the supervisory experience and its distinction from a therapeutic experience come into play. It is not possible to analyze the supervisee, to obtain his or her free associations, and to rely on an interpretive approach for the resolution of a supervisory crisis. Instead, the supervisor must turn to an analysis of the supervisee's interventions and his or her extraneous comments in supervision, and especially to the patient's unconscious perceptions of the supervisee and his or her own supervisory and therapeutic endeavors. These observations supplement the analysis by the supervisor of his or her own supervisory work. The insights derived in these ways—as long as they are not highly personal or inappropriately self-revealing—can then be shared with the supervisee. On this basis, corrective measures can be undertaken in addition to the salutory effects inherent in this type of candid consideration of the supervisory difficulties at hand.

A final type of supervisory crisis is a mixture that involves some disturbance in both the treatment experience of the patient and in the supervisory experience of the supervisee. This particular type of problem is acknowledged by the supervisee to involve his or her own personal difficulties in learning to do effective psychoanalysis. There is a direct appeal for help from the supervisor who is not seen as an antagonist or as significantly contributing to the problem, but who is seen as a potential ally. Even so, the supervisor has the responsibility to engage in a period of self-analysis in order to be certain that in substance he or she has not, indeed, inadvertently contributed to the problems at hand. Here also, adequate resolution of the issues depends on the insightful understanding of the supervisor, and it will often entail some measure of direct discussion with the supervisee, apart from the presentational material. This type of response is justified only at times of supervisory crisis, and it should always be supplemented by further supervisory work based on the patient's derivative responses to the analyst's difficulties in the primary treatment situation.

Dreams of Supervisees

Given the definitive supervisory ground rules and boundaries described previously, no matter how sensitively and loosely applied, the report of dreams from supervisees is quite rare. Since the supervisory situation is structured around the presentation of process note case material and since the supervisory discussions are in no way intentionally therapeutic and seldom extraneous to the clinical material at hand, there is an implicit message that the supervisee should not attempt to utilize his supervisor in therapeutic fashion, nor should he or she offer personal revelations.

At issue here is the extent to which a supervisee's subjective feelings, fantasies, and other reactions toward the patient are utilized in the course of supervision. There are, indeed, many supervisors who actively explore this dimension of the supervisee's experience. The approach described here, however, does not include the specific effort to elicit the subjective reactions of the supervisee, and therefore it significantly reduces the likelihood of the report of supervisee dreams. On the other hand, that supervisory approach that not only explores the subjective factor within the supervisee but also proposes to utilize these reactions in intervening with the patient (e.g., through the self-revelation by the analyst of his or her dreams to his or her patients; Tauber, 1954) will tend, on the whole, to create a supervisory atmosphere in which dreams of this kind are less rare.

In the present approach, no effort is made to discourage either allusions to, or to explore specifically, the subjective reactions to the supervisee. This dimension is left to the presenter. On the whole, this will lead to occasional remarks regarding the supervisee's subjective state, and these tend to appear most often at the time of some type of major or minor supervisory crisis. It has been found that the supervisory experience and process is quite sufficiently educational without more elaborate reports of this kind. To the contrary, a preoccupation with the subjective reactions of the supervisee tends to interfere with the reporting of the essential process note material that is needed for sound supervisory interventions, and it may create substantial obstacles to effective supervisory work.

In the light of the sparse psychoanalytic literature on the details of supervisory interactions and their principles, it is not surprising to find that there are few reports of dreams from supervisees. To my knowledge, there is but one clear instance in which the dreams of a supervisee were utilized in the course of a supervision (Spotnitz & Meadow, 1976), though even here we lack many details of the supervisory transactions and the presented treatment experience.

In addition, the specimen dream of psychoanalysis—the well-known Irma dream (Freud, 1900/1958)—may be viewed as a supervisee's dream. There appears to be no recorded knowledge of whether Freud reported this dream to anyone in a supervisory or semisupervisory capacity (though such a report is likely, and the publication of the dream itself in *The Interpretation of Dreams* [Freud, 1900/1958] has such implications). However, we do know from Freud's own presentation, that on the night of the dream, he had been moved to prepare a case report on the patient who was the subject of the dream. (She is called Irma in the dream book, though we now know that the actual person in the dream was a woman patient named Anna Hammershlag, though Freud immediately understood that she was also a substitute for his patient Emma Ekstein.) Also, it was his intention to review one of these cases with his colleague, Josef Breuer. In this respect, Breuer was clearly marked for a supervisory role, and it is of special interest that Breuer himself appears manifestly in the Irma dream—albeit in a somewhat diminished capacity. Thus, before turning to my own material, I will now present and discuss the two dreams culled from the literature and one from a coincidental discussion.

The Dream Specimen of Psychoanalysis

Freud's (1900/1958) well-known Irma dream—the dream specimen of psychoanalysis—may be considered along with its many other meanings and functions (Elms, 1980) as a supervisee's dream. Dreamed on the night of July 23, 1895, Freud was responding to implied criticism from a colleague who had visited Irma and found that she was not quite well. Freud had planned to give the material he had written to Dr. M.— known now to have been Josef Breuer—in order to justify himself, and, undoubtedly, to obtain some type of supervisory comment from his senior colleague who was the inventor of the cathartic method. Thus, the Irma dream is in part a specific response to a planned quest for supervision. We may therefore consider the dream through which Freud discovered the primary-process mechanisms and the key to dream formation (his theory of wish fulfillment) as being simultaneously the first recorded dream of a supervisee.

More broadly, the Irma dream was prompted by the recent publication of *Studies on Hysteria* (Breuer & Freud, 1893–1895/1958), and was therefore a reaction to the introduction of insight-oriented psychotherapy (later to be termed *psychoanalysis*) to the medical profession (Langs, in press). The dream, as reported by Freud (1900/1958, p. 107), reads as follows:

> A large hall—numerous guests, whom we were receiving.—Among them was Irma. I at once took her on one side, as though to answer her letter and to reproach her for not having accepted my "solution" yet. I said to her: "If you still get pains, it's really your own fault." She replied: "If you only knew what pains I've got now in my throat and stomach and abdomen—it's choking me."—I was alarmed and looked at her. She looked pale and puffy. I thought to myself that after all I must be missing some organic trouble. I took her to the window and looked down her throat, and she showed signs of recalcitrance, like women with artificial dentures. I thought to myself that there was really no need for her to do that.—She then opened her mouth properly and on the right I found a big white patch; at another place I saw extensive whitish grey scabs upon some remarkably curly structures which were evidently modelled on the turbinal bones of the nose.—I at once called Dr. M., and he repeated the examination and confirmed it. . . . Dr. M. looked quite different from usual; he was very pale, he walked with a limp and his chin was clean-shaven. . . . My friend Otto was now standing beside her as well, and my friend Leopold was percussing her through her bodice and saying: "She has a dull area low down on the left." He also indicated that a portion of the skin on the left shoulder was infiltrated. (I noticed this, just as he did, in spite of her dress.) . . . M. said: "There's no doubt it's an infection, but no matter; dysentery will supervene and the toxin will be eliminated." . . . We were directly aware, too, of the origin of the infection.

Not long before, when she was feeling unwell, my friend Otto had given her an injection of a preparation of propyl, propyls . . . propionic acid . . . trimethylamin (and I saw before me the formula for this printed in heavy type). . . . Injections of that sort ought not to be made so thoughtlessly. . . . And probably the syringe had not been clean.

For the present study, the focus will be on the manifest dream and the conditions under which it was dreamed. While Freud offered a series of limited but illuminating associations to specific elements of the dream, these will be afforded only peripheral consideration. Because it is considered technically inadvisable for a supervisor to request from a supervisee associations of this kind, I will concentrate on the understanding that can be derived from a careful reading of the manifest content of such dreams and their most evident and likely implications.

The preamble offered by Freud is rather similar to the general comments frequently offered by a supervisee before reporting a dream to his or her supervisor. While Freud's remarks lack the specificity of the particular sessions with his patient that may have prompted the dream and do not include a direct consideration of the relationship between himself and Breuer—the supervisor and supervisee—they nonetheless offer a general context for the dream report.

Thus, Freud's preamble begins with a reference to the difficulties that are inevitably experienced by a psychoanalyst who offers treatment to a patient who is on friendly terms with the analyst and his family. This reveals immediately that the Irma dream is a ground rule, or framework, dream (Langs, 1979b). In fact, it is the difficulties of a mixed relationship of this kind (social and professional) through which Freud first attempts to account for and excuse his failure to cure his patient. The immediate stimulus for the dream was, as noted, a recrimination regarding the case from a colleague who had recently seen the patient. On the whole, the efficacy of Freud's psychotherapeutic technique had been called into question.

In essence, then, the general stimuli (day residues) for the Irma dream involved deep concerns in Freud with respect to a patient whose treatment was not going well, and more broadly, the value of the psychotherapeutic procedures that Freud was using at the time. A second and interrelated issue concerned the conditions of psychoanalytic treatment, and, quite specifically, a deviation from the ideal framework—the social relationship between Freud and his patient.

It may well be, then, that dreams from supervisees reported to (or intended for) supervisors are stimulated by deep concerns in supervisees regarding their own therapeutic work, their handling of a particular case that appears to be going badly, and issues pertaining to the basic ground rules and boundaries of the treatment experience—the holding and containing, most stable dimensions of the healthy therapeutic symbiosis (Langs, 1982).

In addition (and this is only implied in the dream and is somewhat more evident in Freud's later associations), the biographers of Freud (Clark, 1980; Jones, 1953; Sulloway, 1979) inform us that soon after the publication of *Studies on Hysteria* (sometime in May or June of 1895), the relationship between Breuer and Freud began to deteriorate. It seems evident from Freud's decision to present Irma's case history to Breuer that there was still a professional bond between the two physicians. On the other hand, Breuer is both demeaned and made the fool in the manifest content of the Irma dream (and resented for disagreeing with Freud in the latter's associations—this undoubtedly alluding to his opposition to Freud's overriding belief in the sexual etiology of hysteria and other neuroses), all of which points to a disturbance in the relationship between the two men. By implication, then, another broad stimulus for this particular dream involved tensions between these two individuals—supervisor and supervisee. (Oddly enough, originally, it was Breuer, who in piecemeal fashion, first used Freud as a post hoc supervisor in that he reported to Freud the details of his work with Bertha Pappenheim—the Anna O. patient in *Studies on Hysteria.*)

The Irma dream is one of the longest dreams to be investigated in this chapter. It is therefore necessary to be selective in culling out manifest elements that appear to contain implications regarding the clinical issues that the supervisee and dreamer—Freud—was working over through the dream.

In this regard, we may note first that the patient Irma appears in the manifest content of the dream. This is a clear means of indicating that on one important level the dream itself is an attempt to work over and resolve anxieties, conflicts, and guilt with respect to the treatment of this particular patient. Further, the dream quickly shifts from a social situation to that of a medical examination. Freud reproaches his patient for not having accepted his solution as yet—the word *solution* having an evident double meaning, one that was related to his formulation of his patient's neurosis and the other was latently sexual. Freud then blames the patient for her continued pains, and Irma responds by expressing her wish that Freud know how she was suffering.

To this point there is evidence of guilt in Freud with respect to his failure to cure his patient and a need to blame her for this outcome. On the other hand, the patient's comment that if Freud only knew suggests an unconscious perception within Freud himself that he was missing something—that there was something he did not know as yet and that accounted in part for the incomplete outcome of the treatment. This latter point is reinforced in Freud's later thought that he must be missing some organic trouble—a manifest element that again suggests an unconscious self-perception that something important has been overlooked on a psychological level.

As the dream continues, the patient is recalcitrant, and then she is seen as diseased. At this juncture, Dr. M.—Breuer—is called in for consultation, and he confirms Freud's impression. Here, as has been noted by Whitman and his associates (Whitman, Kramer, & Baldridge, 1969), Freud seeks out a supervisor for support and confirmation of his own efforts.

Next, there is the portrayal of Breuer as pale, walking with a limp, and with a clean-shaven chin (i.e., the loss of his beard). These are hostile and demeaning images that speak about tension in the supervisory relationship. As the dream continues, there is a renewed effort by Freud and his other colleagues to account for the patient's continued symptoms on the basis of an organic lesion rather than some psychological difficulty. In this way, even on a manifest content level, Freud attempts to exonerate himself from responsibility for the treatment failure.

At this juncture, Breuer diagnoses an infection and suggests that the mode of cure will be the appearance of dysentery and the elimination of the toxin. Breuer functions here as a supervisor with an optimistic outlook. Yet the mode of cure is primitive, based on action-discharge rather than insight, and it contains within it a measure of ridicule. Clearly, there is concern here regarding the treatment procedure. This is then followed by a representation of the origin of Irma's illness in a contaminated syringe from another physician, which was given to her when she was feeling unwell. This final note suggests an unconscious perception within Freud that his well-meaning therapeutic ministrations have in some manner been the cause of his patient's symptoms and of the therapeutic failure as well. There is a recrimination—another superego expression—that injections of that sort ought not to be made so thoughtlessly.

The interested reader can review Freud's subsequent associations to this dream—an aspect that I have studied in some detail in another context (Langs, in press). Suffice it to say that these associations center on the themes already evident in the manifest dream, although in addition there are several references to patients who actually succumbed to well-meaning treatment measures. Thus, the material suggests a strong and deep concern within Freud regarding the harmful effects of his psychoanalytic procedures to a degree that extends well beyond a controlled measure of guilt for a therapeutic failure or incomplete treatment result. There is a struggle here with the unconsciously perceived toxic and fatal attributes of the psychotherapeutic effort.

This initial analysis suggests that dreams from supervisees may be reported under conditions of therapeutic failure and tension between supervisor and supervisee. They may well be motivated by guilt over unconsciously perceived hurtful qualities to treatment measures, and they appear to constitute an effort to gain freedom from the pressures of the superego. They may constitute adaptive endeavors designed to gain insight into the underlying conflicts and issues. They seem to occur at times of treatment crisis and to constitute an intense appeal for help from the supervisor. An examination of additional dreams will help us to determine the extent to which Freud's dream specimen of psychoanalysis is indeed the harbinger of general trends regarding the nature and function of dreams from supervisees.

A Dream from a Paradigmatic Psychotherapist

In their volume on the treatment of narcissistic neuroses, Spotnitz and Meadow (1976) include two dreams from a supervisee. They are offered in a section on the self-analysis of countertransference feelings that lead to an incapacity by the therapist to resolve transference resistances. The supervisee was a woman in supervision with a supervisor who appears to have been the senior author of the book. The patient was a young man who is characterized as being in a state of negative narcissistic transference.

The session that preceded the supervisee's dreams involves the patient's reactions to his wife's trying to pressure him into obtaining a better job. The patient threatened to divorce her and states that he should get angry but could not. He feels like taking a knife and plunging it into his head—this is characterized as a narcissistic defense. In response, the analyst queries why the patient did not do it. The patient refuses and says that he wants to grow up.

In the following session, the patient reports that he is starting a new job and is worried that he will not work hard and will get fired, become a bum, and then have to shoot himself. The analyst asks what is wrong with that—this is characterized as joining the narcissistic defense. The patient responds by saying that he feels the analyst is trying to destroy him by having him kill himself. The analyst's rejoinder is to the effect that she does not want him to kill himself but that she just wants the patient to say what comes into his mind. The patient then responds that he does not want to die and that he gets mad at himself because he is not doing enough.

It is the stated goal of paradigmatic therapy to enable a patient to mobilize narcissistic rage directed toward himself and to shift the focus of the rage onto the analyst as a means of modifying narcissistic defenses and pathology. Nonetheless, on the surface, the technique appears to be highly provocative and even assaultive in a manner that risks the sanctioned expression of sadistic countertransferences.

In the context of the supervision offered to this analyst, her comment that she did not want the patient to kill himself and simply wanted him to free associate was seen as a countertransference-based intervention. It was believed to reflect problems in expressing appropriate hostility as a vehicle through which the patient might resolve his own problems.

Virtually nothing is reported about the supervision of these two sessions. Nonetheless, the analyst evidently described a dream to her supervisor that had taken place the night of the second session. In the dream, the patient again states to the therapist that he thinks that she is trying to destroy him. He gets off the couch and stands before her. The therapist is terrified that he will kill her.

In associating to the dream, the analyst was self-critical of her comment that she did not want the patient to kill himself, suggesting that she should have asked the patient what difference killing himself could make since he was destroying himself as it was. The student analyst felt that she had been inhibited because she was unable to be that hostile, adding that the patient standing up in the dream signified that he intended to attack her sexually.

The following night the supervisee again dreamed of her patient. During a session, a stranger walks in and the patient leaves the office with him. The stranger returns alone and tries to rape the analyst. She cries for help but no one hears her, and she wakes in a state of terror. This dream was understood to indicate that the analyst actually wanted to be raped by someone other than the patient.

It is then reported that the understanding of these dreams freed the analyst to use her negative, narcissistic countertransference feelings in the following hour with the patient. Thus, when the patient—in the next session—says that he feels hopeless and that there is nothing to do but to kill himself, the analyst queries as to why he does not do it now. When the patient speaks of the pain, the analyst says that he could die without pain. When the patient says that he did not want to die, the analyst asks why he could not die to please her. Finally, the patient says that he does not want to please the analyst. When his wife nags him about getting a better job, he does not feel like doing so in order to spite her. He gets mad when the analyst talks about his dying. He then asks the analyst how would she like it if he picked up the table and smashed it over her head? Would she like to die then?

In a final comment, it is suggested that the analyst recognized that her difficulties in responding to the patient in harmony with induced feelings of anger were linked to her own unmet needs.

It is beyond the purview of this chapter to discuss the highly questionable technical approach proposed by the paradigmatic position. Suffice it to say that there is reason to suspect the existence of shared countertransference among therapists who propose to resolve a neurosis by suggesting to patients that they should commit suicide and that they should do this to please their analyst.

The reader who is familiar with the interactional approach—through which manifest contents are analyzed as derivative communications triggered by the adaption-evoking contexts of the therapist's interventions and their implications—will recognize likely negative unconscious perceptions of the therapist and her technique in this material.

These begin with the image of the patient's wife trying to push him to get a better job—a displaced perception of the pressure placed on this particular analysand by his analyst. The patient's allusion to divorce suggests an unconscious thought of termination because of these pressures, and there follows an encoded perception of the patient's failure to express his hostility toward the analyst because of her interventions. Then, too, the allusion to failing to grow up might well involve a perception of the analyst's immaturity, and the association regarding the patient's wish to plunge a knife into his head could represent, first, the assaultive attributes of the analyst's technique, and second, the patient's own reactive rage (note the target of the head).

To select some additional highlights, the patient eventually consciously expresses his perception of the therapist as wanting to destroy him, and then later shifts again to encoded responses to the therapist's interventions when he describes getting mad at himself when he is not doing enough—a likely valid commentary on the therapist's efforts. Then, in the last segment, there is the patient's reference again to his wife's nagging, his wishes to spite her, and eventually, his direct rage at the analyst—again directed toward the head—that also contains an evident additional encoded perception of the assaultive qualities of the analyst's own work.

When work of this kind is taken at face value, it can be afforded any type of hypothetical rationale and justification. When it is understood in terms of adaptive context stimuli and encoded responses, the evoked image derivatives reveal a telling and valid commentary by the patient on the harmful nature of the therapist's interventions and the ongoing therapeutic interaction. While the formulations proposed here must be seen as somewhat speculative, they are strongly supported through other studies of this kind that have obtained extensive validation based on the principles applied here (Langs, 1978, 1982).

As for the two dreams reported by this supervisee to her supervisor, there is also a sense of a therapy in crisis, with abundant evidence for the existence of unresolved countertransference difficulties. Both dreams manifestly involve the patient who complains—as did Irma—of his treatment by the therapist. The theme that the therapist wishes to destroy him and an image of murderous, rapacious revenge by the patient are also prominent on the surface. The dream itself ends on a threatening note—without any sense of resolution. This suggests that the supervisee is both plagued with guilt and is unable to resolve a highly sexualized sadomasochistic relationship with her patient, one in which there is unresolved aggression on both sides.

It seems likely too that this dream contains an unconscious perception within the therapist of the highly destructive qualities of her own therapeutic work and of her patient's responsive rage. It is of special interest, then, that the dream was reported in an effort to resolve a supposed countertransference difficulty related to being more hostile and assaultive toward the patient—an effort that had to be made in order to better follow the paradigmatic technique that the therapist was being taught.

Thus, there is evidence of a highly significant split within this therapist, not unlike the split observed earlier within Freud: On the one hand, she strongly believes in the so-called positive aspects of the paradigmatic technique on a conscious level, while unconsciously, her derivative communications suggest an awareness that these efforts are highly destructive and that they could lead to murder or suicide. It seems likely, then, that the dream was reported to the supervisor in an effort to call to his attention through disguise and derivative expressions doubts within the supervisee regarding the nature of the treatment procedure and of the supervision itself—questions that the supervisee either did not experience consciously or that she feared to report directly to her mentor.

This formulation suggests that supervisees report dreams to their supervisors as a means of conveying highly significant perceptions and fantasies that are either entirely repressed within them, or are too dangerous to communicate directly in supervision. For this reason, the supervisor to whom such a dream is told should, indeed, make some effort to understand not only the manifest implications of these dreams, but also should consider them as derivative expressions in need of image decoding. The adaptive context for these dreams must be considered in terms of the material from the patient, the ongoing therapeutic interaction, and the interventions of the supervisor himself or herself.

Thus, we are justified in now shifting to a reading of this dream as an *unconscious* commentary on the supervisory relationship and experience. In keeping with the principles already established (Langs, 1982), we seek out encoded unconscious perceptions before developing formulations of distortion and fantasy formations.

The patient's comment in the supervisee's dream that he thinks the therapist is trying to destroy him may well be an encoded unconscious perception of the supervisee's valid view of the supervisor. There is support for this thesis in the impressions already cited regarding the paradigmatic technique with its highly assaultive qualities, an approach that the supervisor was promoting with his supervisee.

The allusion to the patient's getting off the couch and threatening to kill or sexually attack the analyst would suggest that the supervisor's interventions are seen as nonanalytic and sexually assaultive. In this context, it is well to note that the image of the patient's getting off the couch is a modification in the usual ground rules of psychoanalysis, which require the patient to remain on the couch until the hour is at an end. This is an important allusion to the framework of the treatment (and possibly the supervision) and suggests (again based on prior observations) the likelihood that the therapist is aware of one or more deviations in the ideal set of ground rules in this treatment. We are given no information regarding the conditions of this therapy, though there are some indirect hints that the patient had some awareness that the analyst was in supervision. Still, there is an important ground-rule image in this dream, just as there was a critical issue regarding the basic conditions of Freud's analytic work with his patient Irma. Further, as in the Irma dream, issues of life and death are quite notable. There is a suggestion that this analyst also perceived aspects of her technique as murderous, in a manner similar to the concerns expressed by Freud in the dream specimen of psychoanalysis and in his associations to that dream.

The hypothesis—that this particular dream involves unconscious perceptions within the supervisee of the nature of her therapeutic work with her patient as well as her interaction with the supervisor—is lent considerable support as well through the second dream reported by the supervisee. Here, too, there is a break in the frame: The entrance of a stranger into the session (a third party to treatment, with a resultant lack of privacy and confidentiality) and the patient's leaving the office with this man—the premature termination of a particular hour.

It seems quite likely that on one level the intruder is the supervisee's supervisor. He is, in fact, the stranger who has entered this treatment situation and who has taken over a measure of responsibility for the treatment experience. It is rather striking, then, that the stranger returns alone and tries to rape the supervisee. At this juncture, she directly cries out for help—a clear message regarding the need for supervision—but no one hears her. This strongly supports the thesis that the rapist is indeed the supervisor, and further, that the supervisee's pleas for instruction are going quite unheeded. The result is a sense of terror, drawn, it would seem, in part from an unconscious perception that the supervisor, instead of serving the teaching needs of the supervisee, is in some way disrupting the treatment and behaving (on a derivative level?) in a sexually assaultive manner toward his student.

The supervisor to whom such a dream is reported must seriously reconsider the nature of his supervisory work and teaching. He must take dreams of this kind as being fraught with valid unconscious perceptions of the nature of his supervisory efforts, and he must attempt to understand the sources of these encoded perceptions. Most important, he should suitably modify his techniques in order to remove these qualities from his work. A dream of this kind should also lead to a basic reconsideration of the fundamental techniques involved and to a deep and abiding concern that they are creating serious difficulties in the student analyst and patient alike.

In contrast to the Irma dream, both of these dreams end on a note of hopelessness and terror. While all three dreams share in common likely unconscious perceptions of destructive aspects of the treatment procedures at hand and reflect serious issues of hostility within the supervisory relationship, Freud's dream shows a mixture of condemnation and hope, while this supervisee's dream is filled with nothing but despair.

These dreams were treated in supervision as reflecting the psychopathology and countertransference of the supervisee, and especially the inappropriate needs to be raped and assaulted. No consideration was afforded the supervisee's likely unconscious perceptions of the nature of her own therapeutic technique and difficulties, except for the proposal that the supervisee had simply not been assaultive enough—a proposition that seems to be significantly contradicted by this dream material. Further, no thought was afforded the equally great likelihood that the supervisee's dreams were an encoded commentary on the nature of the supervisory experience (at the very least, the principle that any individual to whom a dream is told is involved in the dream itself should have been invoked). Because of these failures, the supervisee continued with her hostile paradigmatic technique, only to find that the therapeutic interlude culminated with an expression of murderous rage toward the analyst.

Finally, in keeping with the findings of Arlow (1963) and Searles (1962), there is a likely interconnection between the nature of the supervisor's interventions, those offered by the analyst, the experience of the patient, the subsequent responses of the analyst, and the material she then conveys in turn to the supervisor (see also Langs, 1979a). Thus, the material from these sessions and the dreams of the supervisee suggest a sequence of uncontrolled sadomasochistic exchanges in which an assaultive and rapacious type of sadism appears prominent. These seem to be the main qualities of the supervisor's effort, and they lead the supervisee in this particular direction in her work with the patient—much of it is based on a strong and highly destructive supervisory introject (Langs, 1979a). It is the patient who then receives these communications and projective identifications and who seems most capable of bringing them into conscious awareness as is reflected in several of his direct comments to the analyst. Nonetheless, there is no sign of a full metabolism and understanding of these particular qualities of these interpersonal exchanges, and the sequence ends on the one hand with the supervisee's terrifying dreams and on the other—the patient's cry of outrage. Much of this has taken place in part because of the supervisor's failure to analyze properly the supervisee's dream in light of both therapeutic and supervisory adaptation-evoking contexts and to arrive at their likely encoded meanings.

A Dream from a Personal Report

Recently, a young psychotherapist still in training had occasion to discuss his work with me. In the course of that discussion—as he offered a sample of his therapeutic efforts—he discussed the twice-weekly psychotherapy of a young woman diagnosed as suffering from a severe narcissistic disorder. Since the supervisee worked in the Chicago area, he had selected a rather prominent follower of Kohut as the supervisor for this case. In the main, the supervision had emphasized the nature of the patient's narcissistic disturbance and the use of mirroring techniques, the analysis of idealization trends, and so-called interpretations of the manifestations of the patient's narcissistic disorder. As a result, and this was reflected in the case presentation offered to me, the therapist had adopted a therapeutic approach that was in some sense supportive and that tended toward a mirroring and satisfaction of the patient's narcissistic needs and formulations developed almost entirely in terms of manifest disturbance of the self, including the patient's self-image, ideals, problems with control, sense of inner tension, and lack of cohesive identity. Many of the interventions had an evident seductive overtone in that they involved direct efforts to reassure the patient that her problems stemmed from past maternal failures rather than her own inner conflicts. In addition, instinctual drive conflicts were not addressed at all. Manifest contents were the main basis for intervening.

Quite early in the course of this psychotherapy, the therapist had two dreams about a patient. Both were reported to his superior (a male). He was quite certain that the individual under discussion was the person involved in the dream. In the first dream, the therapist was gazing longingly into the eyes of an attractive female patient who seemed to be beckoning him to embrace her. In the second dream, he was lured into kissing a female patient.

While it is impossible to validate any hypothesis developed from this material, it can be stated, nonetheless, that this particular dream may well reflect the supervisee's unconscious perception of the seductive qualities of his supervision as well as the similar qualities in his techniques with this patient. The dream is included here because it contains in its manifest content inappropriate instinctual drive satisfactions of types similar to those seen in Freud's Irma dream and in the paradigmatic supervisee. There is, of course, no indication of renunciation of pathological instinctual drive satisfactions.

DREAMS FROM FOUR SUPERVISEES

We turn now to the dreams that have been reported to me in the context of my own supervisory work. The first of these arose in the early months of my supervision with a young married psychologist who had come to me for private supervision. After attending several seminars at which I was the principal speaker, she contacted me for supervision and began with considerable enthusiasm. In the light of the process-note material presented by this therapist and from occasional comments regarding her personal life, it soon became clear that she had received her major training in a so-called analytic training program that advocated the use of extensive deviations in the ideal ground rules and boundaries of the psychotherapeutic relationship, including the full sanction of physical contact between patient and therapist when deemed necessary. Quite consciously, the supervisee was in extreme conflict with respect to these teachings, and she was deeply concerned about the nature of her therapeutic work. While capable of offering interpretations and other types of interventions, she was extremely dissatisfied with her efforts. There was evidence also of a highly personal struggle with the ground rules and boundaries of her own social relationships. Though married, it was evident she was struggling with temptations to become involved with other men. There was a sense, then, that she sought supervision not only for fresh perspectives on psychotherapy and psychoanalysis but also in an effort to shore up her failing defenses as both therapist and individual.

The early case presentations by this supervisee were characterized by considerable chaos. The supervisee worked both in a clinic and in a private office that she shared with three other therapists in a quasipartnership arrangement. Ground rules and boundaries were loosely established—if stated at all—and framework issues were in strong evidence. Her mismanagement of the ground rules had wreaked considerable havoc with her patients and her therapeutic work.

It was in this broad context that the supervisee began a supervisory hour by stating that she was quite upset with the difficulties she was having in utilizing the adaptive context approach with patients and in securing the framework of her various efforts at treatment. While strongly motivated to make constructive changes (for example, she was investigating ways of getting out of her present office lease in order to have her own private-office setting, and she had rectified many other unneeded deviations), she felt great distress with the slowness with which her work was falling into place. She had recently lost a male patient with whom she had attempted to establish better the ground rules of the treatment and with whom she had had both a therapeutic and personal relationship. (She had once permitted this patient to take her out for a drink after an evening session.) Despite her marriage, she found herself quite attracted to another man, and she felt that any involvement with him would be quite destructive. She was making efforts to discuss these problems with her husband and to secure her relationship with him better. (On the whole, she felt that her marriage was a good one.) In all, though, she felt quite unstable.

In this context, she wanted to tell me a dream. She dreamed that I looked like Alan King. She and I were in bed together, in a hotel, or someplace like that. We were making love, but then we stopped—we interrupted the lovemaking. We shifted to having some kind of a discussion, and we decided it would not be good for us to be involved in that other way. As we continued to talk, there was some indication that I might have been involved with her mother around the time of her birth or that I might have been her father.

This particular dream does not manifestly involve the patient who was under supervision at the time (though it probably does so latently), but instead, it directly concerns the supervisee and supervisor. In a manner similar to the dream from the paradigmatic supervisee, the manifest dream is blatantly sexual, though clearly without a notable sadistic component. Instead of being highly dysphoric, the sexuality is at first gratifying, though eventually it is renounced.

In this context, it is well to note the great difficulty that a supervisor encounters in attempting to formulate a diagnosis based on a manifest-dream report. Thus, there is no inherent reason to believe that blatant dreams of this kind reflect severe psychopathology in the supervisee who dreams them. It is well known that under conditions of extreme distress, manifest dreams may contain open expressions of instinctual drive wishes and other major difficulties. Certainly, one can infer certain psychodynamics from the manifest dream, though here, too, caution is necessary in that such formulations must take into consideration possible unconscious perceptions of the patient and supervisor before accounting for the dynamics and genetics of the supervisee. Utmost caution is well advised.

The allusion to Alan King involves a performer and comedian. The supervisee spoke positively of him; thus the image is one with a positive tone. The central image in the first part of the dream involved being in a hotel and making love in bed together. Thus, the supervisor must first ask himself if he has been at all notably seductive with this supervisee. If so, such trends must be rectified and self-analyzed.

There is also a change in the setting of the supervisory relationship from the supervisor's office to the hotel room. The supervisor must therefore determine whether he has in any way modified the usual boundaries of the supervisory relationship and how he has done so. While, on occasion, the supervisee had not been able to have the supervisory hour in person and had therefore been supervised by telephone, the supervisor was aware of no other break in the framework of the ideal supervisory experience. Furthermore, while the supervisee was, indeed, seen by him as a somewhat attractive woman, the supervisor had no sense of a countertransference difficulty in this sphere nor was he aware of any significant seductive aspects of his work with the supervisee. Nonetheless, the report of a dream of this kind called for an extensive reconsideration of this aspect of the supervisor's relationship with the supervisee. It is only when the supervisor can find no essential basis for the possibility of encoded perceptions of this kind that the dream can be taken as a primary expression of the supervisee's wishes and needs. In this instance, this appeared to be mainly the case, though minor levels of seductiveness were indeed identified and rectified.

It is important to note, however, that the lovemaking stops in the middle of the dream and is renounced in favor of talking and discussion. This implies that whatever seductive elements might have existed in a supervisory relationship, they have been modified in favor of cognitive supervisory efforts. This is a highly favorable shift, one that suggests that the inappropriate needs of the supervisee (and probably the supervisor as well) have been brought under control and modulated in order to ready the situation for sound supervisory work. What is quite important for the supervisee is that an expression of an alteration in the usual and necessary boundaries of the supervisory relationship (seduction on any level is inappropriate) has been brought under control and subjected to renunciation. Once this is accomplished, the highly incestuous qualities of a break in the framework of this kind (whether in supervision or in treatment) is then revealed.

This particular dream was reported by a supervisee who was in a state of acute distress regarding her efforts at modifying the inappropriate qualities of her work with patients and who was struggling desperately to secure the framework of her treatment relationships and those in her personal life. A careful investigation revealed no acute framework deviation in the supervisory relationship, which was cordial and sound at the time of the dream. Thus, the dream appears to reflect in the main an intrapsychic struggle within the supervisee that was far more than an interpersonal problem with the supervisor. The problem had been reflected in her work with patients, which had improved considerably.

For the supervisor, the dream helped to clarify some of the issues with which the supervisee was struggling unconsciously while she was making constructive efforts to secure the framework of her treatment and personal relationship and to become more effective as a therapist. There had been an evident seductive quality to her approach with the supervisor, though with his indirect help this too appeared to be now under better control by the supervisee. The dream suggests that the supervisor had been effective in helping the patient to renounce her pathological incestuous sexual needs, and their acting out. The dream itself appears to have been a further attempt by the supervisee to work on and work through important aspects of these conflicts and issues. The dream's positive cast suggests considerable mastery as well as growth and development—impressions that were borne out in subsequent weeks.

The second dream is also from a woman supervisee, a psychiatrist who was extremely unhappy with her knowledge of therapy, her therapeutic work, and her career as a therapist. She was referred to me for supervision by a friend, and she had little awareness of my publications. However, once involved in supervision, she read avidly and extensively from these works and became deeply committed to the adaptational-interactional approach.

As supervision unfolded, the supervisee quickly experienced a strong sense of inadequacy. She was involved in many forms of deviant therapy—such as family therapy—and she had an office in her apartment. She was involved in the treatment of former drug addicts and saw them individually, with their families, and in groups.

The patient whom she presented in supervision was a woman who was in both individual and group therapy, who had communicated repeated derivatives that reflected her wish for exclusively individual therapy—she complained again and again of the intrusions of others, of being infantilized, and of wanting her independence. The therapist's efforts at interpretation and rectification, while well meaning, were rather disorganized. Nonetheless, the patient was doing reasonably well, though the supervisee remained deeply concerned and somewhat upset regarding the problems she was discovering in her therapeutic endeavors and their mastery. In this context, the supervisee reported the following dream:

> I dreamt I had skin cancer on the palm of my hands. I was surprised I had let it go so long because I knew skin cancer was curable. I showed it to my father who is a doctor, and he just picked the cancer off my palms without anesthesia. He ripped it off my palms and I said: "How can you do this to me?" He said, "It's not cancer."

The supervisee had insisted on telling this dream to the supervisor because she had subjected it to self-analysis. She had experienced the dream following the last supervisory session. It was therefore evident to her that the supervisory experience had been the adaptive context or stimulus for the dream, and that it had dealt with her reactions to supervision. On the whole, her images of her father—a thinly disguised stand-in for the supervisor—were warm and positive. She saw him as a kind man who had been supportive of her throughout her life and who had been a constructive figure.

The skin cancer, she felt, stood for her view of herself as a therapist in terms of her previous teachings, and more broadly, her picture of the field at large as sick, highly destructive, and devouring. And yet, once the self-condemnation had been expressed, there was a sense of self-acceptance, or perhaps mercy, in representing her countertransference in the form of a curable sickness. Here, the supervisee acknowledged that the attitudes of the supervisor had given her a sense of hope in the face of many realizations in respect to her own disturbances and difficulties as a therapist. Further, the curative measure taken by her father was—for the supervisee—a clear representation of her view of the supervisor. She felt that he was, indeed, helping her to get rid of her countertransference problems.

In all, the supervisee felt that the dream was a response to her acute sense of distress in the face of her growing realizations regarding the inadequacies of the therapeutic techniques she had been taught, those in use by her colleagues, and those reflected in her reading of the literature. And yet, while deeply disturbed, the supervisee saw the dream as hopeful and optimistic, and she felt that it validly portrayed her perception of the supervisor and his supervisory work—direct in his diagnoses of the supervisee's difficulties, yet basically helpful and constructive.

The supervisor responded with some general comments regarding the patient's struggles and the common difficulties experienced in carrying out therapeutic work in sound fashion. In order that he was not carried away by the supervisee's idealization, he reviewed the dream to himself and asked such questions as to whether he had in any way been destructive or devouring toward the supervisee and if there was any justification for a split perception of himself—on the one hand destructive and on the other, highly helpful and curative. While he could find little reason to identify himself with a cancerous lesion, he was able to accept a different split image of himself—as gently helpful at times, while a bit more blunt and hurtful at others (the allusion to ripping off the cancer). On the whole, he also felt encouraged by the candid realizations reflected in this dream, and he saw the dream as an affirmation from the supervisee of the positive qualities of a difficult supervisory experience.

The next dream was presented in group supervision. The dreamer—a male psychologist—was married to another psychologist who was also a part of the supervisory group. There were evident tensions because of this arrangement that raised an issue as to the advisability of spouses sharing a supervisory experience. Eventually, each arranged their own separate supervision.

The presentation involved another psychologist who was in therapy with the supervisee and who had quite inadvertently been asked to interview and test one of his therapist's children. The procedure included an interview with his therapist's wife who was aware of the therapeutic relationship, but was concerned about the status of her child. The situation had occurred as part of a school crisis, and there had been little time to consider other possibilities. The supervisee—the testing psychologist's therapist—had found it necessary to speak briefly on the telephone to his patient about his daughter.

While the patient in his sessions had said virtually nothing directly about the incident, his derivative material was abundant with images related to the rupture in the usual interpersonal boundaries of the treatment relationship, the sudden exposure of the therapist's family to the patient, the powerful and curative role into which the patient was actually placed in regard to the supervisee's daughter (he had, in fact, proven to be quite helpful), and the highly uncertain and seductive contacts that had occurred in the contaminating situation (latently both homosexual with the supervisee and heterosexual with his wife).

Nonetheless, despite an overabundance of material of this kind, the therapist had failed to intervene in this sphere and, instead, had commented rather superficially and manifestly on other self-evident aspects of the patient's material. Through further derivatives, by talking about people who failed him and refused to listen and help him, the patient revealed his unconscious perceptions of the therapist's difficulties in this regard. The situation was complicated further by a major regression in the patient and the reemergence of rather severe depressive symptomotology.

Because of the crisis nature of the situation, the supervisee decided to present this case when it was his turn to offer material. Because the supervisor had worked with the group for more than a year and in the light of the crisis nature of the situation, the supervisory comments had been rather strong. They involved an extensive formulation derived from the patient's material of the many critical ramifications of the testing incident. The necessity for intervention, the ways in which it should have been carried out in the sessions reported in supervision, and the need for future therapeutic work were discussed in some detail.

The supervisee began the next supervisory hour, in which he was to continue his presentation, by indicating that belatedly he wanted to mention the dream that he had the night *before* his last presentation. The dream had been prompted, he was quite certain, by his decision to discuss this patient in supervision. An additional stimulus had been an expression of interest from his wife in having some type of sexual contact with him. Exhausted, he had fallen asleep. The dream was reported as follows:

> I fell asleep during a session with this patient while he was talking about his relationship with my wife. He saw that I was asleep. He tells me: "This is important. Here you are falling asleep." I wake up and try to straighten things out. I'm nervous and embarrassed and I become rather active.

Here also the supervisee offered his own interpretation of the dream. Even before the supervisory presentation he had begun to realize that he had developed a significant blind spot in his work with the psychologist patient and that he had failed to deal with the testing incident and had probably missed important opportunities to intervene in this area. He realized that he had represented this problem in his manifest dream by alluding to his wife and to his being asleep. On the other hand, his waking up and trying to straighten things out, alluded, he felt, to his own wishes in this respect and to his anticipation of help in supervision. He had decided to mention the dream because the previous supervisory hour had been so helpful and because he had, indeed—in the session with the patient that had followed—begun to respond interpretively to these issues.

To these comments, we may add the observation that once again a supervisee has dreamed manifestly of a patient with whom he was having an acute crisis. While the supervisor does not appear in the manifest dream, his latent presence is suggested when the patient himself adopts a supervisory role in endeavoring to wake up the therapist. This is a constructive intervention that leads to the mobilization of the therapist. It implies a positive image of the supervisory experience—this, in addition to the split in the supervisor—sleeping at one moment and attempting to straighten things out at another.

Of course, the question must be raised about whether the supervisor had in any way justified an image of himself as split and as missing certain important supervisory interventions. This could not have occurred in connection with this case because the dream had been dreamed before the supervisory experience. However, the kernel of truth in this image may involve the presence of husband and wife therapists in the same supervisory group. It seems evident that on a second level this also is the subject of the dream and that the supervisee's encoded, derivative message is to the effect that the joint supervision is in some way disturbing to him and to his therapeutic efforts. While the supervisor had raised questions regarding this particular problem, in the absence of clear material, he had not taken a definitive stance in this regard. An issue of this kind is certainly difficult to handle in the supervisory situation. As noted before, data accumulated over many months suggests that this type of arrangement is far from ideal and should be avoided.

Finally, we may note a trend shared by each of the two previous dreams: All three begin with a representation of some type of problem in the supervisee, and each ends with a constructive effort to ameliorate the difficulty.

The fourth and final dream was reported by a male supervisee who was a resident in psychiatry. Having worked a half year with the present supervisor, he had now been assigned to new supervision. He began his last supervisory hour by indicating that he had had a dream about supervision. It proved to be embedded in a three-part, lengthy dream. The following synopsis condenses the middle segment:

> We are in an informal setting. I am aware we are not going to be working together anymore, and that you place your hand on my shoulder. You have an expression on your face; you are placating me. You tell me, "You really haven't gotten it yet, but keep hanging in there. It takes time and I think you'll find it's gonna come." You mention your son and you say: "My son has a very similar background to yours. He had a serious separation problem to deal with when he was very young. It took him a long time to get this as well, and now he's got it." And then, kind of joking, you said, "There's hope for you."

In brief, in the third sequence the patient is in a large boat in the middle of a racetrack with an attractive and flirtatious woman. He is attracted to her and she is quite high-powered. They strike up a conversation and the race goes off. They have an excellent view of the race. The lead horse falls down and the crowd gasps. In slow motion, all of the other riders are able to turn their horses away without serious injury. The riders get off their mounts and help their horses get up. It is all rather pleasant.

Finally, in the first segment the therapist receives a call from a physician who has promised to refer patients to him when he completes his training. In reality, he is rather crazy. In the dream, he is going to refer someone to the therapist. They are standing together and he speaks of something's driving him crazy. There is something about medical tests and his feeling overwhelmed with all the knowledge he is supposed to have and the amount of work he is doing. He says something about straightening things out by winning some money, and he then leaves to go to a card game. The supervisee feels pity for him.

In brief, the supervisee spoke extensively of his regrets at having to terminate supervision. He felt he had struggled hard with the adaptation-interactional approach, and he experienced a sense of hope recently in both the interventions from the supervisor and in his own sense of his work. He found the dream of the supervisor rather reassuring.

For the supervisee, the second dream suggested that he had an image of the supervisor as being rather powerful and yet interested in the supervisee. The racing accident reminded him of a recent newspaper story about an accident in which a horse had been impaled on the side railing and had thrown the rider. The supervisee has a special love for horses and was very upset by the story. The dream seems to have eliminated the terribly upsetting qualities of the actual experience.

The dream material also reminded the supervisee of several recent family losses. These were connected to his father about whom he had ambivalent feelings—intense love mixed with some measure of disillusionment. The final dream seemed to reflect the supervisee's own feeling that he had been overwhelmed by the task of learning the communicative approach and by his own struggles in trying to integrate all that he had learned into a sound treatment technique.

At the time of this dream the supervisee was presenting his work with a young woman who had a physical disability. His therapeutic efforts were somewhat erratic in that he alternated between rather sound interventions and those that appeared to be based on countertransference. Thus, while the present dream dealt manifestly with the supervisory relationship, it might also have important latent implications for the supervisee's relationship with this patient—much of it in terms of his own bodily concerns, his struggles with the patient's seductive attitudes, and his responsive erotic countertransference.

In supervision, the supervisor emphasized the optimistic outlook reflected in these dreams, and he complimented the supervisee directly on his work. To himself, he saw the possibility that each of these images involved some perception of his work as supervisor—it was he who may have failed to work in an integrated fashion, who had been flirtatious, who had been attacking to the point of creating bodily anxieties, who had been crazy in some fashion, who seemed overwhelmed, and who had provided an image of uncertainty and a gamble. On one level, each of these images could be justified in some minor fashion. In substance, however, the supervisor could find little to support the idea that these dreams dealt primarily with unconscious perceptions of his supervisory efforts. Instead—once again—it seemed likely that the supervisee was indeed attempting through this dream material and its communication to the supervisor to work over further and to work through his own anxieties and fantasies as influenced by the supervisory experience. It is to be stressed that in keeping with the three prior dreams, the central dream here of supervision once more ends on a hopeful note—this in strong contrast to the other dreams of supervisees presented in this chapter. This finding suggests that despite the arduous nature of supervision from the communicative approach, its underlying positive and constructive qualities are clearly experienced—consciously and unconsciously—by its supervisees.

Discussion

The material presented in this chapter indicates that in a relatively structured supervisory situation that concentrates on the process note presentation of case material—in which the supervisor does not ask for dreams or free associations from the supervisee—dreams are reported by some student therapists at times of crisis. At issue as a rule is an acute problem with a particular patient and at times with the supervisor also. In Freud's dream about Irma, there is evidence of difficulties in both spheres as there is in the dream from the paradigmatic therapist.

In the four dreams reported to me as supervisor, the major crisis was either with a particular patient or reflected a struggle within the therapist to resolve countertransference-based and educational difficulties in his or her own therapeutic work. The sense of supervisory crisis arose primarily in response to the traumatic qualities inevitable in learning about one's significant problems as a therapist and confronting the difficulties inherent in their modification. Supervision from the adaptational-interactional vantage point, with its necessary emphasis on the patient's unconscious perceptions of the therapist's errors and other difficulties (Langs, 1979a, 1982), tends to increase the likelihood of this particular type of supervisory experience.

However, in all instances in which a dream of this kind is reported, it is essential that the supervisor not simply account for those aspects that deal with the supervisory experience in terms of a supervisee's inevitable anxieties and difficulties but also to search carefully for possible countertransferences and errors of his or her own. It is a tentative affirmation of the communicative approach that careful self-analysis in this regard did not reveal significant supervisory errors, and it could attribute much of the patient's concern to the expected difficulties inherent in learning this arduous treatment modality.

Of interest is the finding that the patient appears manifestly in four of the seven dreams, while the supervisor appears manifestly in three—though his presence is in evidence in all instances studied. This strongly suggests that the relationship between the supervisee and supervisor constitutes a major stimulus (adaptive context) for each of these dreams.

Some type of ground-rule issue is evident in six of the seven dreams reported by these supervisees. These pertain mainly to the treatment situations—though perhaps surprisingly—in all but one of the dreams (the exception being the dream about skin cancer). That dream also concerns a significant issue regarding the ground rules and framework (conditions) of supervision. This finding lends support to the previously recognized critical role played by the ground rules and boundaries of the therapeutic situation (Langs, 1979b, 1982), while offering a comparable finding regarding the supervisory relationship.

By implication, then, careful attention should be paid to the structure of the supervisory experience and relationship, and should an issue arise in this area, it deserves the careful attention of the supervisor. Since he or she is dealing with actualities frought with unconscious implications, supervisory interventions in this regard should involve both the *rectification* of unneeded deviations (e.g., the actual separation of the husband and wife in joint supervision) as well as some type of limited comment based on the supervisee's direct communications to the supervisor and any relevant material from the patient under supervision.

It is well to realize that the manner in which the supervisor structures the supervisory relationship will reflect his or her attitudes and needs in respect to, and as organized in terms of, the seven basic dimensions of therapy (Langs, 1982). These include the following:

1. Frame management.
2. The type of cure in which he or she is invested (insight versus action discharge and pathological merger).
3. The mode of relatedness between supervisor and supervisee (which may be *pathologically autistic* in that it fails to deal with the true meaning of the supervisee's communications. It may be *pathologically symbiotic* in that it provides pathological instinctual drives, superego, and merger satisfactions for either or both participants in supervision rather than true understanding. It may be *parasitic* in that the supervisor or supervisee exploits the other member of the supervisory dyad, or a *healthy symbiosis* in which there is a clear supervisory framework and sound teaching and learning).
4. The mode of communications between supervisor and supervisee (from truly meaningful to defensive and falsifying or destroying the truth).
5. The actual dynamics and genetics of their relationship.
6. To whom these dynamics and genetics mainly allude (supervisee or supervisor—because of countertransference).
7. The realm of self-identity and narcissism—as influenced interactionally by both participants to supervision.

Several other findings are of importance. First, five of these supervisees offer a derivative, unconscious representation of the treatment experience that takes on either highly destructive qualities (e.g., a toxin that can cause death or a form of cancer) or involves uncontrolled sexuality and incest. (While latent to the Irma dream, this theme is strongly portrayed in the dreams of the paradigmatic therapist and my own first supervisee.) Thus, dreams from supervisees tend to reveal the unconscious meanings of doing psychotherapy or psychoanalysis as unconsciously and validly perceived by a particular supervisee. Because access to this level of fantasy and perception is extremely difficult from observations of the supervisee's conscious thoughts and therapeutic work, the report of these kinds of dreams can be a source of insight along these lines to both participants in supervision. Often, a particular supervisee's difficulty in doing therapeutic work is meaningfully illuminated in this fashion. In the main, however, the supervisor should offer little in the way of interpretive response, but should instead encourage or advise the supervisee to engage in efforts directed at self-analysis or to bring up these problems in the course of his or her own personal psychotherapy or psychoanalysis.

The sequence of the dream events in the dream of a supervisee is also of importance. Should the outlook be pessimistic, the problem of the dream unresolved or aggravated, or should there be signs of adaptive failure and hopelessness, the supervisor should be quite concerned regarding the mental state of his or her supervisees as well as with the disruptive qualities of his or her own supervisory work. In general, dreams that convey adaptive failures should be cause for considerable concern and reevaluation in both spheres. This type of dream is especially in evidence in the report from the paradigmatic therapist. In contrast, Freud's Irma dream, while containing moments of pessimism and adaptive failure, ends on a note of guarded optimism—dysentery will intervene and rid the patient of the toxin.

On the other hand, a dream that begins with some type of direct and/or encoded statement of a problem in the supervisee's work with his or her patient and/or a supervisory issue and that proceeds to some form of renunciation, resolution, sense of hope, and evidently adaptive response appears to be a sign of constructive functioning in the supervisee and in the supervisor as well. Such dreams seem to be a part of highly adaptive efforts to deal with a treatment and/or a supervisory crisis. They tend to involve statements of inevitable countertransference and expected problems in learning to do psychotherapy or psychoanalysis and to crystallize definitive efforts at resolution. The consistency with which supervisees report dreams of this kind may be taken as a measure of affirmation of the supervisor's teaching efforts.

SUMMARY

This chapter presents the dreams from seven supervisees. Two are from the literature, one is from a clinical discussion, and four are from the author's personal experience. In each case, the supervisee appears to have been motivated to report a dream to his or her supervisor because of a crisis in the therapeutic work with a particular patient or in his or her general therapeutic endeavors and/or in supervision. Two types of supervisory dreams have been identified. In the first type there is no manifest sign of resolution for the problem posed in the dream. In this instance, the supervisor is well advised to reconsider the nature of his or her supervisory work and to be concerned as well with the failing capabilities of the supervisee. The second class of dreams states a supervisory or therapeutic problem and subsequently represents some type of adaptive solution. This type of dream is viewed as a part of relatively sound efforts to adapt to a crisis situation, and it tends to affirm the supervisor's work. Although this chapter does not propose that supervisors seek out dreams of these kinds and, in addition, suggests a rather restricted response to these communications, their value in better understanding a supervisee's work, his or her conflicts and anxieties, and problems within both therapy and the supervisory experience have been highlighted.

REFERENCES

Arlow, J. The supervisory situation. *Journal of the American Psychoanalytic Association*, 1963, *11*, 576–594.

Breuer, J., & Freud, S. Studies on hysteria. In J. Strachey (Ed. and trans.), *The complete psychological works: Standard edition* (Vol. 2). London: Hogarth Press, 1958. (Originally published, 1893–1895.)

Clark, R. *Freud: The man and the cause.* New York: Random House, 1980.

Elms, A. Freud, Irma, Martha: Sex and marriage in the "Dream of Irma's Injection." *Psychoanalytic Review*, 1980, *67*, 83–109.

Freud, S. The interpretation of dreams. In J. Strachey (Ed. and trans.), *The complete psychological works: Standard edition* (Vols. 4 & 5). London: Hogarth Press, 1958. (Originally published, 1900.)

Gill, M. The analysis of transference. *Journal of the American Psychoanalytic Association*, 1979, *27*, 263–288.

Jones, E. *The life and work of Sigmund Freud* (Vol. 1.) New York: Basic Books, 1953.

Kanzer, M. The communicative function of the dream. *International Journal of Psycho-Analysis*, 1955, *36*, 260–266.

Little, M. Counter-transference and the patient's response to it. *International Journal of Psycho-Analysis*, 1951, *32*, 32–40.

Langs, R. Day residues, recall residues and dreams: Reality and the psyche. *Journal of the American Psychoanalytic Association*, 1971, *19*, 499–523.

Langs, R. The patient's unconscious perceptions of the therapist's errors. In P. Giovacchini (Ed.), *Tactics and techniques in psychoanalytic therapy* (Vol. 2). *Countertransference*. New York: Jason Aronson, 1975.

Langs, R. A model of supervision: The patient as unconscious supervisor. In R. Langs (Ed.) *Technique in transition*. New York: Jason Aronson, 1978.

Langs, R. *The supervisory experience.* New York: Jason Aronson, 1979. (a)

Langs, R. *The therapeutic environment.* New York: Jason Aronson, 1979. (b)

Langs, R. *Interactions: The realm of transference and countertransference.* New York: Jason Aronson, 1980.

Langs, R. *Psychotherapy: A basic text.* New York: Jason Aronson, 1982.

Langs, R. Freud's Irma dream and the origins of psychoanalysis. *Psychoanalytic Review,* in press.

Searles, H. Problems of psycho-analytic supervision. In H. Searles (Ed.), *Collected papers on schizophrenia and related subjects,* New York: International Universities Press, 1965.

Searles, H. The patient as therapist to his analyst. In P. Giovacchini (Ed.), *Tactics and techniques in psychoanalytic therapy* (Vol. 2) *Countertransference.* New York: Jason Aronson, 1975.

Spotnitz, H., & Meadow, P. *Treatment of the narcissistic neuroses.* New York: The Manhattan Center for Advanced Psychoanalytic Studies, 1976.

Sulloway, F. *Freud, biologist of the mind.* New York: Basic Books, 1979.

Tauber, E. Exploring the therapeutic use of countertransference data. *Psychiatry,* 1954, *17,* 331–336.

Whitman, R., Kramer, M., & Baldridge, B. Dreams about the patient: An approach to the problem of countertransference. *Journal of the American Psychoanalytic Association,* 1969, *17,* 702–727.

8

Supervision
Illusions, Anxieties, and Questions

RUTH M. LESSER

> Whatever the merits of our high degree of . . . education, we have lost the
> gift for being puzzled. Everything is supposed to be known—if not to our-
> selves then to some specialist whose business it is to know what we do not
> know. . . . To be puzzled is embarrassing, a sign of intellectual inferiority. To
> have the right answer seems all-important. To ask the right question is con-
> sidered insignificant by comparison. (Fromm, 1951, p. 3)

Most psychoanalytic supervisors view their roles in the supervisory process as being substantially different from their roles in the psychoanalytic process, and they stress the dangers of blurring the distinctions.
Levenson's (1982, p. 13) directive to "stay out of the supervisee's analysis" is generally adhered to in principle, although not often in practice.

Supervisors attempt to facilitate the supervisee's analytic work by
elaborating technique, by elucidating transference manifestations, by
proposing the direction and thrust of the inquiry, and by suggesting
appropriate dynamic formulations about the patient or the process. A
major aim is to increase the supervisee's ability to observe and explore
significant patterns. When the supervisor becomes aware of resistances
and/or countertransferences that rest primarily in the supervisee, the
supervisee is usually advised to "take it up in analysis." The prevailing
notion is that the supervisee's countertransference may be alluded to
but not be directly explored.

Portions of this chapter were originally presented at the William Alanson White Society
Meeting, February 1981.

RUTH M. LESSER • Clinical Professor, Training and Supervising Analyst, New York University Postdoctoral and Doctoral Programs in Psychology, New York, New York 10003
and Guest Lecturer, William Alanson White Institute of Psychiatry, Psychoanalysis and
Psychology, New York, New York 10023.

Fromm-Reichmann (1950), Tauber (1954), Searles (1961), and other authors have discussed and elaborated on the positive value of utilizing the analyst's personal reactions to the patient. These unique reactions are viewed as important to a more complete understanding of the patient's way of living. Epstein and Feiner (1979) summarized the current thrust by subtitling their extensive compilation of writings on countertransference as follows: *The therapist's contribution to the therapeutic situation.* These ideas can be usefully extended to the supervisory relationship; like the analytic interaction, the effects of each participant's personal characteristics on the other are crucial.

The reality and value of maintaining traditional distinctions between the psychoanalytic and the supervisory situations are questionable. Many presumed differences prove to be illusory and probably serve defensive purposes. If anxieties inherent in the supervisory situation are not appreciated, they may interfere with the goals of supervision. An understanding of the dynamic similarities of both situations should enhance the supervisory process for its participants.

ILLUSIONS IN SUPERVISION

Illusion: The Supervisor Knows Best

An underlying assumption in the supervisory relationship is that the supervisor knows best. This belief probably encourages methods that hinder, rather than facilitate, the supervisee's development as a psychoanalyst.

The usual roles assumed by each member of the supervisory dyad foster the idea that the supervisor knows and the supervisee does not know the nature and roots of difficulties in the work. What is rarely acknowledged is the supervisor's advantage of being a "Monday-morning quarterback" in the privileged position of listening to the consequences of a supervisee's interventions. Both participants expect and respect the supervisor's ability to evaluate critically and to insure the quality of the analytic process.

The primary focus is on helping the supervisee aid the patient. Both need the supervisor to fulfill the helper role, and both need to maintain the hierarchical order within the relationship. As a result, the supervisor often feels pressured to make knowledgeable remarks, and the supervisee needs to present material naively. Failure to fulfill these traditional roles may lead to the disturbing experience of anxiety.

Unless a supervisor refuses to accept the conventionally assigned roles, he[1] enters into a gentleman's agreement similar to the one that frequently characterizes the analytic enterprise: "The patient [supervisee] comes, talks, and pays, and the analyst [supervisor] listens and 'interprets.' The rules of the game are observed, and the game is agreeable to both of them" (Fromm, 1970, p. 3). Both collude in encouraging the supervisee's passive-dependent stance and the supervisor's stance of superiority.

Resisting the role of *the supervisor knows best* creates different expectations. In this context, the supervisee is encouraged to become a more active contributor and to frame the critical questions. Consequently, he is given the opportunity to become more aware of the effects of his participation in the analysis and to develop a better sense of his own expertise.

Illusion: The Supervisor Is Objective

The contract between members of the supervisory dyad differs from the contract in the analytic dyad. The main task in the supervisory situation is to study and help a third person, the patient. The supervisor responds to material about the patient as presented by the supervisee. This one-step-removed aspect presumably allows greater objectivity about the patient and the process in which the supervisee is engaged.

To be sure, the analyst often feels more certain as a supervisor than as an analyst. Levenson (1982, p. 1) stated that there is "something oddly infallible about the experience of doing supervision." Bromberg (1982) pointed out that the stance of questioning one's personal reactions as a supervisor is not built into the supervisory process in the same way that it is into the analytic one. He believes that this nonquestioning stance may serve security needs.

The recent emphasis on the analyst's being transformed by the patient's needs (Levenson, 1972; Searles, 1961) has perhaps diverted attention from the ways in which the analyst transforms the patient. Analysts are not always aware that patients begin to speak their language and even present dreams in symbols that are congruent with their predilections. It is not entirely coincidental that the reported dream contents of Freud's patients differed from those of Jung or Fromm.

---

[1]The content of this chapter refers to both sexes; the generic use of the male pronoun is employed in the interest of simplicity.

Supervisors also tend to ignore their influence on the supervisee when they use the concept of participant observation primarily, if not exclusively, in their analytic work.

Information about the patient is necessarily contaminated by the supervisee's participation and way of conceptualizing the material. It is also mediated by the supervisor's participation and his conceptual organization. One must question the supervisor's experience of objectivity that is based upon such complex processes. The supervisor "has an inescapable, inextricable involvement in all that goes on in the interview; and to the extent that he is unconscious or unwitting of his participation in the interview, to that extent he does not know what is happening" (Sullivan, 1954, p. 19).

If there is no exploration of the supervisee's transferences and countertransferences, important sources of information about his work with patients are lost. Similarly, the supervisor's lack of awareness about his own transferences and countertransferences and their effects on the supervisee can result in even less information about the supervisee's work and the illusion that the supervisor is objective is reinforced.

Illusion: Parallel Processes

Systematic examination of the unconscious factors influencing the supervisor has been largely limited to the description and discussion of parallel processes (Caligor, 1981; Doehrman, 1976; Gediman & Wolkenfeld, 1980; Searles, 1955, 1962). Parallelism occurs when the supervisor unconsciously identifies with the supervisee. The supervisor's reactions presumably parallel the supervisee's unconscious identification with the patient's defenses against anxiety. Searles (1955, p. 159) stated that through this process "the supervisee communicates the obscure difficulties besetting the patient–therapist relationship." He considered this phenomenon to be a powerful tool in supervision that offered important information about the patient (Searles, 1962).

Gediman and Wolkenfeld (1980) criticized the idea that parallel processes are initiated by the patient. They emphasized the "multiple identifcatory processes" within the supervisor–analyst–patient network. Indeed, the supervisee's identification with the patient may represent an effort to resolve his own personal issues that have not been sufficiently explored in his own analysis. Similarly, the supervisor may be dissociating anxiety-provoking aspects of the interaction with the supervisee. Searles (1955, p. 172) acknowledged that the supervisee may be behaving similarly in the therapeutic and supervisory situations. However, his emphasis was on the supervisee's response to the patient because of "a stirring up of . . . anxiety with regard to the comparable areas of his personality." He did not refer to the supervisee's stirring up a supervisor's anxiety because of comparable areas in the supervisor's personality.

It is evident that the supervisee is an independent variable in the analytic and supervisory situations. Although the interaction between supervisor and supervisee may appear parallel to that between the supervisee and patient, it is not the same because different people are involved in each dyad. The supervisor's experience of parallelism is useful because it provides a clue to selectively inattended aspects of the supervisor's and supervisee's personalities as they are unwittingly expressed in the interaction. When the supervisor relates to the supervisee primarily vis-à-vis the patient, potential anxieties for both participants may be avoided; but one loses the opportunity for a shared, in-depth inquiry into "distortions occurring in supervision" by the supervisor as well as the supervisee and "working through participation toward individuation" (Wolstein, 1972, p. 168).

ANXIETIES IN SUPERVISION

Psychoanalytic thinking has evolved to the point of acknowledging and accepting the analyst's anxieties, and this awareness has allowed their constructive utilization in the analytic enterprise. However, the supervisor's anxieties are generally unrecognized, perhaps because anxieties are less acceptable to the supervisor than to the analyst. Awareness of the supervisor's anxieties is essential for fulfilling the supervisory task.

The supervisor's responsibility to evaluate the candidate is anxiety provoking for both members of the supervisory dyad. No matter what efforts are made to minimize it, both are aware that the supervisor's judgment may affect the candidate's career in the professional world. The anxieties of evaluation are complicated further by a supervisor's status and prestige within the hierarchical organization of the training institution, a factor of no small significance to either participant. The supervisor is bound to be affected by the potentially serious consequences for the supervisee of a poor evaluation. Certainly, participation as a co-equal becomes strained.

The burgeoning of peer supervision groups may be seen as an attempt by candidates to alleviate the inescapable anxieties of the evaluative aspects of the traditional supervisory situation. Despite such inhibitory dynamics as rivalry and fear of ostracism, candidates often experience greater freedom to articulate personal reactions and to share mistakes without having the anxiety of a supervisor's evaluation.

There are many potential anxieties that may affect each supervisor differently, depending upon his character. Overt and covert criticism or praise may evoke anxiety. *Failure* with a supervisee or the supervisee's *failure* with a patient can be disquieting. There may be shame at becoming aware of one's grandiosity. There may be discomfort about one's sadistic or masochistic tendencies. Anxiety may result by exclusion from the "deeply pleasurable, preambivalent symbiosis" between the therapist and the patient, by losing the candidate's therapeutic help, or by not feeling needed when supervision is terminated (Searles, 1962). It is stressful to experience one's limitations after the enormous emotional, intellectual, and economic investments have been made to achieve the position of supervisor.

Doubts arise in the supervisor about whose needs are being served because supervisors need supervisees to maintain their statuses and reputations. The supervisor's economic needs and concerns also relate to the need for supervisees. Supervisors need approval, acceptance, and nurturing. The need to cure the supervisee as well as the patient may entice the supervisor to become unnecessarily involved with the supervisee's similar need to cure. A need for personal or metapsychological converts may conflict with the wish to develop the supervisee's uniqueness and autonomy.

The supervisor's competitive feelings with the supervisee and with the supervisee's analyst are discussed by Searles (1955). Competition between supervisors is also of consequence; supervisors value being sought after by candidates and feel some pride when they "modestly" let it be known to their colleagues that their supervisory time is booked for a number of years. This statement reflects the need to be respected by one's colleagues and to maintain status within the institution. Similarly, the extent to which the supervisor helps his supervisee become successful may relate not only to his evaluation of the supervisee but also to his own competitive needs. There is a sense of disappointment if a highly esteemed supervisee is not similarly regarded by the next supervisor or by the training committee. How well the supervisee performs in relation to the institution, to the next supervisor, and with his patient all may reflect upon the supervisor.

It is important to be aware that the supervisory room is crowded with all sorts of "persons" who create anxieties for both the supervisor and the supervisee. The supervisory room is often even more populated than the analytic room. Each participant must consider his own multiple transferences, which include the patient, colleagues, training-committee members, and others in the institution. Certainly, the supervisee is influenced by the training analyst's attitude toward the supervisor which may limit his freedom to engage in a mutual inquiry. The supervisor's attitude toward and relationship with the supervisee's training analyst, whose "presence" the supervisor feels, also may be a limiting factor for the supervisor.

Finally, and perhaps most importantly, one must consider the supervisor's anxieties about intimate relatedness, with its attendant struggles and disappointments. The usual structure of the supervisory relationship and the accepted roles and rules allow a relatively comfortable, trouble-free mode of interaction. The supervisor's experience of uncertainty may be resolved by assuming the expert role. Focus on the patient may serve as a screen behind which each participant's individuality is hidden and may represent a resistance to intimacy with a significant other. The supervisor may attempt to resolve some of these ubiquitous anxieties by using distancing and intellectualization as defenses. As a consequence, the supervisor may not only dissociate aspects of himself but also aspects of the supervisee and the patient.

To Teach or to Treat?

Several authors have strongly advocated the importance of mutual inquiry into the analyst's countertransference in the psychoanalytic context (Levenson, 1972; Searles, 1965; Wolstein, 1972). However, in the supervisory situation, these authorities caution against the supervisor's pursuing an in-depth inquiry into the supervisee's personal reactions. Searles (1962, p. 602), for example, stated that "analyzing of the student's countertransference" should be done "sparingly, if at all," implying that only teaching, not treating, is appropriate in supervision. DeBell (1963) noted that the teach-or-treat issue in supervision is false and suggested a form of collaborative analysis. This form, however, maintains the traditional distinctions between supervision and analysis. He recommended that the supervisor and other training faculty members collaborate with the training analyst by meticulously reporting their observations to him. This information is considered useful because the supervisee's ego-syntonic character traits can be elusive and perhaps impossible to detect in the training analysis. DeBell's recommendation seems limited in that it minimizes the importance of the analyst's direct experience of significant characteristics in the immediate, actual context in which they occur. Fruitful inquiry can take place only when important interpersonal and intrapersonal phenomena are experienced, not simply talked about or intellectualized.

A collaborative analysis that takes place within "the two-way field. . . of two particular coparticipants" (Wolstein, 1981, p. 400)—the supervisor and the supervisee—seems more useful. This necessitates an in-depth inquiry into and analysis of each member's transferences and countertransferences that are directly experienced by and are observable to one another. A collaborative and co-participant model recognizes that the supervisor is an observed as well as an observing member of the dyad. Being observed, the supervisor offers the supervisee an important opportunity to experience the supervisor's willingness to be self-aware and genuinely responsive to the supervisee's observations—even in the face of potential anxieties. This may well encourage the supervisee to do the same.

It is an interesting paradox that analytic training institutes value one-to-one supervisory relationships, although strictures are expressed against pursuing personal issues in supervision. It seems that, at some level, the critical importance of providing a supervisory structure in which intimate matters may be explored is implicitly recognized. The requirement for several different individual supervisors demonstrates an underlying belief that the supervisee's growth depends upon relatively intense experiences with different people. It also implies that each supervisory relationship has its own particular character that reflects the individual personalities of each participant.

Despite conscious views regarding what is appropriate or inappropriate in supervision, there is undoubtedly a close parallel between how one functions as a supervisor and as an analyst. It is difficult to imagine that the supervisor's interests, concepts, and values are not revealed during the course of supervision. The supervisor's awareness and direct expression of these in the supervisory relationship may allow the supervisee to become clearer about his own unique perspectives and their consequences on his work. As a significant other, the supervisor contributes to the personal and professional growth of the analyst-in-training. The practice of collaborative analysis in supervision, which includes the supervisor's therapeutic participation, does not necessarily interfere with the training analysis, but may serve as a useful addition.

It is relatively easy to teach or to learn any particular metapsychology. When traditionalism is highly valued by both society and its substructures (e.g., psychoanalytic institutes), unconventional and potentially controversial individual reactions can be avoided. However, traditional parameters of the supervisory relationship are not in the interest of promoting awareness, and therefore limit the goals of analytic training. The supervisory relationship offers the analyst-in-training another important opportunity to participate in a mutual inquiry into his and the supervisor's unique psychological patterns.

Sullivan's statement (quoted by Levenson, 1982) "God keep me from a therapy that goes well!" can be extended to "Keep me from a supervisory relationship that goes well!" *Going well* may mean that there is more superficiality in the relationship but less anxiety; a more comfortable atmosphere but limited interpersonal engagement; a greater sense of certainty but complexities are dissociated; more interpretations but little structural change in the relatedness between participants; more efforts to preserve the status quo but less opportunities for experiencing new dimensions of oneself and the other; that disappointments and struggles have more likely been avoided, but the potential richness and joy of a significant relationship is lost.

REFERENCES

Bromberg, P. The supervisory process and parallel process in psychoanalysis. *Contemporary Psychoanalysis,* 1982, *18,* 92–111.

Caligor, L. Parallel and reciprocal processes in psychoanalytic supervision. *Contemporary Psychoanalysis,* 1981, *17,* 1.

DeBell, D. E. A critical digest of the literature on psychoanalytic supervision. *Journal of the American Psychoanalytic Association,* 1963, *11,* 546–575.

Doehrman, M. J. G. Parallel processes in supervision. *Bulletin of the Menninger Clinic,* 1976, *40,* 3–104.

Epstein, L., & Feiner, A. *Countertransference: The therapist's contribution to the therapeutic situation.* New York: Jason Aronson, 1979.

Fromm, E. *The forgotten language.* New York: Holt, Rinehart & Winston, 1951.

Fromm, E. *The crisis of psychoanalysis: Essays on Freud, Marx and social psychology.* New York: Holt, Rinehart & Winston, 1970.

Fromm-Reichmann, F. *Principles of intensive psychotherapy.* Chicago: University of Chicago Press, 1950.

Gediman, H. K., & Wolkenfeld, F. The parallel phenomenon in psychoanalysis and supervision: Its reconsideration as a triadic system. *Psychoanalytic Quarterly,* 1980, *49,* 234–255.

Levenson, E. *The Fallacy of understanding: An inquiry into the changing structure of psychoanalysis.* New York: Basic Books, 1972.

Levenson, E. Follow the fox. *Contemporary Psychoanalysis,* 1982, *18,* 1–15.

Searles, H. F. The informational value of the supervisor's emotional experience. *Psychiatry,* 1955, *18,* 135–146.

Searles, H. F. Phases of the patient–therapist interaction in the psychotherapy of chronic schizophrenia. In H. F. Searles (Ed.), *Collected papers on schizophrenia and related subjects.* New York: International Universities Press, 1961.

Searles, H. F. Problems of psychoanalytic supervision. In H. F. Searles (Ed.), *Collected papers on schizophrenia and related subjects*. New York: International Universities Press, 1962.

Searles, H. F. (Ed.), *Collected papers on schizophrenia and related subjects*. New York: International Universities Press, 1965.

Sullivan, H. S. *The psychiatric interview*. New York: Norton, 1954.

Tauber, E. S. Exploring the therapeutic use of countertransference data. *Psychiatry*, 1954, *17*, 331–336.

Wolstein, B. Supervision as experience. *Contemporary Psychoanalysis*, 1972, *8*, 165–172.

Wolstein, B. The psychic realism of psychoanalytic inquiry. *Contemporary Psychoanalysis*, 1981, *17*, 399–412.

9

Follow the Fox

EDGAR A. LEVENSON

AN INQUIRY INTO THE VICISSITUDES OF PSYCHOANALYTIC SUPERVISION

One might well wonder why a chapter on the problem of psychoanalytic supervision would carry such an odd title. But there may be more similarity between supervision and riding to the hounds than at first appears evident. Oscar Wilde—my favorite aphorist—took a particularly dim view of fox hunting. It was, he said, a marvelous example of the *unspeakable* in pursuit of the *inedible!* With a very slight shift, much the same might be said about the process of supervision. It is a marvelous example of the *infallible* in pursuit of the *ineffable!*

This may appear to be a rather strained bit of punning, but I have something quite specific in mind. First, there is something oddly infallible about the experience of doing supervision. Second, as we would all agree, there is something ineffable (or beyond words) in the process of doing therapy. In the ordinary course of my work, I spend (as I am sure we all do) a very considerable part of my time being perplexed, bored, confused, and at sea. Sometimes I dream of a midlife career change to something simple, clear-cut—say dermatology. But when I supervise, *all is clear to me!* With the rare exception of the supervisee who is so con-

This chapter was first presented at an April 1981 country weekend meeting of the William Alanson White Psychoanalytic Society. As it happened, the meeting was held in the heart of fox-hunting country, thus rendering relevant the foxy title. The chapter was then published in *Contemporary Psychoanalysis*, 1982, *18*(1), 1–15, and is reprinted by permission of the William Alanson White Institute.

EDGAR A. LEVENSON • Fellow, Training and Supervising Analyst, William Alanson White Institute of Psychiatry, Psychoanalysis and Psychology, New York, New York 10023 and Clinical Professor, Graduate School of Arts and Sciences, New York University, New York, New York 10003.

fused or inchoate that I can capture no sense at all of what he is doing, the problems that the supervisee is having with a patient, the difficulties—technical and theoretical—seem to me to be surprisingly clear most of the time. As far as I can tell in reports on other people's supervision, this phenomenon is not so very unique. People whom *I* have supervised, who seem confused to me at the time, seem to be perfectly clear when *they* are supervising other people. And I have had the experience at a White Institute class of presenting my own adumbrated clinical material and having a class of seven or eight candidates seeming to be perfectly lucid about what is wrong with what I am doing and what I should be doing instead. I do not think this is a consequence of any obvious pecking order in psychoanalytic institutes, but rather, it is some odd, seductive aspect of the phenomenology of the supervision process itself. It is extraordinarily out of synchronization with our own clinical experience, and it is misleading to our supervisees, inasmuch as they are led to believe that when they "grow up" all will be clear to them also. It also creates considerable discord in the supervisee's own training analysis, where obviously no such coherence or clarity of concept and purpose can exist. Of course, this claim that doing supervision breeds infallibility may simply be my own grandiosity, or, in the preferred pejoration of the times, narcissism. However, I consider it to be an issue worthy of further examination. I think it does exist and that it is the consequence of what Bateson called, following Bertrand Russell, a "failure in logical typing"; that is, a failure to understand that supervision is of an entirely different level of abstraction than therapy (Bateson, 1979).

Briefly, the theory of logical typing posits that a class and the members of the class are of different levels of abstraction. In other words, a class cannot be a member of itself. Applied to the process of supervision, it follows that what we are doing is discussing a *class* of transactions of which the particular patient is a *member*. We are never really discussing a specific patient in supervision, but a class of transactions applicable to *all* patients and illustrated by a specific patient. The apparent clarity is a consequence of this step up in abstraction level, and as Count Alfred Korzybski noted, clarity increases with the level of abstraction (Korzybski, 1954). If the supervisor really participated in, for example, "parallel process,"—that is, to become part of the therapy—he would be largely rendered speechless because it would become evident that the interactions were so complex that the supervisor could say nothing. The moment one moves from the general category of patients for whom this patient is an example to the actual patient, one has plunged into a complex interpersonal morass that is now no longer limited to the three participants but encompasses all the usual ramifications that proliferate in any analysis. Now there are three participants in a poorly controlled and delimited field. The number of persons symbolically present in the room increases exponentially, and the field becomes virtually chaotic. One is left with a psychoanalysis run wild.

Lee Caligor quotes Doehrman on parallel processes as saying that "one is struck by the multifaceted nature of what on the surface seems to be a simple, and even limited, relationship" (Doehrman, 1976). To repeat, the ramifications of supervision, transference, countertransference—all the orchestrations of the patient–therapist–supervisor triad could become so complex as to defy any real understanding. In a word, I am suggesting that supervision is possible only because it is *not* therapy. It is something altogether different, operating at a higher level of abstraction.

I do not think that the second referent of my aphorism—the *ineffability* of psychoanalysis, that is, the difficulty of putting it into any kind of words—requires much elaboration. It seems perfectly clear that in any process that is both performed and talked about, what is said and what is done are not in a direct relationship to each other. One cannot learn to do anything exclusively by being told how to do it, and no one who knows how to do something well can transfer that knowledge by telling the other person how to do it. Anyone who has practiced a physical activity, a sport, a craft, or an art is perfectly aware of this discrepancy. *The art of teaching operates in the interstices between the word and the act.*

So, we are confronted with an apparent paradox: We feel very clear about what it is we wish to teach, and we are equally clear that we do not know exactly how to formulate it. From this perspective, there is nothing unique about the problems of teaching psychoanalysis, or for that matter, psychoanalysis itself. The psychoanalytic act seems to me to be a very special case of human discourse, and its effectiveness lies, not in any esoteric distinctions, but in a rigorously maintained, focused attention. I will elaborate on that, but for the moment I want to simply suggest that—in golf, skiing, tennis, playing the piano, or painting a picture—the same paradox operates. We have, most of us, learned (at least, those of us who have any friends left) to avoid supervising in nonanalytic situations. Somehow, our wives, our children, our tennis mates, and our skiing partners seem to become oddly angry and resistive if we point out to them the obvious shortcomings in their techniques. Why do people have such trouble listening to good advice? Well, maybe because it is irrelevant.

Now, if it is true that we are not helping the supervisee with a specific patient, but rather, abstracting the analytic process, it would be most useful to have a classification of supervisory interventions; that is, different styles of intervening in supervision. As an attempt at classification, I have delineated a number of rough categories:

1. Holding or confirming
2. Teutonic, or by-the-numbers
3. Algorithmic
4. Metatherapeutic
5. Zen, or opening-the-fist, supervision
6. Preceptorship

I shall briefly review each of these rather arbitrary—and surely incomplete—categories of ways of teaching psychoanalysis, or rather, supervising psychoanalysis.

HOLDING

Erwin Singer and I were in joint supervision in our candidate days at the White Institute with Clara Thompson. Many of you may remember Clara and may have had a similar experience with her. Erwin and I were in supervision with her for, I think, well over two years. During this time she hardly said a word to either one of us. She would sit quietly, scratching her crossed forearms, with her deceptively mild, brown eyes looking vaguely over our heads, nodding occasionally. Erwin and I would have coffee later in the Croydon Hotel, absolutely convinced that she had not listened to one word that we had said. However, when trouble came up, when we were blocked or confused, she could—with a couple of casual sentences—pick us up and set us back on our wheels. It was, in many ways, an extraordinary experience. She was not warm or maternal or benevolent or supportive. Nor was she critical, derogating, or obstructionistic. She did not seem to want anything from us—to be reassured that she was a terrific supervisor and theorist, lovable, nurturing—anything. She was like the Matterhorn—simply there. I do not know exactly what happened, but it was one of my better supervisional experiences, and I learned a great deal, although I could not tell you what I learned. It was, I think, technically a holding atmosphere. She established (in the psychiatric sense, not in the derogatory sense) a "playground" in which she let us find ourselves. If we asked, we received advice, but otherwise we were left alone to explore our own idiosyncratic styles and talents. It may be a wonderful way to do supervision. It was certainly a catalytic process—in the literal sense of the word—but it takes someone of very considerable presence and reputation to do it successfully. It establishes no structure to the supervision at all, but it allows the therapist to listen to and feel for the *movement* of therapy. (I will elaborate later on this.) It also allows the therapist to fall by the way, and being supervised by Clara was somewhat like having an eagle for a mother: She took you out of the nest and dropped you; if you flew, fine; if you did not, *tant pis!*

TEUTONIC, OR BY THE NUMBERS

This method of teaching operates on a manual of prescribed situations and responses. It is also inevitably "lock stepped" into a metapsychology that is both authoritarian and omniscient. For everything the patient says and the supervisee does, the supervisor has a theoretical formulation and a corresponding piece of behavior. The patient is explained to the supervisee in terms of the metapsychology, and the therapeutic intervention follows automatically, to wit: "This patient is narcissistic and unable to . . . and therefore one must . . ." I confess that I find this process as abhorrent as painting by the numbers, and I think the outcome is about as predictable and esthetically miserable. This neat fit between theory and practice is, I believe, the last resort of the unimaginative. However, it has considerable appeal, and it tends to make the supervisor rather popular among psychoanalytic candidates who wish to believe that *someone* is clear about what they are doing. Moreover, this genre of supervisor radiates great confidence and cheer—the unjust reward of the true believer. Sullivan once said, "God keep me from a therapy that goes well, and God keep me from a clever therapist!" I think this is what he may have had in mind.

THE ALGORITHMIC APPROACH

This method is superficially like the authoritarian, or by-the-book way of teaching psychoanalysis, but it has some extremely important and subtle differences. An algorithm is defined as a series of systematic steps that lead to the solution of a problem. The algorithm is so designed that one step leads to the other. Now, here's the important distinction: The algorithm simply claims that, if one follows the steps, the outcome results. It does not claim that it has an intrinsic relationship with the problem itself. Let me clarify that. The book method, the interpretation-by-the-numbers method, claims that therapy works because the theory is right, and if the theory is followed correctly, applied correctly, and timed correctly, the outcome will be correct. Therefore, a successful outcome demonstrates the validity of the metapsychology. It is a tautological device. In contrast, an algorithm is simply an operational series of steps. It may or may not have a theoretical idea behind it, but it makes no claim that the theory is necessarily related to the outcome. As a very simple example, in the Middle Ages there was an algorithm for preventing the ague. People knew then that you had to close the windows at night (i.e., avoid night air), build your house on high land, and make sure there was no stagnant water in the house or surrounds. Now, these ideas were based in some way on the assumption that there were evil effects from humors and night air. People did not know about the anopheles mosquito, and they did not know about the malarial protozoan. But they had a stepwise procedure—an algorithm—for preventing malaria, and if one followed it, it worked. Now, this is essentially the position I am going to develop later—namely, that the function of supervision is essentially to supply the supervisee with an algorithmic approach to the analytic process, with the caveat that this algorithm facilitates treatment only through an indirect relationship to how treatment works. I suspect that the algorithm very probably taps into some deep structure, as does the treatment for ague, but that our hermeneutics, our explanatory systems, really may be irrelevant to that. In other words, therapy depends not on the rightness of the hermeneutics but on the relevance of the algorithm. I think the metapsychology one chooses—whether it is interpersonal or Freudian or object relationship—is really more a matter of personal aesthetics. I would prefer the supervisee to find his own system of belief, as long as he recognizes that successful therapy does not depend on the supervisee indoctrinating the patient with his beliefs or translating these theoretical beliefs into systematic action. Nor, obversely, does it prove his metapsychology is correct.

THE METATHERAPEUTIC APPROACH

This approach, it seems to me, consists largely of seeing the supervision as an extension of the supervisee's analysis—that is to say, the supervisor works with "countertransference." This usually means that he feels entitled to inquire into the therapist's personal problems and sees the supervision as an opportunity to help the therapist to expand his self-awareness and to see where his anxiety points are located. Thus, supervision becomes the analysis of countertransference, either (in the classical sense) to minimize it, or (in the interpersonal sense) to utilize it. The supervisor sees himself in the role of a special catalyst for the supervisee's personal psychoanalysis and psychological growth. My objection is not that it does not help the supervisee's therapy with the patient (because I think it does), but that it does not advance the basic issue of supervision as I see it. This is not how to get the supervisee to learn what we already know, but how best to facilitate, or at least not to interfere with, some ineffable process of learning by which he or she settles into professional competence.

THE ZEN METHOD

The technique is one in which the supervisor confronts the ineffable by creating an atmosphere of creative disorganization. He harasses, raps, and interferes until the therapist, the supervisee, in the Zen term *opens the fist*—that is, lets go all of his preconceptions and tightness out of a sense of despair. It may appear as if I am ridiculing this method, but I have been on the receiving end of it both in psychoanalytic supervision and in learning other activities. It really works, particularly with tight, obsessional people. If one is screamed at long enough, one becomes despairing and suddenly lets go, stops thinking, and to one's absolute amazement, discovers that the activity now seems natural and easy.[1] Anyone who has had a by-the-numbers, Class II supervisor should certainly have a "Zen," or Class V, supervisor as an antidote. In fact, I think they sometimes make a useful team, like the hostile-and-kind interrogator teams used by the police. One first learns the rules, and then gets them knocked out of one's head. It is a combination worth considering.

PRECEPTORSHIP

Here the therapist learns by watching what the supervisor does with the same situation. This is the technique that Searles, Caligor, and Bromberg wrote about as "parallel or reciprocal process" (Bromberg, 1982; Caligor, 1981; Searles, 1955). The supervisee brings the therapy into the supervision process by playing out (albeit unconsciously or automatically) the interaction with the supervisor in such a manner that the therapist plays the role of the patient. The supervisor can then, at firsthand, experience the intersubjective psychoanalytic situation and

[1]See Kvarnes's book on his supervision with Sullivan (Kvarnes, 1976). It is a wonderful example of Sullivan's devotion to this process.

react to it. It has the value of showing the supervisee the homeostatic power of systems. But I do not much like this method because, although it illuminates the therapy for the supervisor so that he can formulate more clearly what is going on, it seems to me to be quite passive-submissive, inasmuch as it treats the supervisee as something of a conduit. I think it is quite interesting in this style of supervision to note that the patient frequently dreams of the supervisor, usually quite accurately gauging sex and age and other details—thus unconsciously acknowledging the presence of a superadvisor. The patient is marginally aware that *his* therapist, the supervisee, has become an intermediary for a supertherapist in a supertherapy.

This is, of course, an arbitrary and hasty delineation of supervisory styles, and it is, I hope, more for stimulating discussion than for closing the debate. All these different methods of teaching have considerable values in different circumstances and with different supervisees. Still, my own proclivity is toward an algorithmic concept because I would like supervision not to encourage the therapist's submission to superior wisdom or skill. It is seductively easy to impress a supervisee with your perceptiveness, only to leave him with the feeling that he is inept and that he can never know how you arrived at your conclusions. It is a very common experience in doing supervision, for instance, to have a supervisee passed from one supervisor to another, with the report (at, say, training-committee meetings) that, with every supervisor he seems to begin knowing nothing and that by the end of the supervision period he is really quite competent. Then, he starts all over again with the next supervisor, as though—somehow—none of the supervision had any impact. I think there may be a way of simply defining an algorithm of therapy for the supervisee, showing him how to work, defining his lapses from the algorithm and then letting the supervisee find his own way of defining and using insights.

The algorithm that I would like to elaborate consists of essentially three steps. The first is the establishment of constraints and limits—those arrangements that are made in psychoanalysis about contractual commitments—time, money, frequency, cancellation of sessions, vacations, and so forth. There is also a much more subtle structuring by the therapist within the first few sessions of the patient's motivations for being in therapy, goals and expectations for the therapist. Moreover, in the process of inquiring, the therapist defines and frames his *own* limitations and areas of competence.

A patient who has just been separated from his wife and is depressed is not necessarily a candidate for psychotherapy of any sort, and even less, a candidate for psychoanalytic therapy. A therapy in which the patient wanders in, states his complaints vaguely, and extracts a tacit agreement from the therapist to treat him has already violated the rigorous constraints of the algorithm. To repeat, the first step is essentially a definition of limits. That means not simply the physical framing of the therapy but defining the limits of possibilities, the limits of commitment, and the limits of interest. Having established constraints, the therapist goes to the second step of the algorithm that is, in the Sullivanian sense, the extended inquiry. That is, the therapist listens to the patient's story, gets a background, looks for what are essentially the lacunae—the holes in the Swiss cheese, the gaps in the continuity and coherence of the patient's life story. When the therapist finds these gaps, he inquires into them further and, at the very least, delineates them. In the classical psychoanalytic sense, with the patient on the couch, this is simply done by encouraging the free-floating fantasy—in other words, fantasy fills the gaps. In a more Sullivanian, pragmatic inquiry it is more factually and realistically oriented. Nevertheless, this *textual enriching of the data* is the second step of the psychoanalytic algorithm.

The third step has to do with the transfer of the issues under inquiry into the transference; that is to say, those issues under inquiry in the therapy become played out in the transference between the therapist and the patient. This is in Freud's strictest use of the word *playground* (Freud, 1914/1958). It is this last step—the use of the transference, the fantasy or real exchange between the patient and the therapist—that distinguishes psychoanalysis from psychotherapy. In other words, a rational, detailed inquiry, in which the holes and inconsistencies are pointed out to the patient and in which an attempt is made by the therapist to interpret distortion is not really psychoanalysis in anybody's terms. It is simply a rational, directive, Meyerian psychotherapy. It is the carry-over of the material into the relationship between the patient and the therapist that defines the unique area of psychoanalytic inquiry.

I have presented a simple three-step algorithm for doing therapy. One notes that it promotes no metapsychology, no manual of tactics or timing. I want to emphasize that I think this algorithmic three-step process is at the core of *any* psychoanalytic position—from the most conservative to the most extreme. The therapeutic leverage lies in the resonance of the second and third steps that are made psychologically tolerable for both participants by the containments and constraints of the first step.

How the transference is perceived varies greatly between psychoanalytic groups. In the Freudian system, the patient's problems are projected *onto* the analyst. In the object–relationship position, the problems are projected *into* the analyst. In the Sullivanian position, a much more complex mélange of distortion and accurate perception occurs, and it is the function of the therapist to aid by consensually validating and sorting out the patient's perceptions. There is also considerable diversity (and no small acrimony) in the debates about how active the therapist may be, and where the therapeutic leverage lies. The therapist may see himself as a nonparticipant purifying the field, as providing a holding environment, providing a corrective emotional experience, involved in a heroic struggle for authenticity, for the patient's sanity, or explicating a homeostatic system that can be only shifted by increased awareness.[2] In other words, there are many different ways of perceiving one's participation.

For me, the transference is not particularly a place of projections, projective identifications, or parataxic distortions, but it is, rather, a real transaction. In the course of a detailed inquiry into the patient's life—including his fantasies and dreams, within the constraints of the therapeutic agreement that limits and contains the anxiety of both participants—something relatively simple happens. As the therapist inquires into the patient's life and as the events that are reported become more complex, it becomes evident that it is possible to view them from a variety of perspectives. That is to say, anything the patient tells one is subject to an almost infinite number of observational perspectives—a veritable "Rashomon." Indeed, it is virtually impossible to say anything to anyone—even a stranger accosted in the street—that is not, from some perspective, true.

Thus, it seems to me very unlikely that the therapist can listen to anything that the patient is saying and be perfectly clear that there is only one possible explanation. It therefore follows that, however the therapist sees or understands what he is listening to, whatever questions he asks to extend the data, whatever interpretations he makes represent a posture or position about what he is hearing. He is therefore—willy-nilly—participating in what he observes. This participation is both called out by and calls out some response from the patient who will color and select his data, either obligingly, defiantly, or whatever. This dialectical exchange constitutes the act of participant observation and consensual validation—not listening to and then helping the patient sort out what is real and what is not real, but this much more complex dialectic between what the patient is saying and what you are selecting to hear and to respond to. Both participants can and will respond to that exchange (the transferential exchange) from an almost infinite variety of

---

[2]See Epstein and Feiner (1979) for an extended discussion of uses of countertransference.

positions, and they will choose those that are most consistent with their life experience and security needs. To put it succinctly, *the transference is the way that the patient and therapist will behave around what they are talking about within the framework established by the constraints of the therapy.*

Analyzing the relationship between what is talked about and the behavior that goes along with what is talked about constitutes the psychoanalytic process, as I see it, and it is what distinguishes it, essentially, from all other forms of psychotherapy.[3] The transference from this perspective is seen as a dialogue of two real people who are interacting in a real way out of their own particular interests and experiences and investments. Therapy is rooted in a matrix of a real relationship that is defined by the terms and agreements of the psychoanalytic setting. The traditional psychoanalytic view is to see the therapeutic leverage as lying somewhere in the correlation of the transference and the patient's infantile life; that is, in a transformational correlation between what happens in the transference and what has happened early in the patient's life or what he has fantasied as having happened early in his life. I would prefer to see the therapeutic leverage as lying in the resolution of a redundant interaction with much homeostatic power. The therapist and the patient struggle through to a different kind of engagement against the pull of the homeostatic system. This, then, permits the patient to review and enrich his perception of his earlier life and permits him a wider range of participation with people with whom he is currently involved. I do not believe a therapy works unless it is authentic and unless both participants are engaged and changed by the experience.

To return to the issue of supervision: With beginning therapists I would work on structuring the therapy, delineating it, helping the therapist to pace and control the flow of material and to learn how to do an inquiry, and how to visualize what he is being told so that if he cannot see it and he does not know it, then he can ask more questions about it. I tell supervisees that, if they were directors with a script and they could not show their actors how to play out a particular part, they really do not understand the whole matrix of metacommunication that is taking place. Psychoanalysis, in this sense, is the science of omissions. Last, I would introduce the therapist to the notion that—while he is examining the patient's life—he is also interacting with him or her. I would tell the therapist also to notice the extent to which parallel or isomorphic interactions seem to take place in the patient and in himself in the process of the therapy. The next level of supervision would have

---

[3]See Levenson (1979) for an extended discussion of this issue.

to do with elaborating the nature and intentionality of interpretation; that is, to indicate to the therapist that every time he interprets, he is taking a position about the material and that this is only one of many positions that can be taken about it. Also this position represents a participation with the patient that is both isomorphic and resonates to the patient's life experience, but also comes out of who the therapist is and what his real life experience is. Simply examining the expanding ramifications of this network of interactions enriches the therapy and, as Sullivan pointed out, it is like widening the beam of a flashlight on the patient's life.

The third level of inquiry that I would reserve for more sophisticated and senior analysts and particularly for those who are working in the termination phases of therapy is to begin to examine their realistic participation with the patient. In this sense, the therapy is seen as genuinely being in the intersubjective realm—that is, it occurs between the patient and the therapist, and it is a situation in which they are equal coeval participants. Herein, the distinction between doctor and patient becomes blurred. I would reserve this inquiry for the termination periods of therapy, not because I think that it is limited exclusively to that time, but because it requires a certain amount of experience and familiarity with the psychoanalytic technique to be able to use this methodology. Like all learning procedures, one begins with a set of rules and then learns to violate the rules for virtuoso purposes.

You will note that the supervisee is not instructed on how or why this works, how he should *use* the transference, or *how* to make the patient change. The supervisee is not supposed to figure out what is wrong with the patient or how to change him. As Bion put it, each session is entered without memory or desire; that is, without conscious intention or direction (Bion, 1970). Most supervisees have extensive experience doing psychotherapy. They are used to goal-oriented, defined, purposeful therapies, and they are disconcerted by the loose, floating quality of what I am suggesting. It is only when they hear the material begin to enrich and shift, and when they hear the recurrent themes emerging through the material and experience the extraordinary recapitulation of the material in the intersubjective realm that they come to see that *some* process is going on that they have not initiated or energized. There is the remarkable experience of being carried along by something larger than both therapist and patient: A true sense of an interpersonal field results. *The therapist learns to ride the process rather than to carry the patient.*

I do not think that steering the therapist by helping him clarify his countertransference or showing him how to do it or giving him an interpretative, metapsychological armature on which to rest his interpretations is ultimately very useful. It may well be political because it reduces anxiety and is very endearing to supervisees. Let me use a brief example: Suppose a therapist comes to me for consultation, a single session, about a patient with whom he has been working for some time and with whom he is having difficulty. As usual, it all seems perfectly clear to me. I tell the therapist the way it looks to me, and he seems relieved, leaving happy and grateful. It is indeed the *infallible* in pursuit of the *ineffable!* The real question is, why, if it is so clear to me, then why is it not so clear to him? Does he not see something because he has a "countertransference"? Is the therapist dumb? Is he bound by theory? I think you are telling the therapist what he is telling you to tell him. At this point one has entered a very complicated hall of mirrors, and, I think, violated the constraints of the psychoanalytic process.

What can one do? First, one can maintain the constraints of the supervision, which is not to violate the privacy or limits of the psycho-analytic inquiry. In a word, stay out of the supervisee's analysis. Second, one can listen to the data, show him how to expand blind spots, and point out that in the process of doing so the supervisor is taking a position about the therapist's position about the patient—not that this position is necessarily clearer or closer to the real truth. It is only more explicated. Hopefully, this would permit the supervisee to detach himself from the supervision and look at his own position vis-à-vis his own patient. It is the exploration of this engagement that is the leverage of psychoanalysis. And for that, the therapist must go back and work with his own patient—not with the supervisor.

To be sure, I have set up a whole series of artificial boundaries and distinctions. Clearly, in the actual process of supervision, as in therapy, these categories overlap and often become indistinct. Nevertheless, what is appealing about the algorithmic approach is that it is useful to have a method that works, even when you can not be sure why. I would like to think that this algorithmic approach would work with any meta-psychology. If the patient spends an hour talking about bad mothering, has a dream in which she is lying in a bathtub and finds that the water is floating with cockroaches, looks under her legs and sees that her little dog is drowning under her feet, then tells you that she spent the entire night lifting the real, aging dog on and off the bed every two hours because it would jump up and then be unable to get down, and that she is planning to have a baby in a year, one would certainly hope that the therapist would see this as a continuous, recurrent theme having to do with mothering and nurturance. If the therapist points this out, it is psychotherapeutically useful and, above all, reassuring. It says to the patient that "by naming this, I indicate that your fears about mothering are only fantasy expectations." If the patient then proceeds to explore her own experience with mothering as a child, her own fantasy systems, and so forth, one is enriching the contextual field. However, I still do not think it is psychoanalysis. If the patient calls out in the therapist an unnurturing, hostile response or if the patient acts with the therapist in a cold and unnurturing way, the transferential dimension has been introduced, and one would hope that the therapist could correlate what he has heard with what is being played out between them. If mutual warmth emerges or if either participant is called upon to be excessively nurturing, another transferential perspective is being played out. There is an infinite variety of ways the dyad can engage the issue, but until they are aware that what they are talking about and expanding is simultaneously being enacted between them I do not really see it as psychoanalysis. There are, beyond that, all sorts of extrapolations of how one does that and how one participates, but I believe they largely constitute variations in technical approach and are not so central to the psychoanalytic principle.

As I mentioned earlier, Harry Stack Sullivan once said, "God keep me from a therapy that goes well!" No one seems to say that about supervision. Supervision is not therapy. It operates, I repeat, on an entirely different level of abstraction. To confuse supervision with therapy is—in Korzybski's famous aphorism—to confuse the map and the territory.

We should find another name. I think it is not supervision. It is really *continuous consultation*, which is something else altogether. The moment the supervisor violates the consultant role and becomes the supervisor, he drops out of the class and becomes one of the members of the class. In other words, he then stops treating the class of events and begins to work on the specific therapist–patient event, at which point the constraints have been completely violated, and one has an uncontrollable situation. If the therapist becomes passive, he can become the conduit for the supervisor, and the therapy can go relatively well. He will likely receive a good supervisory report. But, as I have said, I think these are the people who tend every year to start over again right from the beginning, as if nothing had been learned.

I think we can grapple best with the process of supervision by focusing not only on the value of what we are teaching but on the phenomenology of learning as well. To do that we have to involve the supervisee in the process. What is his experience? Not only how do we teach, but how does he learn? If we are the infallible in pursuit of the ineffable, we are "following the fox." Our problem from this perspective is how to teach the supervisee what we know but simply cannot clearly say. We are in hot pursuit of the elusive truth. Rather, I think the problem is closer to how to teach the therapist a *procedure* that calls forth a *process* that carries us all—supervisor, therapist, and patient.

REFERENCES

Bateson, G. *Mind and nature, A necessary unity.* New York: E. P. Dutton, 1979.

Bion, W. *Attention and interpretation.* London: Tavistock Publications, 1970.

Bromberg, P. M. The supervisory process and parallel process in psychoanalysis. *Contemporary Psychoanalysis,* 1982, *18,* 92–111.

Caligor, L. Parallel and reciprocal processes in psychoanalytic supervision *Contemporary Psychoanalysis,* 1981, *17*(1), 1–27.

Doehrman, M. Parallel processes in supervision and psychotherapy. *Bulletin of the Menninger Clinic,* 1976, *40,* 3–104.

Epstein, L., & Feiner, A. *Countertransference.* New York: Jason Aronson, 1979.

Freud, S. Remembering, repeating and working through. In J. Strachey (Ed. and trans.), *The complete psychological works: Standard edition* (Vol. 12). London: Hogarth Press, 1958. (Originally published, 1914.)

Korzybski, A. *Time-binding, the general theory.* Lakeville, CT: Institute of General Semantics, 1954.

Kvarnes, R., & Parloff, G. *A Harry Stack Sullivan case seminar.* New York: Norton, 1976.

Levenson, E. Language and Healing *Journal of the American Academy of Psychoanalysis,* 1979, *7*:2, 271–282.

Searles, H. The informational value of the supervisor's emotional experiences. *Psychiatry,* 1955, *18,* 135–146.

10

Teaching the Psychoanalytic Method
Procedure and Process

Zvi Lothane

LEARNING AND TEACHING AS INTERPERSONAL NEXUS

All learning is a labor of love between a student and a teacher. Teacher and student, master and apprentice, trainer and trainee, tutor and tutee, preceptor and preceptee, or, as of late, supervisor and supervisee? Which is the proper model in psychoanalytic education?

All organized education has its academic function—imparting knowledge and skills—and its administrative function—passing on the student's performance and personality. At some point the words *supervision* and *supervisee* acquired citizenship in the jargon of psychiatric residencies and psychoanalytic institutes. In the institutes these words, which are not in the spirit of the tradition of medical education, have replaced the older terms *control analysis* and *control analyst*. What is in a name? A convenient label, a content, and an intent. These names, old and new, indicate a greater concern with control and surveillance than with teaching and guidance. In this chapter, at the risk of appearing whimsical, I will continue to use words *teaching* and *teacher* and *student* where others use *supervision* and *supervisor* and *supervisee* to refer to the job of training a person to become a psychoanalyst. This choice of name reflects an intent of separating tasks of education from those of administration.

Learning and teaching are reciprocal processes: Students and teachers learn from each other. "I have learned much from my teachers, more

Zvi Lothane • Clinical Assistant Professor of Psychiatry, Mount Sinai School of Medicine, City University of New York, New York, New York 10029; Training Analyst, Institute for Psychoanalytic Training and Research, New York, New York 10028; National Psychological Association for Psychoanalysis, New York, New York 10011.

from my friends and most from my students," says the sage in the Talmud. The same spirit pervades the Socratic method of teaching in the dialogues of Plato. The psychoanalytic experience itself is also a process of learning. In *Studies on Hysteria*, it can be seen that Breuer and Freud (1895/1958) taught their patients and learned from them. Later Freud called the psychoanalytic experience an aftereducation (*Nacherziehung*).

Teaching implies that there is a subject matter and a method to be taught. The subject matter in psychoanalysis as a therapeutic discipline is the treatment of disorders of behaving or acting by means of the psychoanalytic method. *Behaving* is what people think, say, and do to each other, whether the other is present in the flesh or only in the imagination. It is also a reciprocal action, and it takes place in dyads. It is transaction—action carried from one person to another. A person is a monad, a self-contained system, only insofar as he is a physiological system.

The fact of reciprocity of human behavior is relevant to a requirement that there should be a congruence between a theory of disordered behavior, a theory of a treatment method applied to the disorder, and a theory of teaching that method. Freud's psychoanalytic method, his own original discovery, was from the start applied to dyads—the analysand and analyst who were engaged in the psychoanalytic process. By contrast, his theory of disordered behavior was formulated largely in terms that were applicable to monads. Thus, there has persisted in Freud a perennial tension between the theory of disorder and the theory of treatment. Sullivan (1964), on the other hand, even though he was influenced by Freud, developed a transactional and dyadic theory of disordered behavior as a disorder of interpersonal relations. He was influenced by Bridgman's operational approach. Bridgman (1959, p. 3) defined an operational analysis as "an analysis in terms of activities . . . doings and happenings . . . [rather] than in terms of objects or static abstractions."

Applying the operational principle of activities and doings to mental symptoms and disorders, Sullivan viewed both hysteria and schizophrenia as meaningful in an interpersonal context (1962). These disorders were not like the natural diseases of the body, but they were strategies in adaptation and communication learned in the course of living in the family and in society. This is why Szasz (1961), following Sullivan, called mental disease a myth. He was misunderstood as denying the reality of mental disorders, when what he meant was to define them in terms of behavior and communication and not in terms of bodily happenings.

What follows is a highly condensed statement by Sullivan (1964) about the "interpersonal situation, this rather discrete if transient entity."

> Every interpersonal context seems, then, to include two or three human organisms, and/or reverie toned simulacra or illusions thereof, integrated into a single more or less discrete entity by forces tending to produce cooperative, collaborative, antagonistic and/or disjunctive movements.

While falling into the habit of energy and entity words, Sullivan is not describing physical or metaphysical entities or forces but people in a transaction, trans-action, or action carried from one to the other. Such transactions may take the form of a communion, as if the two persons interacting formed one fused state of being, or a transient entity. Or they may occur in the form of communication, in thoughts, words or deeds. Furthermore, such communing or communicating may take place in the real waking world or in the imaginary world of reverie, illusion, and dream. These latter distinctions follow Freud's delineation of external reality and psychic reality and their relation to human expressive behavior (Lothane, 1983).

The preceding statement by Sullivan is also true of the collaboration in the psychoanalytic setting. It embodies a distinction relevant to the application and teaching of the psychoanalytic method—the distinction between *procedure* and *process*. Operationally, the psychoanalytic situation consists of a dialogue set within a relation, and both are governed by specific rules of conduct. The rules governing the relation, the procedure, and the process are defined technically as *reciprocal activities*. In addition, the rules governing the relation and the procedure are also defined ethically.

Operationally, the psychoanalytic situation means maintaining and observing the *intra*personal and *inter*personal operations, procedures, and processes that constitute it. Operationally, the *intra*personal processes of thinking and feeling (images, emotions, and sensations) in one person—the speaker—become *inter*personal when, as acts of speech or expressive gestures, they *evoke* responses of thinking and feeling (images, emotions, and sensations) in another person—the listener. This conjoint figure of speaker-and-listener is fundamental to all the varieties of communication, whether in the marketplace, in the private space of lovers, or between analysands and analysts. Buber (1958) called it the dialogical principle of the I–thou or me–you relation. Thus, interpersonal is synonymous with communicational.

Whereas it is difficult to determine where procedure ends and process begins, it is useful to think of these as separable and interrelated events. It is also useful to think of them as being causally related. Adhering to the requirements of the psychoanalytic procedure sets in motion the psychoanalytic process, both as an unfolding and as a cure. I will consider procedure and process separately.

TEACHING THE PSYCHOANALYTIC PROCEDURE

Teaching the psychoanalytic procedure and its technical and ethical ground rules should be the first order of business in any psychoanalytic institute. As a matter of fact, teaching the procedure has been overshadowed in most institutes, both in bulk and emphasis, by the emphasis on various theories, which are mostly of a monadic or hybrid cast (Lothane, 1980, 1981a, 1981b), at various removes from the dyadic nature of the psychoanalytic transaction.

The transactional and ethical definition of the psychoanalytic procedure and process is fully developed in Freud's 1912–1914 papers on technique. Earlier in his career, Freud was concerned with self-analysis as a solitary pursuit employing solitary free association. By contrast, analysis proper is the collaboration of two participants—both employing free association. Like the dialogue itself, free association is both procedure and process.

Man is a rule-following animal and procedure means following rules. In these papers Freud described "the rules which can be laid down for the practice of psycho-analytic treatment," or the "rules of the game" (Freud, 1913/1958). He compared the psychoanalytic practice to "the noble game of chess."

Sticking to the rules of the game is ipso facto tantamount to creating the very conditions that are essential for the existence of a psychoanalytic-therapeutic setting, or the frame, to use the graphic metaphor of Robert Langs (1978). Moreover, since a viable therapeutic setting is only possible when both players—analysand and analyst—play by the rules, it follows that the analytic game, or any social game of living for that matter, requires that there be mutual agreement, or a contract, to stick to the rules.

The basic ground rules that comprise the mutually binding therapeutic contract include the persons (the parties to the agreement and no third parties), place (a comfortable and quiet space to work in), periodicity (fixed schedules and promptness), payment (setting and collecting of adequate fees), privacy (policy about confidentiality for both partners), and procedure (an understanding about the right to talk and be silent, *both* agreed upon as modes of communication). All these are clearly spelled out by Freud in the technique papers, which should be read and reread by every beginner and old-timer practicing psycho-analysis.

The push in the analysand for self-expression, self-revelation, and self-awareness and the complementary pull of the conditions of the psychoanalytic-therapeutic setting will act as both propelling forces that will set in motion processes of unfolding (undoing of repression and recall) and cure (emergence of insight and change). The analyst's role is to be receptive, noninterfering, and nonsoliciting in order to allow procedure and process to take their effects. Such an attitudinal prescription for the analyst dispenses with the emphasis on analyzing resistance. Resistance, whether as an issue of the analysand's defensiveness or an issue in collaborativeness versus antagonism, is left to the decision and choice of the analysand. The analyst proposes—the analysand disposes.

The ethical rules of the game have been stated by Freud no less clearly than the technical rules: "psycho-analytic treatment is founded on truthfulness. Since we demand truthfulness from our patients, we jeopardize our whole authority if we let ourselves be caught out by them in a departure from truth" (Freud, 1915/1958). The sexual abstinence rule, a derivative of the prohibition against incest and also demanded by the Hippocratic oath, is the most self-evident application of such truthfulness. Freud also said that "for the doctor the ethical motives unite with the technical ones to restrain him from giving the patient his love" (1915/1958). But carnal gratification is only a special case of using the patient instead of serving him. According to Freud, "educative ambition is of as little use as therapeutic ambition" (Freud, 1912/1958, p. 169), especially because it is prone to masquerade as altruism. The caveats combine with a positive message: "The welfare of the patient alone should be the touchstone" (Freud, 1915/1958). The analyst should be moral—not moralistic. Another powerful implication is that safeguarding truthfulness is also an advocacy of the patient. But in the teaching situation there are two advocacies—that of the patient and that of the student.

The ethical position advanced here is that while both advocacies are important, in the teaching situation the advocacy of the student takes precedence over the advocacy of the patient. By adhering to this principle, the needs of both students and patients will be met adequately.

The opposite has been common practice in psychiatric and psycho-analytic education, and in this both have differed from medical education. Since medicine deals primarily with the body and secondarily with behavior and character, it is easier to reach consensus on approaches, performances, and skills, because the practice of medicine is primarily a technology. Because psychoanalysis as a practice deals with character and behavior exclusively, because it is less a technology and more an art of interpretation and moral suasion, it is easier to clash with the characters and behaviors of others—patients, students, and teachers. There is more room for likes and dislikes, for arguments ad hominem than ad rem, for hatreds bred by the narcissism of small differences. There are also sociopolitical differences between medicine and psychoanlaysis. Medical graduates embrace a profession defined by the law, they often migrate far from the alma mater, have the privilege of open enrollment in medical societies, and are policed by the law. Psychoanalytic graduates practice a profession that is not regimented by the licensing authorities. They often stay in the therapeutic community that grows around the institute and its society. Their graduation and access to the local society, often acting as an elitist club, are passed on by people who are members of both society and institute. Furthermore, psychoanalytic malpractice, which is more difficult to define than medical malpractice, does not come to litigation as often as does the other. Whereas organized medicine has been run as a professional guild, organized psychoanalysis acquired the characteristics of a family-run business, with a lot of family dynamics thrown in.

In such a climate it is tempting for the psychoanalytic educator to arrogate to himself the powers of quality control and surveillance under the guise of the advocacy of the patient. This is often facilitated by the fact that students treat clinic patients, and the teacher, who is pressed into service as an overseer, naturally comes to regard the patient as his own property, thus taking an adversary position toward the student. It is only to be expected that under these conditions, as in an institutionally sponsored training analysis, the student cannot pursue truthfulness but must instead resort to hypocrisy in order to survive. Years ago Greenacre referred to the "convoy phenomenon" in psychoanalytic education—a metaphor referring to navigating in mine- (or shark?) infested waters.

The student–teacher relation, like the analyst–analysand relation, should be based on truthfulness. There is a requirement for a mutual pursuit of truth and honesty with respect to communicating about the student's behavior. The student should be able to confide in the teacher; the teacher need not be self-righteous.

To say that the advocacy of the student comes first implies that the student is viewed as having the same rights as a patient in private—not institutional—analysis. The student is entitled to adequate service for adequate compensation to the teacher. In therapeutic analysis, advocacy of the patient does not mean that the analyst forms a conspiracy with the patient against his family and against society—he needs to have a balanced view of all the people in the patient's network—but that he is first and foremost attuned to the needs of the patient. *An analyst for a need is an analyst indeed.* In a deeper sense, the psychoanalytic-therapeutic space is a sanctuary from judgmental attitudes. Such attitudes are subject to an *epoche*, a temporary bracketing, to facilitate the conditions necessary for the emergence of all the manifestations of psychic reality, as contrasted with external reality (Lothane, 1983). Similarly, the teacher should be first and foremost attuned to the needs of the student, while keeping the needs of the patient and the teaching institution in reasonable perspective. The teacher should not intervene or intrude in the relation between the student and his patient, or compete with the student or preempt him in any way, just as the practicing analyst should not intervene between patient and spouse. Private domains are off limits to third-party intruders.

The writs of habeas corpus have not been the same in medical and psychoanalytic education. All too often the psychoanalytic student has been viewed as being prima facie neurotic, in countertransference, and being abusive of the patient until proven otherwise. Such things do happen. But there is no need for moralistic *a prioris*. These have often been justified by the ethic that hardship and harshness build character. However, such an ethic can easily slip into lovelessness, lack of fairness, and an undermining of an identification with psychoanalysis. Low morale, burn-out, and defections have become endemic in the psychoanalytic profession.

The student needs to have a supportive, friendly teacher who will teach him how to be strong in the face of the patient's onslaught, who will show him how to be free from guilt in upholding the ground rules and the integrity of the psychoanalytic frame, and from therapeutic ambition greater than the patient's own drive—or ability—to be cured. In short, the teacher will first teach the student sound procedure and process. If this is achieved, the rest will be added. The student will be brought to realize within himself any other shortcomings of a personal nature and will work on them in his own analysis.

As in the analytic-therapeutic setting or in the teaching setting, the reality of the patient–student interaction has to be perceived clearly and acknowledged *before* one gets to dreams, fantasy, or transference. Operationally, who publicly and consciously did what and to whom and where and when need to be known before any assumption of unconscious motivation. Observation of the clues precedes the catching of the culprit. Because the conscious includes the unconscious and the unconscious does not include the conscious, the order of procedure is from the conscious to the unconscious, from the explicit to the implicit, from act to thought, from thought to what is yet undisclosed, or still latent, or preconscious thought.

Time and again students have come to me—beginners and advanced candidates—who have not been taught how to set up and maintain a therapeutic contract. They have been taught a lot of theories, both clinical and metaclinical, and much empathy, but they have been taught only sparingly about ground rules. Consequently, such students have rushed headlong to the bigger and better things, such as interpretations of the patient's behaviors based on clinical theories and other clichés, glossing over the requirement for a foundation of a solid frame. The situation may be likened to a couple who rush into marriage out of love without giving much thought to how compatible their life goals are or what they are going to live on. One day they awake with a start to the harsh economic realities, and there is hell to pay. Neglect in areas of the therapeutic contract vitiates analytic process and cure. Uncorrected lapses of omission or commission linger on as obstacles to learning for both participants. A warm heart cannot make up for the lack of a cool head.

A woman graduate of a psychoanalytic training program presented a patient in the third year of his analysis. She had not established mutually accepted ground rules about the rights of silence and speech for analysand and analyst. She repeatedly felt that the patient's silences were nothing but resistances, and she experienced recurrent guilt, self-doubt, helplessness, hopelessness, and rage about her own and the patient's silences. This often resulted in feelings of stalemate.

In the session presented, she described her state of mind as follows:

> I walked into the waiting room wondering what kind of a session we would have today. I said to myself: "Keep neutral and relax." I opened the door, Mr. R. stood up, nodded and walked through the corridor into the consulting room. He lay down on the couch and was quiet for quite some time. I was thinking: "Oh, shit, it's going to be one of those silent, drawn-out sessions. Oh, God, now my supervisor will hear and see what goes on." I also thought: "If only I was a better analyst, I wouldn't be stuck, and Mr. R. would not be in this predicament." I then felt I was beginning to get angry. I said to myself, "This will get you nowhere. Why don't you think of the issues in this analysis?" I also thought of you [meaning the teacher] and how you would handle it and what we had discussed about ground rules. My thoughts returned to the patient. I am taking one week off next week, so he has got to be working this over. Since he was 7 or 8 years old he would lie still on his bed in silent anger toward his mother. He is hurt and angry now toward me. I began to relax and he started speaking. "A couple of nights ago I had a dream." At this point I was able to be silent in a relaxed, contempla-

tive way. He continued: "Too bad I do not remember more details. But it was with a Great Dane." Here, in addition to visualizing a biting dog, my association was: "great dame," alluding to myself. "The dog was hurting me, he wounded me on the arm, scratched me like my cat would do when I was a little kid." I was now better able to relate his anger to my going away. What I found most interesting is that he started his next session as follows: "I finally reached my orthopedist yesterday." For the longest time he had delayed making the appointment with the surgeon for needed corrective knee surgery.

This vignette could be discussed in a number of ways, but I will focus on aspects of procedure and process. Whereas it may not be possible to determine where procedure ends and process begins, these two aspects of the method can still be separated both for practical and didactic purposes. In this session the communication within the analysand–analyst dyad is at first blocked, both due to feelings within the analysand and those within the analyst. Without making hypotheses about the analysand's motives for silence, it is suggested that the analyst's preoccupation with herself, her uneasiness, and her feeling pressured to generate the process—instead of calmly waiting for the patient to generate it—are all blocks to the process getting started. Maybe the patient was getting around to speaking anyway, but it is hypothesized here that the analyst's on-the-spot self-analysis and the restoration of her own capacity to listen receptively and contemplatively were important facilitating influences. With the passing of the analyst's depressive thoughts and mood, with the reaffirmation in her consciousness of the rationality of silence as a fundamental communication, a different aura prevailed, and it was transmitted to the patient. That opened up communication within the dyad.

The analyst's "great dame" response to the patient's "Great Dane" illustrates a basic lawfulness of human mental activity—the action reaction, or transaction nature of communicating in thought, mood, and word (Lothane, 1981b). Moods are said to be contagious, and words have the power of evoking in the listener the images that were in the speaker. Every stimulus of word or mood in one calls forth an echo of image, association, memory, and mood in the other. It happens in every dialogue.

What makes the psychoanalytic dialogue unique? What is the proper method of teaching what is unique to that dialogue? It is that *both* interlocutors—the analysand and analyst—follow the fundamental procedure of the psychoanalytic method—free association. I would like to refer to this basic communicative activity in the psychoanalytic setting as *reciprocal free association.*[1] This concept was inspired by Isakower's "analyzing instrument" and Reik's "listening with the third ear" (Lothane, 1981a).

Free association is an ingredient in ordinary conversation. However, in ordinary conversation it is dismissed as irrelevant or as intrusive. In the psychoanalytic setting it is fostered and pursued as a means to an end—the task of analyzing. This is Freud's fundamental discovery.

RECIPROCAL FREE ASSOCIATION AND THE PSYCHOANALYTIC PROCESS

Free association is the instrument of the psychoanalytic method. Following Bridgman, we can say that we are using the instrumental-operational approach when we specify a procedure and the results obtained by it. Procedure, method, and instrument are interrelated. As a methodologist, Freud understood the centrality of this conception. "Psychoanalysis is a method of research, an impartial instrument, like the infinitesimal calculus, as it were" (Freud, 1927/1958, p. 36). It is also the tool of discovery in the setting of psychoanalysis as therapeutics.

Much has been written about free association as the instrument of the analysand (Lewin, 1955). Isakower was unique in consistently applying free association in all its instrumental implications to the analyst as well. He coined the term *the analyzing instrument* and applied it to the activities and attitudes of (1) the analysand; (2) the analyst; and (3) the analysand–analyst transaction. Isakower's views on the analyzing instrument were described by others (Malcove, 1975; Balter, Lothane, & Spencer, 1980; Lothane, 1981b), based on personal communications and quotations from a double set of presentations by Isakower to the faculty of the New York Psychoanalytic Institute (1957, 1963). Recently, I was privileged to get hold of some of Isakower's unpublished, undated, handwritten notes.

Like Sullivan, Isakower defined the analyzing instrument in two distinct terminologies, viewing it as an entity and as a process.

> The concept of the "analyzing instrument" recommends itself primarily on the grounds of its heuristic value, as a point of reference for the clarification of the *psychic processes* which constitute the foundation of the *specific analytic*

---

[1]*Reciprocal* according to the *Webster's Third New International Dictionary* means returning the same way, alternating, a combination of *recus,* backward, and *procus,* forward. It conveys the idea of mutual and shared relation and action, felt or shown by both sides, and of corresponding, equivalent or complementary functioning as a return in kind.

activity . . . in its activated state [it is] . . . a composite consisting of two complementary halves. It will be remembered that in Freud's description . . . both halves function together as *one unit in continuous communication.*

The analyzing instrument represents a constellation of the *psychic apparatus* in which its *constituent structures* are tuned in a way that makes the apparatus optimally suited for functioning in a very specific manner. (New York Psychoanalytic Institute, 1963b; italics added)

Apparatus or activity? Structures or speeches? Parts or persons? Entities or enactments? Which is the better name, the truer vision? As a neurologically trained psychiatrist and heir to Freud's own dilemmas between theories and terminologies (Lothane, 1981a), Isakower oscillated between monadic and dyadic formulations. Defining the operations for the analysand, Isakower stated the following:

The analyst conveys to the analysand the desirability of letting images emerge; the analysand is encouraged to acknowledge and to behold visual contents in his consciousness, and to put these into words, in addition to the contents which are already verbalized.

When this happens, the patient's attention is simultaneously directed to that detail, and his *own*, the patient's analyzing instrument is being activated. (Isakower, unpublished notes)

In the last sentence Isakower provides the clearest definition of the interpersonal and conjoint nature of the analytic process. As a result of this interlocking mental activity, the analyst comes to experience the patient in a specific way:

The analyst's frame of mind when analyzing: While listening, he suspends conscious intellection (reflective thinking) and permits his own unconscious to arrive at a preconscious level. There, influenced by stimuli arriving from outside—the patient's productions—compromise formations arise between what the patient is communicating and the contents of the alert and receptive "analyzing instrument" of the psychoanalyst, the ultimate result being potentially verbalizable statements.

The communications of the patient are bound to "create" in the analyst's *receptive* mind [=mind, which is presumed to be in that receptive state], an integrated entity—image—or assemblage of partial images which are being modified and readapted continuously, while at the same time the analyst's "trained" state of mind is capable of leaving *loose* ends *loose,* but is aware of the quality of incompleteness. (Isakower, unpublished notes)

These quotations describe the three previously enumerated uses of the analyzing instrument—the operation of the analysand, the operation of the analyst, and the conjoint operation. Both participants share an experience, and they resonate to each other in a reciprocal mode of wakefulness, receptivity, and evocation of thoughts and feelings. It is an experience akin to dreaming—both nocturnal and diurnal—and it is governed by the conditions of dream psychology. When such a mood is fostered, there is an increased accession of imagic and metaphorical thought forms, which are particularly suited for taking hold of repressed memories, encoded latent meanings, and representations (dramatizations) in fantasy, word, and act. As shown elsewhere (Lothane, 1983), these modes of thought and feeling are manifestations of psychic reality as contrasted with external or material reality, and the workings of imagination. To grasp psychic reality, it is better not to use ratiocination and not to aim at closure but to give oneself over to temporary looseness, incompleteness, and uncertainty—a state of mind Keats defined as "negative capability, that is when a man is capable of being in uncertainties, mysteries, doubts, without any irritable reaching after fact and reason" (Keats, 1817/1955). Such a negative capability is the precondition for the latent incubation of preconscious thought processes that leads to a spontaneous emergence of images, recall, and understanding, such that the person is taken by surprise and amazement—a point tellingly made by Theodor Reik (1937).

Isakower untiringly stressed the importance of imagination images, all images, but especially visual images and the capacity for visualization, which is the preponderant mode of representation in dreams and daydreams. As the analyzing instrument is the core of the psychoanalytic process, so visual imagery—for that matter, all varieties of imagery—is the core of the analyzing instrument.

When the operation of free association in the analysand is matched by the corresponding free association of the analyst, which Freud called evenly hovering attention, the latter will be,

> hovering between what comes from the outside, from the patient, and what is approaching from the inside, from the analyst. Elements of both will more easily converge and, optimally, coincide [in the analyst's mind]—like, by analogy, in a rangefinder focusing device—within an area where visual images participate in representing a given visual content. Visual representations, those from outside and from inside, lend themselves much more easily to mutual adaptation, or, put differently, to blending into one formation (New York Psychoanalytic Institute, 1963a), to meeting half-way on a common, communicable plane, than do verbalized ones. (New York Psychoanalytic Institute, 1963b)

This blending is not a demonstrable operation. It is a metaphorical description, taken from an optical instrument—the range finder—of preconscious processes of evocation and association in the analyst's mind. Operationally, as Russell (1921, p. 206) put it, images in the speaker evoke images in the hearer:

> And this is really the most essential function of words, namely that originally through their connection with images, they bring us in touch with what is remote in time or space. . . . Images may cause us to use words which mean

them and these words, heard or read, may in turn cause the appropriate images. Thus speech is a means of producing in our hearers the images which are in us.

The process of becoming aware of images is expressed in a variety of postperceptual metaphors—that is, words created or an analogy to sense perception. As vision is the master sense, so visualization is the paradigm of all imagination. Thus, *intro-spection*, *in-tuition*, and *in-sight* all refer to the use of a metaphorical or mental eye for looking into the metaphorical interior of one's consciousness, to observe a parade of images, as in a film strip, or, as in Freud's (1912/1958) train-ride simile:[2]

> as though . . . you were a traveller sitting next to the window of a railway carriage and describing to someone inside the carriage the changing views which you see outside. (Freud, 1912/1958, p. 135)

Using the train-ride simile, Lewin (1970) described the convergence or blending of images or the analyst's mental activities in the following way:

> So far in this essay attention has been directed mainly to the man in the window seat with apparent neglect of the person inside who cannot see the landscape directly. Freud's advice is addressed to this person and there is much to say about the history of his mental processes and evolution, even in terms of the metaphor. He had his own infancy and conflicts and his own store of visual memories, some of them reactivated in the professional setting. Of the many possible things that might be said about him in terms of the analogy, I shall point out that there are two sides to the train, therefore a second window and corresponding landscape. The passenger at the window in the original figure, concentrating on his side of the road, would not perceive the second window. The inside passenger, passively attentive to the verbal messages, would be inattentive to this window too—but not unaffected. He would be subject to an "internal" Poetzl phenomenon and he would register images received from the window through the corner of his eye; that is, by "indirect [peripheral] vision," which, then, he might or might not combine with the messages from the other passenger on the train, while they are travelling companions on the terminable or interminable journey. (Lewin, 1970, p. 49)

---

[2]During his course, The Dream in the Practice of Psychoanalysis, which I took at the New York Psychoanalytic Institute, Isakower called attention to a precursor of the train-ride simile in Freud and to Strachey's mistranslation of it. In the case history of Fräulein Elisabeth von R., Freud (1958a) describes the patient's collaboration with his method of "evoking pictures and thoughts":

> It was as if she was reading from a *long* picture book (*als läse sie in einem langen Bilderbuche*), whose pages were *pulled before her eyes* (*vor ihren Augen vorübergezogen wurden*) (author's translation).

Isakower explained that Freud's analogy was to what is called in German a *Leporelloalbum*, an accordionlike folding string of picture postcards, or a similarly printed children's book, like Leporello's famous catalogue of Don Juan's mistresses. Compare *Standard Edition*, Vol. 2, p. 153.

Arlow[3] (1969) commented on Lewin's previously quoted passage:

> Lewin refers to the pictorial nature of the individual's stores of memories. In connection to a patient's response to a construction he says: "It is as if the analysand was trying to match the construction with the picture of his own." Each analyst has a different capacity for visual memory or fantasy representation. But following Lewin, I think it is correct to say that some form of visual thinking occurs in the analyst's mind as he thinks along with the patient's free associations. The joint search by patient and analyst for the picture of the patient's past is a *reciprocal process*. In a sense, *we dream along with our patients*, supplying at first data from our own store of images in order to objectify the patient's memory into some sort of picture. We then furnish this picture to the analysand who responds with further memories, associations, and fantasies; that is, we *stimulate* him to respond with a picture of his own. In this way the analyst's reconstruction comes to be composed more and more out of the materials presented by the patient until we finally get *a picture that is trustworthy* and in all essentials complete. (Italics added)

Lewin and Arlow refer back to the same phenomena that Isakower described—communication consists of a *reciprocally evocative activity* between the analysand and the analyst.

A special class of imagination images deserves to be emphasized— kinesthetic and visceral sensations evoked in the analyst while listening to the patient's narrative. Jacobs (1973) has reported on awareness of posture, gesture, and movement evoked in the analyst in the process of unconsciously mimicking the patient's enacted or described motions. He says that monitoring such responses within oneself enabled the analyst

> to put himself more finely in tune with his unconscious reactions. This increased self-awareness can then be used, either in the service of providing clues to the meaning of the patient's communications, or in facilitating the recognition of previously undetected attitudes and feelings in the analyst himself. (p. 92)

In this connection, it is of interest to note that, according to the *Oxford English Dictionary*, the word *imagination* is etymologically related to the word *imitation*.

---

[3]Arlow does not identify the last words in this paragraph as a paraphrase of Freud (1937/1958), although he mentions the paper in his references: "What we are in search of is a picture of the patient's forgotten years that shall be alike trustworthy and in all essential respects complete." Arlow has, of course, along with Lewin and Isakower, elaborated and refined Freud's description of the analysand–analyst dyad in that paper: "The work of analysis consists of two quite different portions, that is carried on in two separate localities, that it involves two people, to each of whom a distinct task is assigned."

Many critics of Isakower's ideas, even those favorably disposed (Arlow, 1969; Reich, 1966) have tended to discuss the analyzing instrument as a manifestation of transference and countertransference. Isakower saw it as a superordinate principle and phenomenon, which was not subsumed under the category of transference.

> After Freud the problem of the [analyzing instrument] has been dealt with . . . mainly in terms of vicissitudes of "transference." The concepts of [transference and] countertransference do not cover and comprise what is to be elaborated as the analyzing instrument.
>
> The analyzing instrument, denoting a specific psychological entity, is an *invariable* element in the analytic procedure, the variable elements being the countertransference, the situations that involve empirical devices considered adjuvant, and diverse "interventions." (Unpublished notes)

The purpose of the preceding review of Isakower's views on the analyzing instrument was to lay the ground for operationalizing reciprocal free association as a fundamental process for the enlarging of consciousness, knowledge, and understanding. Again, it plays its role in ordinary conversation, but it is more frequent in the psychoanalytic setting.

From the beginning, free association was promoted by Freud as an instrument for opening the door into the dreamworld and the remembering of the submerged past. Both the dream and the remembrance of the past may emerge in consciousness in visual and other imagery—the image is the message. Getting hold of images requires fulfilling certain preconditions that are operationally the same for daydreaming, solitary free association, and reciprocal free association—withdrawal of attention from the outside world, lifting of self-criticism and self-guidance, immersion in an altered state of waking consciousness, and calm contemplation of the images spontaneously rising to consciousness—the organ of observing and knowing.

Such a state will prevail when the technical rules of the psychoanalytic procedure are scrupulously maintained. Any departure from the correct procedure is transference on the part of the patient and countertransference on the part of the analyst. From the beginning, Freud defined transference in a twofold manner: (1) as a manifestation of the resistance to the process of free association; and (2) as a reliving of past relations. Both these forms belong in the realm of the interpersonal relation and the procedure, or the frame. Playing fair with the procedure versus playing foul with it will bring out the various qualities of character and habits of love, and these will be enacted—or acted out—in the arena of transference and also find their way to become represented in the spontaneously emerging images. Thus, such images, in addition to being windows into dream life, will also offer visions of transference as reliving, or as dreams, acted out. Acting is a form of communicating. To know is to understand all communication in act and in image.

To illustrate reciprocal free association and the connection between procedure and process, I will now describe a teaching session with a student analyst. He presented a second session of the analysis, which was the first he discussed with me.

In the first session the patient, an ordained priest, outlined his current life conflict—a secret affair with a nun. The analyst proposed the terms of the analytic contract, and the patient accepted it. There was some vague reservation about something that the analyst remembered dimly as having heard but that was not discussed with the patient. The patient had previously seen an analyst in consultation who charged high fees. The student set the patient's fee, following an inquiry into the patient's financial situation, at a rate lower than what he felt entitled to by virtue of his level of experience and standing in the community.

In the second session, the patient gave further details about the love affair. He and the woman had been in love since they were in high school, but it was the woman who broke off the relationship to join a nunnery. The patient later went to a seminary and took the vows. As the story was being told in all its poignancy, the analyst experienced the patient as dangerous in some ways—as potentially violent. The analyst could not explain the source of such feelings, and he remained engrossed in the patient's story.

I listened to this account for some time with a comparable degree of absorption. Presently, the thought of Abelard and Heloise—the ill-fated lovers—came to me. This image referred to passionate love, to forbidden love, and to the conflict between the flesh and vows of chastity. I conveyed this image to the student. He responded to this by a visual memory of having seen the play about Abelard and Heloise some time ago. The student dimly recalled not so much the details of the powerful ending of the play as its menacing atmosphere, which was related to Abelard's punishment by emasculation. He also had a personal reminiscence of a forbidden love affair of his own about which he chose to remain silent. The student's reticence was, of course, fully respected. But, in this context, I asked him how he defined free association. He said it meant saying everything that came to one's mind. Here I made a distinction between saying everything, which is never possible, and allowing oneself to think everything that comes up—opening oneself up to evocative processes. The intention of free association in response to the patient's narrative was to allow everything to rise to consciousness— even something as seemingly peripheral or intrusive as one's personal life—for the sake of the patient. Thus, thinking of oneself would not be pursued for the sake of indulging oneself or serving oneself—this would be relegated to one's own analysis—but only as a means to an end: for the purpose of resonating in sympathy to the patient's material.

I used my own image as an example of such a use of free association. Of course, whereas the analysand is enjoined to say everything without any restraint, the analyst who free associates is urged to use analytic judgment about what parts of his free association to convey to the analysand and how to convey this information. The student found my image useful: One of the effects upon him was to place the patient's situation in a wider context of culture and society. It also helped him to sympathize with the patient's predicament.

As the student continued to report the patient's narrative, it now struck me how engrossed he had been by it. It could be said that he was *fascinated* by it, or under the *spell* of it, terms that evoke the quality of being in a hypnotic trance. I did not immediately tell the student about this perception.

After the formal termination of this session, on his way to the door, the patient engaged the analyst in a new transaction. He said he needed to bring something up that had slipped his mind. The analyst expressed a readiness to listen, whereupon the patient announced that he would not be in for the next session due to a commitment made prior to the beginning of this analysis. The analyst said to the patient that he would see him when he next came in. The mood of the analyst after the patient had left was a mixture of unhappiness, of having been had, not to say raped.

The didactic task in this presentation was defined for the student and for me by the material of the hour, the here and now of the patient with the student and the here and now of the student with me. In the context of the procedure I pointed out that the way in which the fee was set had a potential of disrupting the frame, due to the analyst's burying the hatchet of his discontent and the patient's feeling he might be getting a second-rate deal. These presumptive perceptions would be held in abeyance until further evidence was forthcoming.

One frame rift had already taken place—the extension of the analytic session to conduct additional business. Ground rules about time are most frequently abused. There was also a potential for the analyst to collude tacitly in this disruption and to muddy the issue of financial responsibility: It was unclear whether the patient was let off the hook, or whether he was expected to pay for the canceled session.

Returning to process issues, I defined *reciprocal free association*. I felt that voicing my image of Abelard and Heloise was not a totally random occurrence. There are many other famous lovers in the world literature: Tristan and Isolde would be another famous pair. The spontaneous emergence within me was both a result of the student's narrative of the patient's story, and also a stimulus for the unfolding of further evocative processes in both the student and myself. It thus showed a concatenation, a sympathetic vibration, between patient–student's and student–teacher's thought processes. This is what is meant by reciprocal thought processes. The reciprocal interpersonal processes, after a period of preconscious incubation, emerge as nodal points of communication. This is what Freud meant when he said that the analyst gets the drift of the patient's unconscious with his own unconscious (Freud, 1923/1958). The emergence of the spontaneous image is the final common pathway of such preconscious processes converging to materialize as an image, a vision, or an insight.

As the result of this reciprocal give-and-take between me and the student, which, paraphrasing Isakower, I might call the "teaching instrument" (i.e., setting in motion reciprocal free association between us), I was led to a further realization—how engrossed the student had become in the patient's saga and how he was entrapped by it into a deviation from correct procedure at the end of the session. This trapping of the analyst by the patient to act out something out of the patient's or the analyst's life, other than being a deviation, is also part of the analytic process in action. The patient had enacted an abandonment scene, he had materialized something as a transference, and he made a transfer of his past (possibly the abandonment by the girl in the face of earlier promises) into the analytic setting, thus turning the analyst into an unwitting victim. Also, the very cancellation of the third session due to a prior commitment could be an enactment of the life conflict—breaking the vows of chastity in favor of the previous vows of love. The point was not to deplore such events, but to become aware of such transferred, or induced, reactions (Roland, 1981), and to use them for their heuristic value, both for the analysand and the analyst.

Art is long and life is short. An analysand can only tell so much in a session, to cover so much of the multitude of events, thoughts, and dreams that have occurred in a given time. An entire analysis is but a fraction of lived time. Yet, owing to the capacity of the mind to reveal itself in a fragment of creation, the microcosm of the analytic hour is quite sufficient to mirror the macrocosm of life.

Similarly, an hour of teaching can only encompass a fraction of what the patient and the student have lived through in an hour of analysis—let alone a number of hours. However, teaching is not a customs inspection, and if it were it would require several hours to go over the material of one hour in all its ramifications. But then, teaching need not be pursued as a sequential, seriatim sifting through mounds of material to get pay dirt, but as a selective focusing upon a significant segment of transaction to meet the needs of the student—not the needs of the teacher or the administrator.

Recently, I have started trying out a new method of teaching that is but a logical extension of the concept of reciprocal free association. Accordingly, I first suggest to the student that he select for discussion an hour or a segment of an hour that he has defined as posing a problem for himself. The student is thus not merely reporting, but comes with an awareness and a formulation of something that calls for clarification and learning. I then ask the student to give me both texts (the patient's and the student's) of the hour or of the segment. By this I mean the text of the patient's free association and the analyst's running free-associative response, the actual thoughts, images, emotions, sensations, and commentaries, both silent and spoken, that have been evoked in him by the silent or spoken behavior of the patient at every turn.

Usually, while the patient's free association is made manifest, the analyst's free association remains hidden. Clearly, reporting such a reciprocal process cannot reflect the entire scope of the free association of both patient and analyst. Like the patient on the couch, the reporting student will also not be able to reveal everything. But when courage, trust, and openness of communication prevail, a vista of the material comes into view that is quite different from what is seen in the course of customary teaching where the bulk of what is viewed is a run of the patient's narrative interspersed with occasional interventions by the analyst. In this new way, both student and teacher become privy to a transactional mosaic, to a different quality of interpersonal exchange between the interlocutors, to a glimpse into the analyst's mental workshop. The material viewed this way often takes on new and unexpected meanings, such as the cropping up of uncannily near-telepathic communications between analysand and analyst. Alongside the reportage of the patient–student reciprocal process, there takes place the new student–teacher reciprocal process. These combined processes may result in an image, an insight leading to a greater understanding of the patient, the student, and, hopefully, the teacher.

Reciprocal free association is the instrument of the analytic setting, but it is not the entirety of the setting. Many other interpersonal communicative exchanges take place in it, albeit all are informed by a therapeutic intent: chatting, education, and information, depending on the nature of the patient and the stage of the analysis. Also, reciprocal free association does not occur with the same intensity at all times. But it is always there. Similarly, teaching by the reciprocal process is not all of teaching, but it is a basic instrument. Even if it is not possible for the student to say to the teacher all that came to him in response to the patient, at least he can say it to himself. He has been given a tool that has the potential of raising his awareness of and openness to aspects of the interpersonal and intrapersonal that have been hitherto not sufficiently considered. Just as analysis is only a means to self-analysis, so teaching is a means to self-teaching.

SOME CONCLUSIONS

Community, communion, and communication go hand in hand. *Community* is the sharing of common interests, goals, beliefs and ethical principles, and even common traits of character. It is a condition of collaboration. *Communion* is that shared state of being that binds two minds and bodies into one. When community and communion prevail, communication occurs as a shared and reciprocal activity between two interlocutors who alternate as sender and receiver of messages in thought, word, and deed. This is the operational paradigm in ordinary relations, pathologically altered relations, the analytic-therapeutic relation and the student–teacher relation. In all these relations, the participants engage in transactions at the level of procedure and process. Such transactions are relational, complementary, dialectically balanced, and reciprocally evocative. *Dialectically balanced* implies that the more there is of one the less there is of the other, as for example, between the share of participation and the share of observation, that is, self-reflective awareness.

In the interpersonal setting of patient–therapist or student–teacher, interacting observation is participant observation, as Sullivan put it, as distinct from naturalistic observation of inanimate phenomena. No more is the patient a specimen for the analyst's observation than is the student a specimen for the teacher's observation. Each of the participants is both acting and being acted upon. Analytic neutrality does not mean that the analyst does not act upon the analysand; it only means that his actions are subject to the technical and ethical rules of the game.

Procedure and process are phenomenally and conceptually separable, although it is not possible to tell where procedure ends and process begins. They also go hand in hand. *Procedure* is in the realm of action, which can be defined politically (who does what and to whom) and ethically (which action is right and which wrong). *Processes* are activities in the realm of contemplation and are definable esthetically and formally. Thoughts, ideas, and images engendered by action are forms of knowing and avenues to knowing. In the psychoanalytic setting, in addition to knowing that is acquired through sense perception and discursive thinking, knowing is also acquired through imaginal, or representational, thinking that taps the life of memory and the dream—both nocturnal and diurnal. To analyze, in one sense, is to achieve knowing through the interplay of discursive and representational activities of thought.

The image is the core manifestation of representational thinking. As vision is the master sense, so visualization is the master capability of imagination. Image, idea, pictorial thought, insight, and intuition are related concepts. To see the picture means to understand. Contemplation of the image, like poetry in Wordsworth's words, "takes its origin from emotion recollected in tranquillity." This is but a restatement of the Aristotelian theory of *katharsis*, which originally, in medicine, meant purgation. Applied to tragedy, it meant effecting a purgation of the affects of pity and fear. The concept of *catharsis* in Breuer's and Freud's method of the treatment of hysteria was undoubtedly influenced by these classical ideas through Jacob Bernays—Freud's wife's uncle—who wrote on Aristotle's conception of tragedy. The notion that the psychoanalytic setting is akin to the theater has also been discussed (Loewald, 1975).

By contrast, emotion recollected in turmoil or emotion relived as commotion is either pathological action or acting out in the transference. Transference (and countertransference) is a repetition of the past foisted upon another. Other manifestations are also loosely referred to as transference: (1) unreflected reliving of emotions; (2) deviation from the rules of the game; and (3) dreaming (Lothane, 1983).

Depending on whether one chooses a narrow or broad conception of transference, imagery has often been classed as a manifestation of transference. This is a misunderstanding. Rather, transference—like any other experience—is represented in the image. To clarify this misapprehension further, it is necessary to distinguish between acting, acting out, and enactment as expression and imagination. *Acting* is the final precipitate of thinking, feeling, and intending. It is a carrier of power and love in relations, and it is living by virtues versus vices of character—autonomy versus dependence, honesty versus deceit, and obedience versus rebellion. *Acting out* is merely a way of labeling actions that are inappropriate by the arbitrary but contractually binding analytic rules of the game. *Enactment* is expression through the enactive mode of thought (Horowitz, 1975) or through the bodily sensations, gestures, and posture (Jacobs, 1973). These distinctions should be a hedge against an indiscriminate use of the concept *transference* as a negative label, while at the same time not obscuring the fact that unreflected action is also potential communication. Isakower viewed acting out as part of the analyzing instrument, as communication that has escaped through the outlet of action.

The teacher–student relation, like others, is ruled by the ethical norms of love and truth. Power politics and prestige are perennial pedagogic pitfalls. As in any other situation, any deviation from sound norms will result in interpersonal turmoil. The pitfall is to jump to the conclusion that the turmoil is the result of the student's past or transference, or that it has little to do with the teacher's present. It may be that a large share of disturbances in the student–teacher dyad labeled as *acting out* (Arlow, 1963) or *parallel process* (Caligor, 1981; Gediman & Wolkenfeld, 1980) is due, among other things, to unclarified student–teacher tensions in the present. We are mostly told about the student's, not the teacher's, acting out or transference. A portrayal of parallel process, in the strict sense of the word, would require the consideration of the contributions from both participants. Caligor (1981) is a remarkable exception, and he is an example of a teacher who candidly describes his own reactions.

The matter is further complicated by the fact of institutions. Institutions notoriously place their own needs before the needs of the individuals whom they serve and whose money they take. It may be an unavoidable evil, but it should be minimized. Raising awareness about the needs of the student, upholding the advocacy of the student before that of the patient, and matching students and teachers of compatible outlook and temperament might help. People who intensely dislike each other need not be together. Life is not long enough to deal with superable obstacles. One should be spared the insuperable ones.

The process of reciprocal free association has been demonstrated as an instrument of communication, both in the patient–therapist dyad and in the student–teacher dyad. The emergence of an image that leads to insight is not limited to dyads but also occurs in triads and other polyads. It has been described as a manifestation of the group mind in the course of the teaching seminar (Malcove, 1975). I have observed it repeatedly in free-associative interviews of surgical patients with groups of medical students. Questions that were asked under the inspiration of spontaneously emerging associations to the patient's material—whether in the mind of the teacher or the participating medical students—very often led to the emergence of illuminating new material.

It is customary to contrast the rigor and precision of science with the alleged ambiguity of art and thought in general, and the image in particular. This dichotomy is deemed false. Imagic thought can be precise both as personal experience, for example, as a memory, and as interpersonal communication in the course of reciprocal free association. *The image is a fact of thought.* Some images are vague, others, as Freud observed, are ultraclear. The vagaries of opinion have been extrapolated onto the alleged vagueness of images. But the problem of validity of interpretation, which is in the realm of opinion, should not be confused with the validity of the image as a fact of thought. Imagic emergence in the course of free association follows its own lawfulness. Thought arises in response to thought; thought mirrors thought. It is the beginning of insight and prelude to understanding and interpretation. It is a product of the psychoanalytic process, and it moves the process along.

REFERENCES

Arlow, J. The supervisory situation. *Journal of the American Psychoanalytic Association*, 1963, *11*, 576–594.

Arlow, J. Fantasy, memory and reality testing. *Psychoanalytic Quarterly*, 1969, *37*, 28–51.

Balter, L., Lothane, Z., & Spencer, J., Jr. On the analyzing instrument. *Psychoanalytic Quarterly*, 1980, *49*, 474–504.

Bridgman, P. W. *The way things are.* New York: Viking Press, 1959.

Buber, M. *I and thou.* New York: Charles Scribner's Sons, 1958.

Caligor, L. Parallel and reciprocal processes in psychoanalytic supervision. *Contemporary Psychoanalysis*, 1981, *17*, 1–27.

Freud, S. Studies on hysteria. In J. Strachey (Ed. and trans.), *The complete psychological works: Standard edition* (Vol. 2). London: Hogarth Press, 1958. (Originally published, 1895.)

Freud, S. Recommendations to physicians practising psycho-analysis. In J. Strachey (Ed. and trans.), *The complete psychological works: Standard edition* (Vol. 12). London: Hogarth Press, 1958. (Originally published, 1912.)

Freud, S. On beginning treatment. In J. Strachey (Ed. and trans.), *The complete psychological works: Standard edition* (Vol. 12). London: Hogarth Press, 1958. (Originally published, 1913.)

Freud, S. On beginning treatment. In J. Strachey (Ed. and trans.), *The complete psychological works: Standard edition* (Vol. 12). London: Hogarth Press, 1958. (Originally published, 1913.)

Freud, S. Observations on transference love. In J. Strachey (Ed. and trans.), *The complete psychological works: Standard edition* (Vol. 12). London: Hogarth Press, 1958. (Originally published, 1915 [1914].)

Freud, S. The future of an illusion. In J. Strachey (Ed. and trans.), *The complete psychological works: Standard edition* (Vol. 21). London: Hogarth Press, 1958. (Originally published, 1927.)

Gediman, H., & Wolkenfeld, F. The parallelism phenomenon in psychoanalysis and supervision, its reconsideration as a triadic system. *Psychoanalytic Quarterly*, 1980, *49*, 234–255.

Horowitz, M. J. Modes of representation of thought. *Journal of the American Psychoanalytic Association*, 1975, 20, 793–819.

Isakower, O. Unpublished notes.

Jacobs, T. J. Posture, gesture and movement in the analyst: Cues to interpretation and countertransference. *Journal of the American Psychoanalytic Association*, 1973, 21, 77–92.

Keats, J. Letter 32 to G. and T. Keats, December 21, 1817. In *The Oxford dictionary of quotations*, Oxford: Oxford University Press, 1955.

Langs, R. *The listening process.* New York: Jason Aronson, 1978.

Lewin, B. D. Dream psychology and the analytic situation. *Psychoanalytic Quarterly*, 1955, 24, 169–199.

Lewin, B. D. The train ride: A study of one of Freud's figures of speech. *Psychoanalytic Quarterly*, 1970, 39, 87.

Loewald, H. Psychoanalysis as an art and the fantasy character of the psychoanalytic situation. *Journal of the American Psychoanalytic Association*, 1975, 23, 277–299.

Lothane, Z. The art of listening: A critique of Robert Langs. *Psychoanalytic Review*, 1980, 67, 353–364.

Lothane, Z. A new perspective on Freud and psychoanalysis: A review of F.J. Sulloway's *Freud, biologist of the mind. Psychoanalytic Review*, 1981, 68, 348–361. (a)

Lothane, Z. Listening with the third ear as an instrument in psychoanalysis: The contributions of Reik and Isakower. *Psychoanalytic Review*, 1981, 68, 487–503. (b)

Lothane, Z. Reality, dream, and trauma. *Contemporary Psychoanalysis*, 1983, 19(3), 423–443.

Malcove, L. The analytic situation: Toward a view of the supervisory experience. *Journal of the Philadelphia Association for Psychoanalysis*, 1975, 11, 1–19.

New York Psychoanalytic Institute. *Minutes of the faculty meeting.* Unpublished manuscript, 1957.

New York Psychoanalytic Institute. *Minutes of the faculty meeting.* Unpublished manuscript, 1963. (a)

New York Psychoanalytic Institute. *Minutes of the faculty meeting.* Unpublished manuscript, 1963. (b)

Reich, A. Empathy and countertransference. In Annie Reich, *Psychoanalytic contributions.* New York: International Universities Press, 1973.

Reik, T. *Surprise and the psychoanalyst.* New York: E. P. Dutton, 1937.

Roland, A. Induced emotional reactions and attitudes in the psychoanalyst as transference in actuality. *Psychoanalytic Review*, 1981, 68, 45–74.

Russell, B. *The analysis of mind.* London: Allen & Unwin, 1921.

Sullivan, H. S. Modified treatment of schizophrenia. In H. S. Perry (Ed.), *Schizophrenia as a human process.* New York: Norton, 1962.

Sullivan, H. S. *The fusion of psychiatry and social science.* New York: Norton, 1964.

Szasz, T. *The myth of mental illness.* New York: Harper & Row, 1961.

A Sullivanian Approach to Supervision
Beginning Phases

RUTH MOULTON

Sullivan had many specific, practical ideas about how to approach the very difficult, schizoid, or borderline patient. As a result, students brought to him their sickest and most troublesome patients who either would not talk or could not explain in any clear, relevant way what had happened to them as they grew up or precisely how they felt about significant issues. Sullivan felt that schizoid patients had often been raised in such an atmosphere of ambiguity and double-talk—where deep feelings were denied or explained away by meaningless chatter— that they were led away from experiencing the truths of their world. Facts that they may have once seen clearly in early childhood were later buried or distorted to fit in with adult needs and prescriptions. The result was a blurring of memory, a forgetting of episodes that failed to fit into family myths, and an apparent acceptance of rationalizations or untruths in order to please significant adults or at least to avoid their rage and threatening disapproval. Words ceased to have real meaning. Other people's ideas could not be trusted, but one's own perceptions were also suspect or dangerous. Without consensual validation or parental affirmation, clear observations and authentic feeling responses were repressed, resulting in vagueness, confusion, and amnesia. This made it very difficult for the therapist to get an accurate picture of what really went on in the patient's past so that he could understand the present. Thus, it was hard to get the thorough developmental history

RUTH MOULTON • Fellow, Training and Supervising Analyst, William Alanson White Institute of Psychiatry, Psychoanalysis and Psychology, New York, New York 10023 and Life Member, American Psychoanalytic Association, New York, New York 10022.

that Sullivan thought was absolutely necessary as a sound background for treatment. He felt that taking a good history was in itself therapeutic, since it led the patient to rediscover and reevaluate his past with an experienced and impartial new person as a guide. The theory could indicate where to dig and help to decipher the archaic language engraved on tablets from childhood in order to disclose hidden truths that would illuminate current problems in living. Old assumptions and myths had to be documented and reexamined with "benevolent skepticism" to see if they fit the new facts. It was like an archeologist's exploration of the past in order to better understand the present.

Sullivan realized that most sick people were unable to give clear, pertinent histories at the beginning of treatment. The initial overview was important for the basic orientation of the therapist. It would give him some idea as to the central problems and help guide the patient's future detailed inquiry—when the patient was somewhat more trustful and the analyst more aware of which troubled areas needed to be investigated first. Whenever the patient "did not know what to talk about" or blocked due to anxiety, Sullivan would suggest that the analyst use the opening to go back once again to ask, "When did this anxiety first occur" or "What was going on in your life at that point in time?" One could always inquire into obscure areas of history that needed to be clarified. This recurrent inquiry was more meaningful to the patient if it was connected with the content of a recent hour or a current problem. History then became more relevant, not just didactic or of theoretical importance. Sullivan felt the patient needed to be shown what kind of material was relevant by the demonstration of its pertinence during therapy. The analyst was interested in just the kind of material that the parents had forced into repression. To pursue obscured data, the analyst often found himself "bird dogging"—sniffing out emotionally laden areas, seeing discrepancies in the available data that needed to be clarified, and sensing that more lay behind a given story than appeared at first. Every explanatory hypothesis suggested by either patient or analyst had to be questioned, documented, tried out in therapy or real life to see if it fit, if it "rang true," "if it elucidated obscure areas of conflict." Constructs had to become useful in a practical, pragmatic, and nontheoretical approach. Preconceived notions were always to be challenged, because they might be camouflage for a more basic issue that caused too much anxiety for the patient to face alone.

When working with either supervisees or patients, Sullivan would accept no cliches, no generalizations, no fancy or ambiguous technical terminology. When one offered a theory about what was happening with a patient, Sullivan would frequently ask, "As illustrated by what?"

or "Precisely what do you mean by that?" "The man says he has an Oedipus complex; did you get him to spell that out for you? What makes you think so? What made him arrive at *that* conclusion?" Or, he would say, "Yes, many people hate their mothers; exactly how was it with him? What did she do? How did he react when she did that? Tell me how the battle developed between the two of them?"

Sullivan felt that precision was necessary to understand the uniqueness of an individual, and that whatever resentment a patient might have at being questioned would be easily offset by the relief that would result from knowing that somebody cared enough about him to inquire and to listen. Then, a *unique* formulation could be arrived at that precisely fit that patient and no one else. Sullivan felt that the basic security needs of individuals were so similar as to be boring. What made the work interesting was to find out exactly how they were lived out by each person.

He did not recommend cross-examining patients in the same critical way he did students, but he certainly recommended very direct ways of collecting relevant data early in the treatment situation, provided that the patient could tolerate that approach. He was acutely aware of manifestations of the patient's anxiety level and, whenever anxiety seemed to be so great as to be disruptive, Sullivan would say to the patient, "Let's put a red tag on that. It's an important area to explore. We will get around to it later when it is easier for you to handle." While the patient would thus be let off the hook, putting the red tag on the problem reduced the likelihood that it would be forgotten. There was little danger of throwing a borderline patient into a schizophrenic panic, Sullivan felt, if one was aware of minor manifestations of anxiety. This did not mean that he believed that one should be reassuring or avoid basic issues. It was, rather, a matter of how rapidly and in what order one approached them.

Sullivan also warned against the disrespect often contained in kindness or sympathy. He would say, "The patient does not need your kindness but your understanding. Many friends and relatives have tried to be kind to the patient before. None of them understood what was important. That's your job." It was clear from knowing him, however, that he was quite kind to sick people, though always in an offhand rather than sticky or smothering fashion. He was acutely aware that schizoid persons were fearful of inappropriate or premature intimacy before they were fully ready for it. He cautioned against overt reassurance because he felt that most sick people were dreadfully suspicious of it and could smell it a mile away as false.

Consistent with this caution about not pressuring patients into anxiety-ridden areas before they were ready, came Sullivan's warning not to get into transference issues too early with a schizoid, evasive patient who felt he needed distance for a long time before he could trust enough to be more "personal," to admit feelings that might lead to ridicule or rejection. In the beginning months or sometimes years of treatment, one respected the patient's need for space, one did not push the you–me aspects until there was more traction, growing trust, and a positive working alliance. One exception to this was when negative transference—such as paranoid distortions—prevented therapy from moving ahead. Even then, one had to point out the parataxic distortions with care, so that the patient could keep his self-respect and not be humiliated by his grandiosity, his mistaken ideas of reference, his twisted judgment in maligning or idealizing the therapist. Not only was it safer to get history first, because that was less anxiety provoking than personal feelings about the therapist, but history gave one valuable clues as to where transference needs originated, so they could be accurately interpreted when the time was ripe. The patient could then feel understood rather than accused or judged. Sullivan saw this method as quite different from what was appropriate with a less disturbed, more nearly "normal" neurotic analytic patient, who could not only tolerate but who even needed a more direct confrontational approach. In general, Sullivan felt that dealing with transference first and foremost put the analyst in the middle of the stage prematurely. This not only robbed him of his participant–observer role, but obscured the possibility of getting a clear history because the factual landmarks got emotionally flooded before they were mapped out. I think he would also have felt that concepts such as parallel process between supervisee and patient and countertransference to the supervisor were refinements that were interesting and worthy of thought but that they should be left to a later stage of supervision when the basics were clearer.

In an effort to illustrate what Sullivan's approach might have been to a particularly difficult, evasive, schizoid patient, I offer the following example taken from my own work as a supervisor, as it was presented to a study group at the William Alanson White Institute in 1973. The student analyst lived out of town and had difficulty getting analytic patients. This was his third case, and it was assigned to him from the clinic as a case appropriate for analysis. He came to supervision feeling anxious, because he was presumably starting with his last supervisor and hoping for a good case that would prove his readiness to graduate. He was upset to find that he was working with a 33-year-old rabbi who was quite isolated and withdrawn, who was terrified of sexual feelings, and who had never even masturbated, much less had any sexual relationship with another human being. The patient was extremely passive and compliant, especially with his mother, but also in treatment where he was unproductive, could not express or define himself, and waited for the analyst to stimulate him. He had a rich fantasy life about physical closeness with boys, and he was afraid that he might be homosexual. The analyst had never treated a homosexual, did not know how to tackle this problem, and feared that the patient was unanalyzable. This was very threatening to the student, with his need to complete his training. Sullivan would have pointed out the dangers involved in having such a large stake in the treatment process and its success. He would have seen this as interfering with the analyst's freedom to do what was best for the patient even if it meant diverging from accepted analytic technique or risking the loss of the patient. The analyst must feel free to do what the situation requires without thought of the repercussions for him, the analyst. Sullivan used to say, "If you need to keep this patient for financial reasons or to prove your ability, don't bring the case to me. I work for the patient's benefit, not yours. It is expected that you are less needy and more mature."

The supervisee started to present the case in the third month of therapy. The history reported was sketchy and simplistic. The mother was seen as a dogmatic, controlling woman who dominated the family. The father was described as a truck driver—cruel and brutish—who stayed away from home as much as possible. The patient was the passive, good boy who did everything his mother asked. He let her cut up his food until he was 12 years old, and she chose his clothes as well as those of his father until he left for rabbinical school when he was 23 years old. He still went home each time she wanted him, which was as often as every second or third weekend. There was a brother, 7 years younger, who was the "rebel," different from the patient, very aggressive, involved in sports, never at home, and who paid no attention to either parent. The patient acted as if his brother did not exist and as if he was not part of the family. The brother had no emotional meaning to the patient. The entire focus was on the mother and himself—with the father as villain and the brother as uninvolved.

An early example of the patient's extreme compliance came from a visit home early in treatment. The mother asked the patient to take care of the laundry. Although he had studying to do, he obeyed and literally sat motionless for 45 minutes while the washing machine worked. The analyst found this discouraging, indicating apathy and emptiness, and indicative of a bad prognosis. I encouraged a more probing inquiry into what actually went on inside the patient. Did he literally "give in" out of fear of her disapproval? What did he assume she would do to him if he was not so silently obedient? Was he trying to show her up as a castrating witch—ridiculous as well as omnipotent—to cover up his own fear of being appropriately assertive? What had he done about his rage? It was humanly impossible not to have had some. This inquiry led to many memories of his acting as her vassal, being her slave because he felt utterly helpless in face of her apparent power that he did not question until later in his analysis.

Early in treatment this patient described his passive, symbiotic relationship with his mother as though it was "all her fault." He felt that he was a helpless victim who played no role. He joined his mother in having contempt for his father, thus identifying with the stronger parent. He accepted his mother's picture of his father as a boor who was cruel, having no interest in the family. As proof of the mother's strange power, he said that even his father was compliant and weak with respect to her. Here was an evident contradiction on which we could work. How could father have been so strong and simultaneously so weak? The patient seemed to have both bought her stereotype of his father and of men in general. He needed to arrive at a more accurate picture of his father and brother. It did not take long for the intense rivalry with his brother to emerge. Not only was the brother "healthier" in his normal relations with peers whereas the patient shunned other boys and felt "odd and ridiculous," but there was the further fact that his mother disliked the brother for being actively out of her reach. The patient sided with her against the brother and father to get her protection. Meanwhile, he allowed himself to be infantilized and isolated. This made him appear so alienated—as if he was half dead without feelings of his own—that the analyst felt he *was* beyond reach. He felt this patient could not be resuscitated, much less analyzed.

The first job in supervision was to try to show the analyst that the patient could be reached. It is hard to explain fully why I could not share the supervisee's pessimism about the patient. From the beginning I had sensed that there was much more life and vitality in him than appeared on the surface. Apparently, the washing-machine episode was narrated in a deadpan fashion. I felt, however, that there was a kind of irony, some black humor, or tongue-in-cheek quality, underneath. The analyst had taken it literally. I listened to it with disbelief, surprise, and a chuckle. The supervisee had thought, "How can a grown man be this way?" I saw the patient as a pseudocompliant adolescent wanting a strong male to help him grow up and get out of his mother's clutches.

There was good evidence that he felt a tremendous need for treatment although he did not know how to use it. He earned too much to be accepted in the clinic, and he was assigned as a private patient. Even with the low fee, he still had to pay more than he had expected, and he experienced some hardship. Despite this, he paid promptly and without complaint, and he was always on time and seemed to be trying hard to become a good patient. It seemed more than just compliance, because when he felt lost and had nothing new to say, he was discouraged—not relieved. But he could not speak up. I sensed that he was very anxious to express himself but that he did not know how to do so. He needed someone to show him. There was also the fact that he was unsatisfied with the conventional work of a traditional rabbi. He became involved with a forward-looking, liberal group of Jewish educators who were interested in new policymaking. He seemed to have good administrative and teaching skills with younger students and was in charge of a summer workshop. He had developed some areas of legitimate self-assertion, offering a solid basis for self-esteem. He had difficulties with both male and female authorities, but he had a good relationship with a humanistic rabbi. This man valued his intelligence, sensitivity, and ability to teach, and he played the role of a good older brother or encouraging mentor. The patient's ability to work well—and at times creatively—within this setting did not support the notion that he was schizophrenic, as the supervisee feared. The environment was somewhat protected—mostly male. There was little competition except intellectual, and the patient felt comfortable. He was certainly undeveloped sexually and might have had deep problems with homosexuality. Or he might merely have had to go through a period of exploration that he had missed in his restricted adolescence. I found myself telling the supervisee what Frieda Fromm-Reichmann had told me when I brought to her for supervision a very talented, anxious male pianist in his early twenties who considered himself homosexual. He had not come to therapy to have his sexual life changed, but mainly to get rid of his severe anxiety. I had never worked with a homosexual, and I wanted to know some specific dynamics to guide me. Frieda Fromm-Reichmann told me to forget for a while what he was doing with his sex organs and see what he was doing with people and what they had done to him. I realized that I had to try to get to know him as a specific human being and see what lay behind his tremendous performance anxiety that had extended into all areas of living—not just the sexual role. This approach kept us working well for a long time, and when he was ready to look at his homosexuality and its meaning, we already had a good picture of his family background, his character problems, and his present life situation. Then it was possible to make relevant interpretations about his sexual behavior. There was no longer an air of mystery or a need for generalized formulations. I was oriented to him as a unique person.

Sullivan would not have been discouraged by the fact that the young rabbi was "schizoid" and might become "homosexual," although he would suggest that an analyst approach with caution anyone so unformulated, vague, and inarticulate with massive areas of hidden anxiety. Traditional analytic methods of listening and waiting would have to be modified; one could not hope to break through the passive facade by being passive. In this case, the analyst accepted the passive facade as though that was all there was to the patient. I felt it was a defensive mechanism to hide strong feelings; that is, the patient was not genuinely passive but had acted that way for so long that he had lost track of other parts of himself. He needed the analyst not to be taken in but to be skeptical and curious about what was omitted—what data had been lost and buried. The analyst said he was afraid to be active with a passive patient for fear of playing into the passivity, leading him, and feeding him answers.

Sullivan's answer to this dilemma would have been that it was the *kind* of activity the analyst engaged in, not just the amount. Open-ended questions could stimulate the patient's memory, encouraging him to be curious about his past as well as his present behavior. He had to be taught the value of memories, dreams, and stray peripheral thoughts by being shown exactly how they were useful to pursuing new answers. The patient could be misled if the questions were posed in an effort to prove that the doctor's theory or hypothesis was correct. The patient might then be in danger of being overly influenced by the analyst's assumptions, although many schizoid and obsessional patients can be very negativistic when directed, and they will handle suggestions that are useless or wrong by "selective inattention." Thus, they may become more difficult to reach, whereas an open-ended, relevant question gets their attention as they begin to feel understood. If one asks a stupid question and the patient says it is irrelevant, no one is hurt. If a patient accepts a suggestion too readily and one fears he is merely being compliant, one can always ask him to illustrate the point and demonstrate how it fits and what it helps to explain.

Here, the analyst was afraid of being intrusive like the mother. I suggested that this could be avoided by using the patient's feelings as indicators for directions to explore, whereas the mother denied his feelings and showed no interest in them. As an analyst, one can offer a variety of possible explanations for a phenomenon; his mother had given him no choice. She did not question. She told him how it was. The patient was very encouraged by the approach suggested before as he grew to see that the analyst was not as afraid of his mother as he himself was. The analyst questioned stereotypes, assumed rage must exist, and did not buy the patient's picture of himself as a passive, empty failure.

Many patients must be taught where to look for relevant data. They may become good at free association near the end but not at the beginning of treatment. Before supervision, the patient sat up, watching for signs of the doctor's reaction—approval or disapproval. This may have been useful at first while the situation was strange and the patient was anxious and less trusting. Since he was so disconnected, it may have helped him to begin to "know" the analyst by facing him. It may also have helped him to focus and to follow a train of thought while the analyst was learning to encourage him to be more curious and to probe further by his questions. Later, while lying on the couch, it was easier for him to talk about anxiety-provoking topics such as sex. At first, he could not bear to say the word *penis*. Lying down also made it easier for him to bring out some of his anger and hidden aggression. He had to discover slowly that the analyst did not want a "good boy" who would follow him, but instead a thinking, feeling man who could begin to find his own way and to explore his psyche without such dread and caution. He was more able to bring in fantasies and dreams when on the couch. He began to free associate on his own at times.

Another fear the supervisee had was that any pressure on the patient might cause a psychotic break. He was, therefore, proceeding with such caution that nothing was happening in treatment except that both doctor and patient were getting discouraged. The patient must also have felt that the increasingly passive doctor was disinterested and indifferent. When supervision started and the analyst began to question more, the patient became more interesting. It was, of course, appropriate to watch for signs of anxiety, and to respect these when they arose in order to prevent a "psychotic break" due to the too sudden emergence of a disassociated system before the patient was ready. But in this case the real danger seemed to be that *no* repressed material would emerge.

At first, the patient was content to blame his mother for his fear of other children. She told him what to eat, what to wear, what to say. Thus, he did not know how to act on his own. He needed to see what his own role was in maintaining the symbiosis and what secondary gains he received from it. He recalled that when it was time for nursery school he was afraid to go and felt his mother was "getting rid of him." He begged to stay home, and she let him do so for another year. This helped him feel even more different from other boys. It may also have served her purposes to keep him home, but he "got his way." He fought her control by controlling her in a fashion that helped him learn the values of passive resistance. He could complain and back out, but he could not speak up or explain himself or ask for the help he needed. Examples of this began to be brought into the sessions. He reported following a man around for an hour before he had the courage to ask a simple question. The answer was easy, useful, and given without ridicule or hostility, but he "forgot" to ask for an additional piece of data he wanted. He could not sleep with the light on, but he feared asking his roommate to turn it off. After discussion of this in treatment, he was finally able to talk about the problem, and a simple solution followed— again without a battle or even disapproval to face. He began to "speak up" with others as the analyst did with him.

Gradually his self-image of being a "good boy"—passive and help- less—began to crumble. He remembered being quite sadistic with his younger brother until the latter became big and strong enough to fight him off. He then used contempt and silence to push his brother aside, as he had done with his father. He had identified with his mother in valuing education, and he developed an intellectual arrogance to put others down and cover up his physical timidity. He used this weapon with younger male students and even with older, "bossy" female au- thorities. It also was quite surprising to him to discover that he used this weapon against his mother with whom he became increasingly and consciously enraged. After feeling tyrannized by a controlling, arrogant mother, he found himself being like her. When he got into a protracted, self-righteous battle with a female teacher, a colleague, it was important to get him to look at his methods of dealing with her as well as the amount of his rage, some of which was carried over from his anger at his mother, underlying his placating exterior. He was compliant in treat- ment only when the analyst was more passive than he, asking no chal- lenging questions and accepting his version.

The dynamics of his homosexuality began to be seen, at least in broad outline. He was so afraid of physical violence from his father, brother, and peers that he craved a kind male teacher and male protec- tion. He was preoccupied with male organs and sexual attitudes, watched men closely in showers, and was fascinated by erections. He was finally able to masturbate at age 33, and he was most relieved to find that his organ actually "worked." His sexual fantasies were mostly about younger boys—admiring students who looked up to him and who needed his protection. He found a replacement for his absent father in an older, liberal rabbi who also was a homosexual and who helped him feel less guilty by stating his own disapproval of the Orthodox ban on sex as being dirty. The analyst discouraged the patient from seeking out only other homosexuals and actively encouraged him to seek closeness with people he liked and could trust—male or female—since they were all human beings. He discouraged the patient from being so concerned about who was homosexual and who was not. This helped the patient socialize and be less self-conscious, but it did not help him to be more friendly with women. His deep fear of the malevolent, castrating, controlling mother figure remained a problem for deeper analysis at a much later point in time and might never be approachable.

Toward the end of the sixth month of treatment and the third month of supervision reported here, the patient had a dream in which he and his father were sitting on a staircase—the father below him with his back to him. The patient held a book with a title of two movies on it that he wanted to give to his mother. The father offered to pay $500 for the book so that the patient would not use it to terrorize his mother. This led to a new exploration of the family equilibrium. The patient talked about the father's fear of the mother, his weakness in bowing to her, while the patient himself would use books and ideas against her. He saw his father as paying anything to be waited upon, and he said his father had put both the house and car in his mother's name. This was first seen only as placating. It did not occur to him that the father was also avoiding responsibility for mortgage and loan payments and might be preparing to desert the family. This idea led the patient to bring in data about how the father pretended to be dumb and inadequate, thus seeming to accept the mother's contempt but meanwhile letting her take care of everything while he neglected his role as either husband or father and sought out male cronies and increasingly escaped as time when on. The patient began to get mad at the father's neglect, indifference, and passive aggression. It was *not* all his mother's fault. The father not only let it happen, but he played a role in the family interaction and noncommunication. He turned his back on the patient and never protected him from the mother.

At this early point in his treatment, the future was difficult to predict. Progress was bound to be slow, and goals had to remain quite limited. But a beginning has been made. The passive facade had been undermined. The transference was in a rudimentary stage. The analyst was the interested, uncritical father who encouraged and sometimes led exploration. The transference may have been "split" by the presence of the "liberal, older rabbi." In such a case, however, one uses whatever help one can get from the environment at the beginning. In addition to understanding past and present feelings, this patient needed encouragement to observe the real world, to explore it, accumulate knowledge, and obtain experience to make up for his tremendous deficit in learning about life. He was like an early adolescent with very little understanding of people or of himself. Sullivan referred to this process of learning about reality in a schizoid withdrawn person as *re-education* and as being necessary to a successful analysis as insight.

This case illustration, based on less than 15 hours of supervision had a very narrow focus—namely, the need to collect data early and to question stereotypes even though the patient was anxious and evasive. The tendency for young analysts to protect the patient from pain can delay or prevent the development of a useful working alliance. Both parties may be too cautious, and clarity becomes only more elusive.

Another short but more dramatic example of this problem was seen in my supervision of the treatment of a 30-year-old female teacher. The patient was mildly depressed, had no friendships with peers, and had never been close to a man—sexually or otherwise. She did well with her third-grade pupils, lived with her mother, but had little adult conversation with anyone. The major trauma seemed to be the death of her father when she was 6 years old. This was shrouded in mystery. No one in the family spoke about it—not her mother, sisters, or aunts. No explanation was given to the patient—the youngest child—when the death occurred. Everything connected with her father had been destroyed, his clothes, books, pictures, even the toys he had given to the patient. She had kept a few articles of his in a locked trunk in her bedroom, and she locked the door to her room so her mother would not be able to destroy these articles while she was away at work. The mother was very intrusive, but the extent of the patient's retreat seemed bizarre. Shortly after supervision began, I challenged the secrecy about the father's death. The analyst thought it too tender and dangerous a topic to pursue, whereas I saw it as a major impasse. Gentle questioning of the patient about it aroused her curiosity, but no one in the family would talk about it to her. She finally came up with an inspiration of her own. She knew the date of her father's death, and she looked up the *New York Times* files. She discovered that her father had stabbed her mother and then committed suicide by jumping out of his office window in the garment district. This explained why her mother had disappeared for weeks at that time. She was in the hospital.

The Orthodox Jewish family was not only enraged, but in a primitive and superstitious way they felt the suicide as a family disgrace and tried to conceal it. There was no sign of concern about the plight of the father, and no mourning was permitted. With the recovery of these data the patient suddenly felt free to *feel* her loss, and she recalled delightful walks with her father alone in the sunshine before his depression. He gave her more warmth and tenderness than anyone else in the family, and she realized that a large part of herself had "died with him." She was able to recapture her feelings about him and saw her bizarre behavior—locking herself in the bedroom with the trunk and other ritualistic objects—as being her hidden equivalent of "sitting *shiva*" for him alone since no one else cared. When she realized this, she was able to complete her mourning and leave the mother she hated. She moved to a small, appropriate apartment of her own that was closer to work and where she could make some friends of her own. The analyst, by encouraging her to explore the circumstances of her father's death, had enabled her to free herself from a life that was unconsciously dedicated to his memory and to proceed with a life of her own. She was not as "fragile" as her analyst had thought. Behind her paranoid fears of male desertion was a deep wish to reexperience male affection and warmth.

There are many more complicated, sophisticated aspects of supervision not discussed here, but few of them are useful without a good history and a resourceful technique for gathering data despite patient resistance, apparent amnesia, or blocking due to the disruptive effects of anxiety. A good working alliance requires that the analyst receives the cooperation of the more mature aspects of the patient to disclose the hidden trauma and buried infantile needs still operant but connected with the distant past.

References

Fleming, J. The role of supervision in psychiatric training. *Bulletin of the Menninger Clinic,* 1955, *17*(5), 157–169.
Grotjahn, M. Problems and techniques of supervision. *Psychiatry,* 1955, *18*, 9–15.
Moulton, R. My memories of being supervised. *Contemporary Psychoanalysis.* 1968, *5*(1), 151–157.
Sullivan, H. S. *The psychiatric interview.* New York: Norton, 1954.
Sullivan, H. S. *Schizophrenia as a human process.* New York: Norton, 1962.

12

Supervisory Session with Discussion

Roy Schafer

DR. CALIGOR: Can I have your attention please, colleagues and guests. Welcome to the 165th scientific meeting of the William Alanson White Psychoanalytic Society. The focus of our 1980–1981 scientific meetings, as we all know, is on the supervisory process.

Tonight's supervisor is Dr. Roy Schafer. The analyst in training— that is, the candidate to be supervised tonight—is Dr. Susan Harris who is a candidate at the Adelphi Postdoctoral Program in Psychotherapy.

Dr. Schafer was given the following guidelines: "Since our aim is to approximate as closely as possible an actual 45- or 50-minute consultation or supervisory session such as you might conduct in your own office, the candidate will be asked to present an authentic question or problem or issue of the intensive treatment of a patient in his or her current caseload.

Dr. Harris was given the additional following guidelines: You are free to present the case any way that you like, but please focus on current material. Try to keep any history or summary to 4 or 5 minutes. And however you choose to discuss the case, please have your material sufficiently well organized that you can present detailed process notes on recent sessions, some key dreams, and earliest memories if the supervisor should request them.

We will have a 45-minute supervisory session, and there will be discussion following that.

ROY SCHAFER • Training and Supervising Analyst, Columbia University Center for Psychoanalytic Training and Research, New York, New York 10028 and Adjunct Professor of Psychology in Psychiatry, Cornell University Medical College, New York, New York 10021.

DR. H.: I'd like to introduce you to a patient of mine, whom I'll call Rob. He is 29 years old, single, living with his mother and his younger brother. He is a graduate student in psychology and is currently finishing up his final year. I've seen him in treatment for over a year. I initially began to see him on a once-a-week basis, and after the summer vacation that moved to twice a week, which continued for most of the year. And starting this September I've been seeing him three times a week.

He comes from a family of three children. He's the middle child. He describes his mother as an extremely overanxious woman, a very, very intrusive woman, somebody who is very much preoccupied with her own worry and competency. Rob is consistently—over much of the time I've seen him—extremely angry with her. He feels that she has been unable to give to him and has been unavailable to him in any kind of way that he has needed her. And her response to him consistently is one of intrusiveness and worry. His father died right before I began seeing him in May of 1979. He describes his father as an extremely critical, overbearing person, very intolerant and very difficult to get along with. He describes the relationship between mother and father as one in which the father was continually criticizing the mother, and the mother was continually setting herself up to be criticized. Only recently has he been able to voice anything positive about his father, and what he came up with is that his father perhaps served as a buffer in some sense between the patient and his mother.

DR. S.: The father was not so critical or overbearing to him?

DR. H.: He was—extremely so. He describes a couple of key incidents over and over again. In learning how to change a tire on a car, his father screaming at him, "Why don't you know how to do this." And his response was tremendous anger and humiliation and upset.

DR. S.: But he was also a buffer.

DR. H.: Yes, that's a new idea to him. About eight or nine months before his father died, he went through what the patient describes as a really dramatic kind of personality change. His father began to become extremely depressed, upset, and very, very worried—very out of character to how he usually was. It wasn't until Thanksgiving time and the whole family was together that it became apparent that he was really struggling to maintain himself. This was the first time in the patient's life when the father turned to him for anything at all. He was in an extremely depressed state and was sort of looking around for psychiatric help. And he went to an orthomolecular psychiatrist, which was rather peculiar. This was something that the father had read and searched for; looking for magic in a way that is consistent in a way with what the patient does—in fact.

DR. S.: What is an orthomolecular psychiatrist?

DR. H.: I don't really know. It's sort of megavitamins and magic as far as I can tell.

    The patient then at this point became somewhat involved with the father. He was working as a therapy aide at a local psychiatric hospital and got one of the psychiatrists to see him, and she prescribed medication, much to my patient's disappointment. The father saw this person twice and was very disappointed, and then went to the Adelphi clinic and saw somebody two or three times and then left treatment. Shortly after that the father died very suddenly of a heart attack.

    The patient's response to his father's death was really to be upset for a couple of days. He was extremely upset for a couple of days, and then sort of almost put that behind him. I don't feel he ever really mourned his father's death in any adequate kind of way. On the session that fell on the anniversary of his father's death, it wasn't until midsession that he mentioned rather casually, "By the way, it's been a year since my father died."

DR. S.: Did you notice anything different about him during that session?

DR. H.: No. And I had been sort of keeping an eye open, knowing it was around anniversary time. But he was very nonchalant. In general, this is a patient who has been—for the most part—very out of touch with his feelings in a lot of ways. He has sort of gone on and on about things in a rather out-of-touch, almost "as-if" fashion.

    Let me present him physically. He is a rather tall and rather thin young man, and I focus on the thinness because there is a quality about him that comes across as deprived, which is consistent with how he presents himself. There's been a sense of deprivation from his mother and father, and this has been in the last eight or nine months a rather consistent thing with this patient. He feels that he is coming to be in touch with these feelings of deprivation for the very first time in his life. In college—he went away to college upstate—and in his sophomore year he went all the way out to California. And he has always had a sort of counterdependence until this past year, an "I don't need anybody, I'm going-to-go-off-to-California" kind of attitude, and would reject any kind of involvement with his family at all. They would go out to dinner and ask him to join them, and he would have nothing to do with it in a rather rigid I-don't-want-to-be-involved, I-don't-care attitude. In the course of therapy—and I think that this is one of the positive things about therapy—he is getting in touch with the facade that this all was. He has done a turn around in just how needy he feels he is and how deprived he feels he is. And I think there is a way he has of using this as a way not to function and yet at the same time it is a legitimate issue for him.

DR. S.: Did he say what he was looking for in therapy?

DR. H.: Well, he first started in the psychological services and was seen by a graduate student for a year. And then when she left, she recommended continuing, and I saw him after he had had therapy for a year. However, when he first came to the clinic, what he was saying he was looking for was to get more in touch with himself; he was in the field, and he thought he should know himself; very general, very vague things. He was really very, very out of touch with any particular problem or any sense of himself. By the end of the year, with that particular graduate student, his kind of closing comment was, "I could never go back to being that blind again." She sort of opened up the way with him in some sense. He spoke very little about his therapist in the beginning, and I would ask about her. He had very little to say.

DR. S.: That's usually very hard material to get to.

DR. H.: Midway through the first year I was seeing him—he was finishing his first semester of the second year of graduate school—he began to have a great deal of trouble in school. He felt he couldn't handle the work; he was very unhappy; he didn't want to do it; he was having trouble meeting deadlines, doing papers, and so on. This was very much inconsistent with the very capable student that he had always been up until then. And he began to talk about taking a year off from school and not going back to school. Simultaneously, he had a great deal of trouble with a field placement, and he felt a great deal of disappointment in his supervisor. His supervisor was, by and large, absent because of other duties, and what Rob was beginning to get in touch with was a sense of deprivation that I think paralleled what was going on with his parents. He began to go into a kind of panic attack at that and got extremely anxious. All he could say was, "I want out. I can't do it anymore. I don't want to do it anymore. I can't do it anymore." He wanted to take a leave of absence.

DR. S.: Was it a male or female supervisor?

DR. H.: A male supervisor. He had been living with, at that time, his older brother, with whom he had a good relationship. He sort of looked up to him although he describes him as being very much like his father. And yet he was able to find a kind of closeness with his brother. Around this time he began to talk about going back to live with his mother. He was vague about it, but the whole general tenor around that period of time was one of regression. As he got in touch with some needs, it was more like, "I can't do anything, I can't; I'm feeling sort of overwhelmed." It very much had a quality, and this is part of what I want to present tonight—a quality of "I won't do it," of being on strike, in a sense. I used that metaphor with him, of his being on strike—as though for better wages, more love, better working conditions—that kind of thing.

DR. S.: He won't do what?

DR. H.: He won't go to school. He was missing days at his placement. He wasn't doing his papers—that kind of thing.

DR. S.: But he was moving back with his mother.

DR. H.: Yes, he was moving back with his mother.
      I was concerned for a time as to the degree of regression that was going on—at that point. And I felt that I had to be careful in terms of not wanting to be the worried, anxious, and intrusive mother, or the critical father saying, "You can do it, you can do it." So I took a rather neutral stand at that time, although pointing out a little bit that this quality was kind of like being on strike. It was my feeling that there was a deliberate quality to his not working—in some sense.

DR. S.: I want to ask you something. It may be anticipating what you are going to present. Did he go on strike in therapy? Or did he make you into an intrusive, overanxious mother anyway? What came up about that?

DR. H.: Well, yes, I think he tried because I went through a time when I was worried about what he was doing. This alternated with a sort of impatience with him: "It's just one more paper that you have to do, for crying out loud; cut it out and be done with it." So he pulled for that in me, and I rather deliberately stayed away from that, knowing that is what the pull was in that sense.

DR. S.: But he didn't complain or skip hours or fall silent.

DR. H.: Never. He was not late; there was no acting out in terms of that. He was not late or miss appointments. There were no prolonged periods of silence.

DR. S.: Then he acted like you were in good standing with him.

DR. H.: Yes. By and large his attitude toward me has really been what I felt was a very idealized one. He was never angry with me. There were a couple of occasions where I had to cancel an appointment for various reasons—it happened twice. And he was just more than gracious about it. "I understand completely; no problem." He very much had the attitude that I understood him just perfectly, and it is a very idealized kind of thing—none of the anger that he expressed continually toward his parents. It's very much a split in that sense. He would call me Dr. Harris all the time in spite of the fact that I called him "Rob," and when I called him on the phone, I would introduce myself and say, "This is Susan Harris." And you know, he was very formal, distant; he had a sort of stiff kind of quality.

Recent issues really have focused on—they are always focusing on his mother—but there has been sort of a change from just being angry and critical toward her, toward a little bit more of a softening and getting to know her a bit. He has been wondering about her past and wondering how she got to be the way she was. He is taking a family therapy course, and he got very interested in that, and that has led into a renewed interest in his family. He is now interested in his mother. His mother had lost a baby between himself and his younger brother, when he was about 3½ years old. He has only a very vague memory about it. This recently came up, and he used this issue to try to get in touch with his mother. It was somewhat of a vain experience for him. He felt something—some warmness—and he had an urge, he said, to hug her, but he couldn't. He felt very distant from her, and he was disappointed once again that she couldn't understand just being together and sharing an unhappy time, that she had to defend against it and wanted to brush it under the rug, so to speak. So he became disappointed in her response to that.

DR. S.: She lost her child during her pregnancy or after birth?

DR. H.: No, after birth—two days after birth.

DR. S.: And how old was he at the time?

DR. H.: About 3½ or so. Then she became pregnant again with his brother. Rob is not sure what caused the problem. It was some sort of Rh problem but not a typical one. The mother was worried about it during the entire pregnancy with Rob's brother. So that clearly she was unavailable to be involved because she was mourning the loss of this baby and then very, very much involved in the anxiety of this last pregnancy. So that there was, I think, a big chunk of time where quite literally she was not available.

This past semester when Rob went back to school, he went back with a sort of enthusiasm. He got involved in another field placement, and this is also a very interesting kind of issue; he switched between first and second years from a clinical practicum to an administrative practicum. The clinical practicum really was a warm experience for him. The people involved, the supervisors that he had, he always felt were warm. He felt he was taken care of by them. The job he had had before he had gone into graduate school was a clinical-type job. He loved it. He was very happy and productive there. But he made the switch to the administrative practicum, which is really a much more political kind of thing. He began to experience feelings of disappointment. What was beginning to come out was his disappointment in others and his neediness and his sense of deprivation and how "I can't go on. I can't continue, I can't produce; I can't." And this was sort of the track that we were on, starting about this time last year and continuing in an increasing kind of way. And at the beginning of this year, as soon as he started field placement, he had a million and one complaints: "It's too far; I can't make it; I can't do it; it's horrible; it's like a bureaucracy; it's cold; and there is no one to talk to. The supervisor is a compulsive person, ulcer prone and not available." And this was kind of like a constant cry of the patient at this time. It had a cranky and sort of *kvetchy* quality to it. And what I began to feel increasingly was a deliberate, willful child—not that he couldn't do it, but that he wouldn't do it. His history is one of competency with a lot of positive feedback along the way, good grades, people thinking well of him. So that this nonfunctioning really began to have this quality of "I won't, I can't. I won't, I can't." It got rather confused.

What he would do—the session I want to focus on tonight—is that in the guise of "look how much I'm getting in touch with my feelings" or "I'm learning how hurt I am and that is a wonderful sort of thing," he was beginning to screw up on his placement again. He was not doing what he was supposed to be doing, and he was increasingly uncomfortable and increasingly saying, "I can't do it, I can't do it." I think this really leads to the dilemma where I feel we are at right now. That is, how to help him sort of move off the dime. I really felt that relief, in essence for him, comes from his needing in some sense to take responsibility. There is very much a way he has of giving away his responsibility and refusing to take responsibility. I should take it for him and the supervisor should take it for him. Somebody else should take it for him; anybody but him. And then he juxtaposes that with, "I'm really beginning to get in touch with my feelings even though they are lousy feelings, but I'm getting in touch." Therefore, he is sort of entitled to go on and on in this fashion. And I feel in a dilemma with him in just that regard. This is a guy who has been consistently out of touch with his feelings, very unaware of himself, very unaware of the impact he has on other people. He has set up many situations that increase his sense of deprivation. He will not take anything from anybody, he will not let his needs be known in any fashion, and that sort of just makes it worse and worse for him. A perfect example of that is that his mother has started dating a man recently whom Rob is extremely angry with because he sees him as very passive and needy, reflecting a lot of things he sees in himself that he feels are negative. On the other hand, this guy has reached out to him, and has bought him a gift—I don't exactly recall what the reason was—but he bought him a gift. And what Rob did was refuse to take it. He told the guy that he wouldn't take it. And he gets sort of like he's got a rod up his rear end; he gets sort of stiff about it. He says, "Well, I can't take it because it's really being hypocritical." He doesn't take it, and he increases his sense of deprivation. But at any rate the dilemma . . .

DR. S.: I'm conscious of the passage of time, since we are on a 45-minute schedule. We have plenty to discuss already, but you apparently want to include some process material?

DR. H.: Yes.

DR. S.: Let me just say that, at this point, I am so far not sure that this is something one would need to do something about. I mean this might be a stage in his development as a patient in which he's getting to the point where he could say no. And in terms of certain aspirations we might have as therapists—that one should go to school and get one's credentials or get in there and work—he may not be ready for that. On the other hand, then, I suppose, this is one of the things you and I have to try to get into. Could it be that he is acting out something there that is some reflection of some problem in the therapy that we could discuss? So I want to listen to it from that point of view, but I don't have my mind made up. When patients regress, if they are schizoid, they may regress to be more crazy, or if they have always been good and efficient, they may regress to be stubborn and negative. And this is not necessarily something you have to do something about right away, because who are you to say that it is necessarily a bad thing? So this is where I am.

DR. H.: This session is a recent session from the 9th of December. It makes it the 120th session to put in the time. It follows: I see him three times a week, on Tuesday, Thursday, and Friday, and I've taken Thursday and Friday off for Thanksgiving and then was out for the following week with the flu. And therefore, I missed five consecutive sessions with him. This was at a time when his supervisor at field placement had called him in and said, "Look, you're not doing so well. You're sloughing off; you're not doing what you used to be doing." And he was feeling devasted and very angry with her and going increasingly on strike. "Now I'm really not going to do anything" in the guise of "I can't do anything." What had happened was that I was going to see him on December 9th, which was a Tuesday. On that Monday I got a call from him in the middle of the day, which was also unusual; there was only one other occasion when he had called me before a session. He sounded awful. And what he said was, "I'm in a terrible way; I'm in a terrible state with my fieldwork. I can't do anything, I can't, I can't. And my supervisor said I should be doing something, I should be doing this work, and I can't." He really sounded pathetic and horrible. And I was not sure what to do with that. I had not seen him, as I said, for about a week and a half, and I made a comment to the effect that I had not seen him, and he must be upset about that, since it seemed that so much was going on. And he acknowledged that. The tack I took was to go to the "I can't and I won't" issue. He was saying that "he can't," and I said that "he can't" and "he won't" are very close, and sort of left it at that and said I would see him tomorrow. And this is the session tomorrow.

Obviously, I don't have time to go through the whole thing. But he walks in again looking just horrible—drawn and pale and droopy, and really awful. And I asked him what the matter was. And in this low, sad voice he said, "I don't know. Yesterday was just so awful, and I felt a little better after I talked to you, but even after I got home last night, I felt awful. I feel awful this morning." And he just goes on about—should I read it verbatim?

DR. S.: I'll listen for a while.

DR. H.: His supervisor from school was called in about this issue of his not producing, and the supervisor said to him, "Well, talk to your supervisor at work to clarify it." And he goes on to say that "the supervisor and I need to discuss whatever our personality conflicts are." And he said, "I'm just feeling I'll go in and say whatever I want to say and that's it. I was so depressed and so anxious—anxious like my stomach was hurting and I haven't slept well in the past few nights. When I heard the news about John Lennon last night, in one way I felt, "Who am I when compared with something like that? My troubles don't mean anything, and I just started feeling shitty about the world and about myself. I already felt shitty about me, and I feel that the world is such an uncaring place."

I commented then that "your therapist was out in the worst week of your life." And he said, "Believe me, I realize that. I realized that last Tuesday. I think in a sense that one good thing that happened this past week is that I made that realization." That's the first thing that bothered him.

DR. S.: Namely?

DR. H.: Namely, that it bothered him that I was not there, as opposed to rationalizing it away completely.

DR. S.: May I make an observation about the question? I noticed that both over the phone and the way you were talking with him, the way you put it was that he was upset about your being away during the time that so much was going on. That tends to put your absence in a secondary place in terms of his being so disturbed. One could just as well turn the thing around and say, "Perhaps it was harder for you during this past week or 10 days because you didn't see me." You

might say to me that at this point you don't know enough to say anything about that, but I suspect that you do. The way you put it, you are already structuring it in a certain way, like, "Where were you when I needed you so much," when in fact his disruption, his decompensation, whatever it is, might have been his way of showing you in a passive-aggressive way what the effects on him were of your being away—of trying to make you feel guilty or whatever he might be trying to do. In that respect I was thinking too about what you said earlier when I asked you about how his relationship with you has come up, and you said that apparently he has been idealizing you. This is an issue now that has come in for a lot of discussion, especially since Kohut has made the point that it might be a good thing for some patients if the therapist tolerates their idealization. But I would wonder if in your case he might not be using idealization in a way that has more traditionally been interpreted as a defense against the transference, by keeping you at a safe distance. And I would wonder, is he keeping you at a safe distance from his hostility, acting it out on the job by feeling deprived with a supervisor, who is not available enough to him? You, after all, have been seeing him three times a week. Or could he be keeping you out of reach also in a romantic or erotic or sexual sense? I get the impression—I realize you are presenting very condensed material—I get the impression that here is a 26-year-old guy who's been meeting with you all this time, and . . . hasn't he become troubled about . . . any feelings about you?
[*Laughter*]

DR. H.: None that he has mentioned.

DR. S.: Now, have you taken that up with him?

DR. H.: No.

DR. S.: He's never blushed or seemed to gloss over something or fallen silent at a moment when he might have felt irritated with something? I mean you haven't seen him become defensive or resistant or something in relation to you when some of these situations develop?

DR. H.: Any time that I've brought up any kind of issues I felt he would be upset with, he would be upset with me or angry, he really kept an incredible distance about it. One time I brought up the issue of the formality of [*his calling me*] "Dr. Harris" in the context of all that we had talked about; in the context also of his general formality and keeping distance from other people; even how his calling me Dr. Harris is so formal. He said, "Yeah, you're sort of right" and proceeded to call me Susan from that point on, without any discussion of it or his feelings about it.

DR. S.: And you let him; you didn't make a second effort?

DR. H.: Not in a . . . no.

DR. S.: It's one of the big problems in trying to deal with these resistances which Freud called *the resistance against the analysis of resistance,* and that's a good example of it. You call attention to something, and you say, "You seem to be keeping back these private fantasies of yours, and I wonder why you are." And then the patient tells you the fantasy, when, in fact, for the purpose of the therapy the important thing is how come he was holding it back. That's what happened when he switched over and started calling you *Susan.* I would think he is trying to circumvent the issue. What function did it serve to call you *Dr. Harris* and then what function was it serving for him to switch to *Susan* once you raised the question? By implication he was treating your question as if it were a directive. So there is a suggestion that there is a fantasy of you as perhaps like his mother—controlling, dissatisfied.

DR. H.: I feel that as a difficulty a great deal. If I make an interpretation, he will take it in and right away and not much in the spirit of exploring it, but in the spirit of complying with it in some way.

DR. S.: And have you brought that up—that he is being compliant?

DR. H.: In the context of how he seems to respond to things almost as though it were a recipe—not exactly the same thing but in that ballpark. He seems to want to follow a kind of recipe at times. And if he does *a, b,* or *c*—it's not quite the same.

DR. S.: But that impersonalizes it. It would be more fruitful if you said, for instance, "You seem to almost have to fall in line with what you think I want or with what you think I want you to do, very quickly, and I think it would be important to understand what that's about." But your formulation, which has its merits, allows him to talk about what his character and personality patterns are, and that's a big hiding place usually. You know, because people are presenting themselves as objects or static or tending to agree with you as, "Yes, this is what I always do." And so it's better to try to keep it personalized in the interactive sense and try to get at the fantasy which was implied by it. I don't think he would come right out with it, but the sense that he is very emotionally involved with you in some way that he is keeping under wraps would probably become more apparent.

DR. H.: My sense is that when I have tried to make it in any way personal, that there is a retreat into tremendous intellectualization with him.

DR. S.: Do you then take it up further? What I referred to earlier as second effort is very often the essential part of taking up a defensive move. Usually the first response is in one way or another evasive or frustrating, or leaves you with the feeling of, "Well, I tried it, and he did the same thing, so let's wait for the next opportunity." Whereas, in fact, I think it can be particularly important that you say, "Now you just did again the very kind of thing I was raising the question about." And I would indicate an interest in staying with it. Then, I think, whatever his anxiety is in relation to you—and I would imagine it is considerable—would be out on the table for discussion and would become a reference point, with no assurance, however, that he could give you a very rich account of what it's about. But it would become a reference point, and my sense is that his relationship with you is not established as a reference point.

DR. H.: I think that's true.

DR. S.: And some of your comments suggest that you may deal with him in a way that—not in any gross way—sort of accepts, perhaps, too much of his need to keep it impersonal.

DR. H.: Yes, I think that's true. I had felt along the way very puzzled in a sense, in terms of how to make it more personal in the treatment, but . . .

DR. S.: It's risky if you just sort of come at him with this didactically; you've got to keep track of this in the kinds of events that you were just referring to, such as the formality. I meant to ask you in this connection whether anything in the way of a historical prototype occurred to you when he talked about John Lennon's death in this little bit of material?

DR. H.: I'm not sure what you mean in terms of a protocol.

DR. S.: Prototype.

DR. H.: Prototype.

DR. S.: Prototype from his life's history. Is anything reminiscent of what he might have gone through and how he might have dealt with it in the way he told you about John Lennon's death?

DR. H.: In terms—you mean in terms of how upset he was about it and what his response is and my sense of what he was saying about John Lennon? He has a tendency to do that, of being sort of taken in and very involved with certain figures in the world and that's sort of a consistent kind of thing. He was sort of enamoured with Thomas Szasz for a while, and terribly upset when Liz Holtzman lost the election, and gets very involved in some sense with figures like that. Figures that he looks at in a kind of idealized way, I think very unrealistically. It's very much a quality of sort of wanting to merge with these idealized figures and in a sense to sort of be one with them and be close to them if he can.

DR. S.: That could be true of a number of things about him, but I was thinking particularly of what he said when he told you about John Lennon's death—of his feelings of relative unimportance with regard to the death of someone so important.

DR. H.: Yes . . . the thing that comes to mind is a situation that he recalls in terms of playing as a youngster—it doesn't involve a death but a loss in a way—of playing with his mother and being involved with his mother in some sense and then his father's coming home and his mother's sort of dropping him when father came home demanding dinner and demanding to be fed and so on. His mother sort of dropped him, and he became the insignificant one, who was just sort of left so that the mother could be with father . . .

DR. S.: What I was thinking about is the death of the next sibling, and the dilemma that young children particularly would feel in a situation like that. What are their claims on the mother relative to how important it was to her to have lost the baby, which, as you told me about the case, you surmised must have been a very disruptive period. And here you were out sick and away from his therapy for a long time. So you were concerned with your own troubles, let's say. There was that, and there was the Lennon thing, and he comes in with a feeling of how unimportant he is. If I were listening to this from the standpoint of the unexpressed transference difficulties and his resistance against bringing those out into the open, I would think that what he was saying pertained not first of all to Lennon, but to his feeling guilty and self-effacing because his needs for you were felt at a time when you were having troubles of your own. And who is he to make claims on you at this time? I would need to get more of the hour, maybe the previous hour; but I think I would have looked for an opportunity to say that I thought he was troubled by more than John Lennon's death and that he was feeling unworthy that he had feelings about why you weren't there to see him, just at a time when you were having troubles of your own. I wouldn't be inclined to bring in genetic material at this point because until there is a little more out in the open about the transference, I think it makes it too intellectual.

DR. H.: Which is very much a tendency of his.

DR. S.: Assuming you started to develop this, and he showed any response to it, I wouldn't be surprised if before long material pertaining to the death of the brother and his mother's reaction would come up. Usually that or something equivalent to it would very likely come up. I would surmise . . . I'm trying to crowd a lot in because we have only one session and we are actually over our 45 minutes now, but . . .

DR. CALIGOR: It's a 50-minute session.
[*Laughter*]

DR. S.: If you think of the position of a 3½-year-old, who . . . I would think, at any rate from the standpoint of my orientation . . . would be probably well into an oedipal involvement with his mother with very deep anxiety and resentment about the pregnancy and who would probably for the rest of his life, unless analysis helped him with it, bear an unconscious guilt about the death of his sibling, which he partly wished and celebrated. Then, his feeling, frustrated by the fact that he didn't get from his mother what he hoped, that he could continue to get by the disappearance of this new rival, and so on. So that the issue of being either libidinally, erotically, or aggressively involved with a woman who is any kind of maternal transference figure would be horrifying to him because there is a murderer in him, or if not a murderer, at least a villain of the worst sort, however a child would conceive of that. And I wouldn't say this explains fully his cautiousness about letting more of the transference—a complicated transference—show in relation to you, but I would think of it as a very strong dynamic. And I think your recent absence and illness and Lennon's death—all this has stirred up some derivatives of this early relationship. That is why he said, "Who am I next to Lennon?" He sounds from that a little readier to talk about the transference than I think you think he is.

DR. H.: That may be similar in some sense to the way he relates to the supervisor he has now in that he does not allow himself to get anything from her. There is that self-deprivation kind of quality. I'm wondering if you see that as similar to what you were talking about in some sense?

DR. S.: Well, my hunch is that he feels he is not getting enough from *you*, and that is the feeling sooner or later that one *has* in relation to one's analyst. But one of the life-historical prototypes would have been this period of mourning, distress, and presumably grief and depression on his mother's part, and quite apart from your illness and absence, I think that his unexpressed feeling of deprivation in relation to you is probably the basis of his reenacting something like what he might have gone through when he was a kid. He becomes helpless, he becomes desperate, he calls you. I'm not saying he's calling you all the time, but in the midst of this, maybe much as a child, regressing under those conditions, he says, "Hey, look, I have needs, too." Children become sleepless; they become troubled; and it is a way of making a claim, especially if they are afraid of coming right out with their complaints and their demands and their seductions. He says, "Look at the terrible thing that just happened." I don't know how much of his present work difficulty is related to the keeping up of his transference involvement without its having been brought in to the therapy along with his resistances against it. But I think a significant amount of it is, and I would expect that although he might not work it through quickly, it would probably help him function somewhat better in a while if you found a way of making more second efforts.

DR. H.: And not stopping at the first answer.

DR. S.: The first answer . . . You don't know what to make of the first answer. People say yes and they mean no; they say no and then the next five hours are filled with productive reverberations.

DR. H.: Yes, and I think if we had time to go more into the session, the basis for that was there.

DR. S.: [*To Dr. Caligor*] Should I say a few things?

DR. CALIGOR: Yes, but first I'd like to thank the two of you for what I think was a most productive session. At this point we would like to follow a procedure where the two of you perhaps carry on a dialogue in any way you see fit—asking each other about any aspect pertaining to the supervisory session. And then somewhere along the line, Dr. Schafer, I'd appreciate it if you would give us your concept of what supervision is all about, any models or focuses, or any point of departure that you may think are important. Thank you.

DR. S.: Would you like to lead off, or . . . ?

DR. H.: I don't know . . . no. [*Laughter*]

DR. S.: I assume you have been having supervision on this case.

DR. H.: Yes . . . yes, that is what I was thinking about.

DR. S.: I may be suggesting a line of approach which is very . . .

DR. H.: Very different; that is what I was thinking mostly about; what we covered here tonight has been a very different line of focusing than what my current supervision has been . . . which is exciting and an awful lot of food for thought. The issues that Dr. Schafer brought up tonight are very different than those that my current supervision has focused on, which are much more in terms of the willful child in this patient, and focusing on the risk-taking aspects . . . sort of getting this patient off the dime, so to speak.

DR. S.: One of the questions is, how do you get somebody off the dime?

DR. H.: Or whether that's worthwhile.

DR. S.: Well, this goes back to my earliest comment. I think one's primary concern should not be to make the patient do anything, but to try to understand what he *is* doing; and if he's suffering with it, presumably we would like, on some level or to some extent, to help him find a way out of it. But the way out of it would be through understanding. So in that sense you *would* want to help him get off the dime, but it's different from *needing* him to get off the dime. Anytime you need the patient to do a certain thing or become a certain thing, you are all set up for a countertransference jam right away. But I, too, was concerned while listening that maybe there could be something done to help free him from what seems to be an accelerated . . .

DR. H.: Because clearly when he—there have been—I don't know how much I need him to get off the dime or want him to do a, b, or c. But there have been those times that he does do something, and does have a feeling of some sense of competency. Those are the times he feels the most relief about things. But anyhow, that has been, for the most part, a great focus in terms of the supervision.

DR. S.: You've had other cases?

DR. H.: Yes.

DR. S.: This is not your first?

DR. H.: No.

DR. S.: Have you dealt in a more active way with resistance and transference issues? So that this is something that is more specific to this patient or this supervisor? [*Laughter*] It is an important question.

DR. H.: Yes.

DR. S.: This is not to say that I know that your supervisor is wrong. But if you feel that you are doing something with this patient that is not the way you would ordinarily do it because your supervisor has a different view, then the question would be, "Are you aware of it and have you discussed it with your supervisor, or are you perhaps locked into something unexpressed with your supervisor that would parallel the outcome with the patient?" It's something to think about. [*To Dr. Caligor*] Should I talk for a while?

DR. CALIGOR: Yes, please. We would very much like to hear you before we open the discussion to the floor. We would like to hear what you have to say.

DR. S.: As I understood it, I was to finish up by saying some things about how I regard what we did here, specifically in relation to what I usually do or think is appropriate.

I did say earlier that I felt I was trying to squeeze things in very fast because of the sense of limited time, and I had a lot of thoughts about the material that I wanted to refer to that I think ordinarily—for purposes of supervision—it would be better to take up piece by piece because it is a lot all at once for a supervisee. Not necessarily in terms of intelligence, but because there are a lot of emotional issues you usually touch on and I think it's a good idea not to overwhelm a supervisee with all the clever ideas that you as a supervisor think you have. This is one of the ways in which I tend to err in supervision. I get very stimulated and sometimes I talk too much, and it can have a deleterious effect on the work of the supervisee. Occasionally, supervisees who are working through the problems of speaking up against authority in their own analyses begin to indicate to me that I sort of make them feel stupid—things like that. But, ideally, what I would like to do and what I sometimes am able to do is to use the immediate material: I try to work very closely with process material, not with taped material, which I tend to regard as a hiding place, but instead work with the way the supervisees summarize and present the material, because they are more present in the summary as far as the interaction with the supervisor is concerned, in my view, than they are in the "liveness" on the tape or their copying the tape into written notes. I know there are different opinions about that, but in any case I don't in general like to discuss issues with supervisees for very long in terms of generalities. It's very easy to get agreement and intellectual understanding on that, and then when you get process notes, you find that the supervisee is still doing the same thing, albeit another version of the same thing. And so, I prefer to spend the 45 minutes covering as much material as one can, and looking particularly at the areas where something in the interaction seems not to be taken up adequately, and a fair amount of that I began to hear tonight. I mean, not taken up adequately *in my judgment*.

There is always fascinating life-historical material one can discuss with the supervisee. One can make developmental or genetic constructions, some of which I included in the discussion, but what I tried to do here is—what I try to do always in supervision as well as in my own work—is this: If there is something in the life history that seems to me to set a significant template for later functioning and also seems relevant to the material that is being presented, I try to find a way of

seeing how it is expressing itself right now in the therapeutic relationship. If I can't do that, I tend to keep quiet about it. And if I can do it,
first of all or mainly, I refer to the here and now of the relationship. As
patients get freer or a little more collaborative and a little less resistant
in talking about that, they often bring up some of the historical material or comparable historical material themselves. It's not necessary
then, for me as the analyst or supervisor, to refer that much to it. But
it's very helpful to think about such things as the death of a younger
sibling or the death of this guy's father before he went into treatment
and other information that we didn't have a chance to hear today.
How could this be playing a part now in what's going on and not
going on between supervisee and the patient, or between me and my
patient, and so on. And to start with that, we have to keep the focus
very much on it. But that doesn't mean forgetting about the life history, by any means. It makes the life history organized. Otherwise, it's
just a jumble of information.

I personally don't tend to discuss the content of countertransference very far with people I'm supervising, especially if they are in
treatment or analysis themselves at the time I'm supervising them.
But I will if I think they are having difficulty dealing with an issue—
like a homosexual transference or rage, or whatever it is. I will also, if
it becomes apparent that despite discussion and intellectual understanding, they just lack facility; or if they become obtuse or are always
saying the same things in hindsight, which indicates that they really
have a problem in this area that's worth thinking about. I think even if
they are not in therapy, it's a good idea not to carry it too far within
the supervision—unlike some other people—because it blurs the line
of what supervision is, and then when you discuss the case with the
supervisee, you don't know whether you are engaged now in some
quasitherapeutic transference dialogue or a supervisory dialogue.
There is always transference to the supervision, but in many cases it's
not of such a disruptive sort that one has to always keep it in the front
of one's mind. If the supervisees are not in treatment and continue to
have trouble with a number of issues or some big issues, it could be
the basis for discussing with them whether they *should* be in therapy.
And I recall a number of instances where I'd been supervising candidates who had completed their training analysis and were having
gross difficulty with certain issues. It became apparent to them that
they ought to have more analysis, and they went back into analysis.
And, as is often the case—it's not the rule, but is often enough the
case—many people have not been that happy with their first analysis;
and if the supervision is going well and the case is unfolding well,

then they see what an analysis can be and what they didn't have. They see some of the difficulties they're having with material that they thought you only read about in books. Sometimes that becomes relevant, but that's not the same as starting to make deep interpretations of the supervisee's countertransference. This is a summary of my views. Supervision is an endless subject. I'll be glad to respond to any questions.

DR. CALIGOR: Folks, we are going to open up discussion from the floor, but please let's try to address our comments to the supervisory process itself and not so much the therapy. Please, any questions? We always start off slow, and then there is a deluge in five minutes. So who is going to open this for us?

DR. 1: I guess I'll start. I must say I find the self-pitying person very difficult to treat. I do think there is a transference problem here. I like to get a history, and I presume a history was taken here. I also find that from Dr. Schafer's questions there seems to be no information that the patient is male and the analyst is a female. And also, I have no history whatsoever of the fact that this man has a sex life or ever had. And I think that that could have been possibly presented in the five minutes that we had on background. And I wonder what is being contributed by both persons in this regard.

DR. CALIGOR: Any comments pertaining to the supervisory process, please? I'd like to see if we could get a focus. Yes . . . Could you come up here and speak so that your voice will be projected to the audience?

DR. 2: It seems to me that the picture of the supervisory process is greatly influenced by the ambience in which it occurs; that is, private supervision versus supervision in the course of a training program. It seems to me that there are many different emotional factors when one is a candidate in an institution or organization where one is assigned or one goes in a sense for enlightenment that one is expected to receive versus a private supervisory experience where one has, in a sense, hired the supervisor and is going seeking personal-professional goals. I wonder if you would comment about that, and how you have found that affects it?

DR. S.: Well, I haven't done a great deal of private supervision, so I don't have extensive experience to draw on in making that comparison. I know that supervision within any kind of training setting, in a sense, always involves a whole set of complicated transferences to the institution. What will get you graduated from the institute? Which analysis will you get credit for? What might get you a staff job, if you're in training in a clinic somewhere. Things of that sort; also, letters of recommendation and future referrals. There is a selling job in supervision when it's being done under institutional circumstances that I think nobody is totally able to avoid as a supervisee: to make a good impression, to try to be receptive or not to be overly critical, or to identify too rapidly with the supervisor so as not to make waves. This is one of the things I think supervisors have to keep in mind, and I think it is a problem in institutes because so much hinges upon getting on with your supervisors and getting good reports into your files. I think there is one place where the initiative of the supervisor is very important. It's a good idea to assume that we are all just a little corruptible by these factors so that the presentations are going to be slanted by omissions, evasions, and so forth. And to listen with a sharp ear for just those points and to be prepared to discuss any indications that the supervisees have a sense of what the supervisor wants to hear when they are thinking something different. Now that's a lot to ask of the supervisee—to be able to sustain a discussion of that sort. But some opening up of the subject can be very helpful. Where one buys supervision, my impression is it is somewhat like buying an analysis after you have satisfied the training analysis requirements of your institution. Many people have commented on this. They feel, "*Now! This* is my analysis." And at the time they were in the first analysis, it *seemed* like it was their analysis and in many ways it was. It isn't a black-and-white distinction really, but I think there is a sense now in private supervision that nothing administrative hinges on it—at least it is on a more neutral or autonomous level of functioning. Nothing hinges on it except increasing one's own professional competence or expertise. Actually, more than that hinges on it because even under those conditions people develop transferences and resistances to the supervisor. That I have seen; I've seen that from fairly senior people. But then . . . it's no surprise. They don't come unless they feel they are having problems with certain kinds of cases. So there is some kind of inadequately worked-through conflict in relation to their case materials.

DR. 3: Do you feel that the supervisory process should primarily be focused upon the therapy of the patient or upon the supervisee's education?

DR. S.: Well, except where very special problems on the part of the supervisee present themselves, I don't make a distinction in the way I supervise between the two. And, again, I know there is variety in this respect among people who have done a lot of supervision. I think one of the things that some supervisors can offer and like to offer and can get excited about, so that what they do has the full force of their own way of being a clinician and a teacher—and in this case it happens to apply to me—is to help the supervisee develop as orderly and progressive an analysis as possible, so that they will see what an analysis can be. And in the course of that effort, there is time to talk about some of the difficulty the supervisee has—either through ignorance or inexperience or emotional blocks that can be talked about. Some of the emotional problems of the supervisee may be too big for the supervisory relationship. But leaving those aside, I think that this is the one place, apart from the personal analysis—and it's very hard to have distance from one's personal analysis—where one can, with help, go through a full exposure to what an analysis can be and the typical technical problems that come up along the way. Assuming you have a reasonably good case, then, this includes the variety of considerations that can be brought to bear on those problems, such as, "You could do this, but maybe such and such," or "You could do that, but maybe such and such," "Let's try this and see if we can follow the consequences," and so on. This is the one place—the several supervisions one has—that is to me the paramount value of the supervisory sessions. Other things, I think, more properly belong with other supervisors who like to use other pedagogical means, such as confronting the supervisee with more problems to think through and not getting as involved as I do in the patient material. Those problems belong mostly with other supervisors of other types or in the supervisee's personal treatment. So I think what the supervisor is particularly turned on to is very important.

DR. 4: I was very impressed with Dr. Schafer's approach to the supervisee because it seemed to me he combined a genuine wish to teach something, and focusing on a few things instead of a whole panoply of things, which makes them so anxious that they can't learn. One could contrast his approach with two other approaches I feel are less effective. One in which the supervisor is so afraid of making the supervisee anxious that he can't say anything that seems to be very useful or incisive, and the supervisee leaves feeling, "I've learned nothing. I got supported, but what's that worth." The other example is the other extreme, in which the supervisor finds total fault with the supervisee, who leaves unable to function at all. Those are two extremes, and something in between seems to be required for learning. Enough teaching to evoke curiosity but not increasing the anxiety level to a point where it's disruptive and the supervisee can't hear.

DR. H.: Can I sort of echo that in terms of sharing what my experience and main anxiety was from doing this publicly and not simply from sitting with Dr. Schafer? As I'm thinking about it and rehashing what we talked about, clearly this has been a different focus for me than where I've been in terms of supervision, but feeling that I've come away with an awful lot of things—good things—to think about.

DR. CALIGOR: Roy, do you have any specific model in your mind pertaining to supervision? There are various people who have given us a model. Is there any central focus that you feel you adhere to, or do you play it by ear in terms of how the candidate presents himself?

DR. S.: Well, I try to adapt to the presentation of the supervisee. Obviously, you get all kinds of self-presentations from the most dull and tedious to the most flashy, to the most frightened, and so you can't start in the same place with everybody. You just use your ordinary clinical common sense. You have to be concerned first of all with whether there is any significant communication block. You're not always sure you are getting any kind of adequate process report of what's going on in the treatment. So that might require a discussion for a certain amount of time. Or with certain people you might decide the best thing is not to discuss the block but hold your horses and let the supervisee discover that you're not always waiting to pounce on every single thing and—as might occur with a patient—gradually they may begin speaking to you more freely and be able to tolerate a question. There you have to improvise. But otherwise, the model for me, if it's a model, is what I was talking about a minute ago, which is that I get very involved in the clinical material and in the therapy and I really become very much of a co-therapist—sometimes too much so. I know that I do. But there is a point to it, which is that there is only so much you can supervise if you don't have a reasonably orderly analysis developing. And that sometimes takes fairly active participation by the supervisor to see that that happens, and then a lot of phenomena develop that illustrate what an analysis is and what the problems of an analysis are. Otherwise, you may take much too long a time sitting with the supervisee and discussing problems that amount to how to get an analysis started. It's very worthwhile to discuss that, but if it's overextended and doesn't get beyond that, then I think something is lacking. But that approach also fits *me*.

13

In Pursuit of the Truth
An Essay on an Epistemological Approach to Psychoanalytic Supervision

JOHN L. SCHIMEL

DIMENSIONS OF THE FIELD

I suggest that a minimal definition of psychoanalysis would indicate a process in which the behaviors of the psychoanalyst would be calculated to influence the present and future behaviors of the patient, including his thoughts, feelings, attitudes, attention, speech patterns, fantasy life, and the like. In parallel fashion, a minimal definition of psychoanalytic supervision would indicate a process in which the behaviors of the supervisor would be calculated to influence the behaviors of the supervisee with his patient.

The supervisor's tools for the task will include the following: some understanding of human behavior as influenced by past and present contexts, including particularly the psychoanalytic situation; some understanding both of the behaviors of the patient being reported to him and of the psychotherapist's reporting on his patient as well as an understanding of the interactions of the two; and finally, an awareness of the transactions between himself and his trainee. The latter requires the self-knowledge one presumes the supervisor to have acquired. These are among the many dimensions of the field and they are formidable.

The supervisor—thus armed—will oversee the student's work with his patient. He will, when indicated, in addition to instruction in the art

JOHN L. SCHIMEL • Associate Director, Fellow, Training and Supervising Analyst, William Alanson White Institute of Psychiatry, Psychoanalysis and Psychology, New York, New York 10023 and Clinical Professor of Psychiatry, New York University-Bellevue Medical Center, New York, New York 10016.

of conducting psychoanalysis, attempt to increase his trainee's under-standing of his patient and of their interactions. In the course of this work, the matter of the student's lack of self-understanding in this in-stance or that may become apparent in his handling of the patient as well as in the manner of his dealing with the supervisor. The central question that is being engaged, however, is the matter of the behaviors of the one influencing the behaviors of the other.

I submit that the basic element in influencing behavior psycho-analytically lies in bringing certain matters to the conscious attention of the other—matters that are either unknown or unsuspected, inattended, or that are noted but that are not considered significant. There are sever-al key factors that focusing on such matters bring to bear on the fate of such communications either in psychotherapy or in supervision and, for that matter, in life in general. There is bound to be some element of surprise on the part of the recipient of such a communication that will have to be dealt with by him. The recipient has to recover from the surprise in order to continue the transaction. His recovery may take many forms, some of which may warrant such labels as *avoidance, denial,* or *resistance,* all of which find themselves in that part of the relationship we prefer to call *transference,* possibly of the negative variety, and the like. The period of recovery may be brief or relatively prolonged. It may result in manifestations of grief, anger, laughter, stony or perplexed silence, and the like. Optimally, surprise will result in the facilitation of associations, amplification, and clarification. I suggest that the processes of recovery from surprise in a psychological sense are quite unexplored. It may be useful to note that synonyms of the infinitive *to surprise* in-clude the following: *to startle, perplex, bewilder, astonish, amaze, astound, confound,* and *dumbfound.* The nature of the psychoanalytic inquiry is such that it provides, when successful, many surprises for both patient and practitioner. For those who can tolerate surprises, psychoanalysis can be a joy and, no doubt, this factor helps account for the popularity psychoanalysis has achieved. Failure in psychoanalysis can often be traced to the opposite of surprise—to dullness in the psychotherapist whether in manner, inflection, or in the use of limited, unimaginative, or jargon-filled speech. The experience of surprise stresses the indi-vidual—a factor that helps shape his subsequent behavior.

The surprising message is generally conveyed by words, sometimes modulated or amplified by inflection, emotional overtone, gesture, or postural change. There may have been some preparation for the mes-sage, or there may have been virtually none. The words chosen may be everyday or technical. They may assume the form of a question or of a declarative statement. The words may, additionally, convey the message in the forms of analogy, metaphor, humor, anecdote, aphorism—even expletive. These matters interdigitate the element of surprise, and they help determine the response of the recipient of the surprising message. In any event, the surprising message is a clear call for the recipient to attend to it. One patient referred to the fact that, "Your voice was quiet enough but I heard what you said like a clap of thunder." Even the most arcane psychoanalytic interpretation contains the metamessage that it deals with a significant matter that must be attended to. The psychoanalytic enterprise may be considered as an engagement in which the unknown not only becomes known but must also be attended to.

The Search

Let us begin with a small foray. A beginning male psychoanalytic candidate is reporting the initial sessions of a male graduate student with study problems who is having an unhappy love affair. The initial interviews seem ordinary enough and are competently handled by the candidate. As soon as the patient begins to use the couch, however, the productions change markedly and deal largely with the patient's homosexual concerns, which had not previously been mentioned by him. The candidate is pleased, believing he has quickly reached concerns that must be a central issue for his patient. He is aware of the fact that the use of the couch may facilitate a freer exposition of repressed material. The homosexual material, however, seems to the supervisor to be too much, too soon, and the transference aspects too intense and too overt in view of the historical data. As the supervisor's perplexity grows, he begins to consider possible explanations for the flooding of homosexual concerns that are not immediately apparent in the material being presented to him. Could the candidate be sexually seductive in his dealings with the patient? The candidate does not exhibit manifestations of being homosexual himself as far as the supervisor can tell—although he cannot rule this out. Could it be something about the psychoanalytic setting? He communicates his perplexity to the trainee, leading to an increase of anxiety in the latter. Impressed by the coincidence of the homosexual flooding with the initial use of the couch, the supervisor asks for the layout of the student's office. He learns that the patient is being seen in a small clinic office in which the couch and the psychoanalyst's chair are necessarily crowded so close that the psychotherapist sits with his thigh in contact with the side of the couch. When the patient moves or gestures, his hand or arm often comes in contact with the therapist's thigh. What is the truth in this situation?

I am also reminded of the behavior of a schizoid young female patient when the therapist's office was moved temporarily, due to repairs, to a suite in a nearby hotel. She did not appear for several sessions but finally called for an appointment. It was learned that she had been terrified by the thought that there might be a bed in the hotel room, and she did not feel she could trust her reactions in such a situation.

FOR THE TRUTH

Let us make another and more extensive foray. A supervisee reports his patient's pained recognition of his dependence on his father and his resolve to change this behavior. The student believes that this recognition of dependency is a form of insight and that his patient's resolve to change reflects a positive motivation toward growth and maturation. Fair enough. But change to what? In what way? At this stage, one does not really know what the patient means or what is valid.

The supervisor asks the candidate to describe the behavior the patient has designated as *dependent*. It is not infrequently found that theoretical formulations abound without sufficient supporting data. The supervisor is in search of an issue that Freud indicated as central to the psychoanalytic enterprise—the pursuit of, and dedication to, the truth. He does not accept or reject the candidate's formulations. He instructs, instead, that they must be documented. The search must be rigorous and go beyond opinion, conjecture, or intuition, which is sometimes referred to as *empathy*, or colloquially, as a *gut feeling* about a patient. Minimally, truth, or in this sense validity, is in general a state of conformity to a fact or reality that can either be external or internal. Truth is, according to Webster, "the property in a conception, a judgment or proposition, a belief, an opinion, of being in accord with what is, has been, or must be." The issue raised with the supervisee is one of validity. The concern is an epistemological one in that what is being raised is the issue of the validity of presumed knowledge. The question is the following: How does the supervisor validate the so-called knowledge of the supervisee?

Optimally, the thrust of the inquiry will result in a heightened awareness, on the part of the supervisee, of the need for careful documentation of the opinions and assertions of the patient, in both the here and now and in the past, by examples of the data needed to support that which the patient alleges. Through diligence the supervisor will learn that the patient's perceptions and the material that the patient uses to document his opinions of them may bear little resemblance to each other. As Harry Stack Sullivan put it, what a person professes to believe and how that person actually behaves may bear little resemblance to each other. He advised against any tacit agreement as to meaning of words or language generally.

The task is, however, not the patient's alone to produce relevant documentation. By the nature of the matter, the patient—however well programmed to report feelings and beliefs bolstered by facts—will be able to go so far and no further without assistance from the psychotherapist. The latter must learn to listen to each and every assertion of his patient with an awareness of the need on his part for reflection as to its meaning (*truth*) and its function both in the content and the necessary or needed form in which it is being presented to the psychotherapist (*transference*).

In a word, the truth is always larger than the matter at hand. The supervisee must be helped to envision more of the patient's experiences than the patient is aware of or is capable of reporting at any particular moment. The process in which the supervisee as psychotherapist must learn requires not only careful listening but also, at the same time, an ability to reflect and speculate, to correlate past and present events with that which is being reported, to theorize, and to synthesize, using his knowledge of the patient and of human behavior in general. The supervisor tries to see in the reported material more than is apparent, and not only speculates to the supervisee, but also provides the rationale for believing that he sees something broader or deeper than the matter at hand. He is demonstrating in his communications to the supervisee how he augments the manifest content. His agenda includes the opportunity to demonstrate to the supervisee how he, too, may manipulate in his own mind the data that is being reported to him by the patient.

Such active or creative listening may subsequently be communicated to the patient by questions, speculations, or interpretations that go beyond the reported material. A new context, perspective, or dimension, is added to enrich the interchange in order to broaden the scope of the inquiry. It may be apparent that an educational process is being described in which hypothesis formation and documentation in understanding human behavior is being conveyed to the supervisee, over time, through both precept and example.

If therapy is successful, the patient's responses to the therapist's interventions will reflect the latter's responses to the former's productions. In a word, the stimulus, by way of precept and example, followed by imitation by the patient, will be to document or disprove the validity of the psychotherapist's contribution. With patients who are designated as being psychologically minded, the patient will additionally emulate the psychotherapist's attempts to see something broader, deeper, or larger than the matter at hand. One may suggest that this is the true psychotherapeutic process in the triadic supervisor–supervisee–patient relation, the heart of the psychoanalytic enterprise, an epistomological exploration. A central task for the supervisor is to convey these matters to his supervisee and to foster his skills in promoting the search for truth both in himself and in the patient.

In the example about the patient's alleged dependency on his father, the supervisee's concern for truth expressed in his search for definition and documentation of this matter may stimulate the patient, in his turn, to listen to himself as he reports, to reflect, to speculate, to question, to strive for an understanding that goes beyond the matter that is concerning him at the moment. It is common enough in psychoanalysis for the patient to be reporting, sometimes interminably and repetitiously, attitudes that have some of the qualities of an oft-rendered lecture, a consistent and insistent exposition of his views and attitudes, even though the reported events may vary from time to time and reflect data from the present and the recent or distant past. It can be documented that attitudes toward a variety of present events have existed and have continued to exist from the earliest developmental stages.

There is generally a presumption that, during the psychotherapeutic process, the psychotherapist will be reflecting on the matters reported and that, sooner or later, he will report to the patient the conclusion of these reflections, that is, an interpretation. In this description, although the patient does, by far, most of the talking, his role is essentially a passive one. With patients being reanalyzed, I have repeatedly heard that the patient, in earlier psychotherapeutic experiences, had talked a lot during the therapy. The inner experience in that situation was often, or usually, one of a desperate hope by the patient that he could finally hit upon something interesting enough to provoke the psychoanalyst to speak. The need for reflection by the patient had not been attended to as a psychoanalytic issue, and indeed, it had been subordinate to the transference need to please the psychotherapist. These experiences have been particularly poignant in the case of so-called borderline patients. Lack of participation on the psychoanalyst's part was regularly experienced as evidence by the patient of his worthlessness. Often enough this feeling was reinforced by such psychoanalytic sallies as, "I respond when you are really working." An exposition of the negative therapeutic effects of various standard psychoanalytic interpretations, such as those regarding avoidance, resistance, and so forth, would require a separate exposition. The essentially passive role of the patient in such psychoanalytic approaches may nevertheless be apparent when studied operationally.

Although the patient, in the preceding paradigm, does most of the talking, the passive psychoanalyst regularly enacts the active role, no matter how infrequently exercised. In fact, one might postulate that the less frequent the psychoanalyst's interventions, the more active and controlling is his role vis-à-vis the patient, an institutionalized and generally invisible but approved countertransference. The foregoing formulation is not a far cry from classical strategies of psychoanalysis—the couch, the rule of abstinence, and so forth, designed to foster the regression of the patient.

The preceding considerations may confirm for some that the objective in psychoanalytic psychotherapy is indeed to foster such passivity, dependence, and regression in patients. For others it may confirm the notion that efforts must be made to transcend the dyadic model of one who speaks and one who listens, reflects, and interprets. In the latter case, the goal is to reach a collaborative endeavor in which the supervisor's active probing, speculating, synthesizing, and openness to a wide variety of data and explanation will rub off on the supervisee who will, in turn, convey such methods and attitudes to his patient in the hope that they will rub off on the patient—a triadic process.

The pursuit of the truth of the patient's alleged dependence on his father as well as the validity of his presumed positive motivation toward growth and maturation followed an evolutionary path during a course of successful treatment—the kind of path it must follow if psychoanalytic psychotherapy is to be successful. The dependency was documented by numerous instances during which the patient turned to his father for help when things became "sticky" for him. Also revealed was his continual exploitation of his father in collusion with his dependent mother. The search led further to an exposition of the patient's narcissistic sense of entitlement in relation not only to his father but also to his mother, wife, psychoanalyst, and the world when he perceived his needs were not being met. The patient's presumed positive motivation toward growth and maturation came to be seen in the perspective of a bright and engaging infantile person's capacity to adapt to the expectations of others, in this case to those of his psychotherapist. In the light of increased understanding of the patient, it became apparent that goals of growth and maturation could have no meaning to him at the onset of treatment because of his fixation at an early developmental level. This is not to say he was unmotivated or out to defeat the psychotherapist or the psychotherapeutic process. His basic and desperate motivation was to find relief from the misery of his existence, utilizing the ancient and largely ineffectual methods that were available to him.

In the course of the treatment, the psychotherapist enjoyed the gratification of being appreciated by the patient at times when the patient experienced him as an ally, really as a partner in collusion against others in his environment—as his mother had been. The supervisee also experienced frustration and sometimes anger when the patient's narcissistic sense of entitlement led to expectations that could not be met by the therapist, and he experienced the patient's disappointment, anger, and demands as unfair, ungrateful, and undeserved. The psychotherapist's preference to be the loved ally was repeatedly dashed. The psychodynamics of the situation were reviewed as frequently as necessary in the supervisory sessions, including an appraisal of the infantile demanding stage of development of the patient and the psychotherapist's wish to be both nurturant and appreciated. The pursuit of the truth suffered from time to time as both patient and supervisee maneuvered to assuage the loss of self-esteem each suffered in the process.

PARALLEL PROCESS

The maneuvering to assuage the loss of self-esteem sometimes took the form referred to in the literature as *parallel process,* in which the patient's disappointment with and anger toward the therapist was replicated in the supervisee's eagerness to get help from his supervisor to resolve his contretemps vis-à-vis his patient. His reporting often had an importuning quality. The same open exploratory approach to the triadic situation was utilized to put this matter in a broader, deeper frame of reference. The supervisee had sufficient detachment, aided by his personal analysis, to experience a perspective that made the situation more tolerable for him, with an ultimate resolution. In terms of the triadic situation one may presume that the supervisor's continued review and exploration of the psychodynamics of both participants provided an environment for his supervisee that the latter, in his turn, was successfully able to provide his patient.

Problems in the triadic situation of difficult patient–supervisee–supervisor relations has spawned reams of literature recently, and I suspect that this will be true of the current volume. There are a number of issues that can be considered. The supervisor's usefulness to this supervisee or that one will depend to a large extent on his ability to tolerate the latter's inexperience, eagerness, nervousness, and what is most important, his mistakes. Again passivity is not the answer. The concerns of the active-versus-passive psychotherapist are reflected in the supervisory process. The passive supervisor operationally plays an often invisible but active role that can be correlated with the apprehensiveness experienced with him by the supervisee. I believe that this is a more central issue than the frequently debated one about whether the supervisor's primary function is to help the supervisee understand his patient or to help him identify those instances in which the countertransference impedes his work. One or the other, I believe, may be appropriate, depending on the stage of treatment, the maturity and readiness of the supervisee, and a host of other matters that reflect clinical judgment on the part of the supervisor. The active supervisor—the one who can freely expose his own mode of developing his thoughts, his willingness to revise his speculations—invites a similar mode in his supervisee's responses to him. In effect, a condition is established in which a dialogue between supervisor and supervisee becomes possible. It provides for the possibility that the student may be able to confront the formidable task of learning the complexities of the psychoanalytic situation while retaining some feeling of acceptance by the supervisor. This formulation is a variation of Sullivan's dictum that the interviewer should incline the interview in a direction of lesser anxiety for the interviewee because of the observable fact that increased anxiety impairs the critical faculties required for psychoanalytic work. In the supervisory situation described previously, such concerns permitted the learning process to proceed despite the difficulties recounted.

Many agree that the supervised treatment of the difficult patient may not provide the best learning experience for a candidate, and yet it occurs often enough. In this context, the notion of *parallel process* may at times be a useful one. It can also be used irresponsibly. The basic observation is a simple one. The patient wants something from the therapist that is not forthcoming. He or she is displeased. This troubles the therapist, who, in turn, looks to the supervisor for help that may not be forthcoming. The therapist is displeased with the supervisor, who, in his turn, may be troubled and displeased with the supervisee and himself. This is a common situation. One has reason to expect, however, with the increasing skill of the supervisee and the accumulating experience of the supervisor that this kind of situation will be recognized early and dealt with by putting it into an appropriate perspective. Notions that such interactions are simply and necessarily reenacted in agonizing perpetuity as a necessary accompaniment to the treatment and supervision of the difficult patient are most readily held by those who are themselves not skilled in the handling of situations that are common enough in the practice of psychotherapy. Such notions are buttressed by explanatory concepts that point to the malevolent intentions of the patient or to the therapeutic benefits of the therapist's rages and outrages—the countertransference. Psychotherapeutic failure is thus dressed in the cloak of understanding.

It is easy enough to recount examples of such failures without cloaking them. One supervisee, for example, experienced constant turmoil with an infantile patient who was insistent with regard to after-hours telephone conversations and emergency appointments. The supervisee was beside herself, feeling that yielding violated her. She cited the rule of abstinence. She felt diminished in her role as physician and healer. Attempts to restrict her patient's demands were unsuccessful.

The final crisis was played out over coffee. The patient was regularly seen at 8 A.M. in a hospital setting. The waiting area contained an electric coffeemaker. Coffee was routinely made at 8:30 A.M. for a group that met at 9 A.M. Coffee was then available to all patients served by the same waiting area. The psychotherapist drank coffee, which she obtained elsewhere in the hospital, during the sessions. So the stage was set. The coffee-drinking psychotherapist faced an infantile patient demanding equal coffee rights with the therapist and certainly with the other patients who followed him shortly. Both were caught. Possible solutions were explored. There was ample evidence that the patient desperately wanted to continue the treatment in terms that he could tolerate. The psychotherapist could stop drinking coffee during the session. She could supply both with coffee or—less graciously—invite him to bring his own coffee. She could not yield. He could not yield either, and the result, as predicted by the supervisor, was a unilateral termination by the patient accompanied by a plethora of complaining and threatening calls and letters to the institution and the media.

The supervisee emerged with a parallel attack against the supervisor. Kernberg, she asserted, would have been more sympathetic to her problem, would have attributed more malevolence to the patient, and would have been less sympathetic to the patient's demands for equal treatment. The supervisor had indeed urged her to let up and tolerate the infantility of her infantile patient. According to some descriptions of the parallel process, the supervisor, at this point, would have been more or less oblivious of the nursery-age transaction going on and, in turn, would have become resentful and censorious. At this level, the concept of *parallel process* can be used in an unpsychoanalytic and irresponsible manner indeed. Is there no room for experience or wisdom in our practice?

REPRISE

The argument is made that psychoanalytic supervision is best conceived in educative terms. There is a pedagogic aphorism to the effect that, in the educative process, the student studies his professor, emulates him, and becomes more and more like his mentor until he supplants him. The candidate, not unlike other students, learns chiefly through observation and imitation. This is not simply a rote matter but ideally is accompanied by thought, reflection, synthesis, challenge, compromise, and accommodation. The teacher not only instructs but provides a model for an open-ended approach to broadening an understanding of whatever universe they are exploring. In psychoanalysis, the mentor's diligence and open-mindedness in the exploration of the roots of human behavior provide a model for the supervisee and for his work with his patient. The final crucible is the patient whose facilitation of living will parallel the process described when he, the end product, has also acquired an ability for an open-minded, attentive exploration of his own human nature. Psychoanalysis should be an interminable process—one that begins during treatment and continues after termination for supervisors, supervisees, and other patients.

REFERENCES

Altshul, V. A. The hateful therapist and the countertransference psychosis. *The National Association of Private Psychiatric Hospitals*, 1980, *11*(4).

Deutsch, H., Roazen, P., & Zaphiropoulos, M. On supervision analysis. *Contemporary Psychoanalysis*, 1983, *19*(1).

Gediman, H. K., & Wolkenfeld, F. The parallelism phenomenon in psychoanalysis and supervision. *Psychoanalytic Quarterly*, 1980, *49*(2).

Gill, M. M. *Analysis of transference* (Vol. 1). New York: International Universities Press, 1982.

Gill, M. M., & Hoffman, I. Z. *Analysis of transference* (Vol. 2). New York: International Universities Press, 1982.

Kernberg, O. *Borderline conditions and pathological narcissism.* New York: Jason Aronson, 1975.

Khan, M. M. Toward an epistomology of the process of cure. In M. M. Khan (Ed.), *Privacy of the self.* New York: International Universities Press, 1974.

Schafer, R. *The analytic attitude.* New York: Basic Books, 1983.

Schimel, J. L. Psychotherapeutic conversations: A linguistic and semantic analysis. *Contemporary Psychoanalysis*, 1980, *16*(3).

Spence, D. P. *Narrative truth and historical truth.* New York: Norton, 1982.

Sullivan, H. S. *The psychiatric interview.* New York: Norton, 1954.

Sullivan, H. S. *Conceptions of modern psychiatry, The first William Alanson White memorial lectures.* Baltimore: The William Alanson White Psychiatric Foundation, 1940, 1945.

Szalita, A. B. Reanalysis. *Contemporary Psychoanalysis*, 1968, *4*(2).

Szalita, A. B. On termination (Symposium: Problems in terminating psychoanalysis). *Contemporary Psychoanalysis*, 1976, *12*(3).

Winnicott, D. W. Hate in the countertransference. In D. W. Winnicott, *Collected Papers.* New York: Basic Books, 1949.

Communication and the Use of the Couch within the Psychoanalytic Situation
A Supervisory Perspective

ROSE SPIEGEL

COMMUNICATION

The person comes to the analyst for help in what Harry Stack Sullivan called *difficulties in living*—whether about discontent with oneself, interpersonal relationships, or in a state of crisis, such as a crisis about one's work, or with some inner ominousness, such as suicidal urges, depression, and anxiety, or with the range of symptoms formulated in the classificatory manuals, but rarely so designated by the troubled individual. The core person, with his potential hidden within, is often obscured by the struggles in life, the disruptive emotions, the miscarriage of coping solutions, or by reaction-formations that are concretized into character and damaged self-hood. The core person may be concealed within an as-if personality, or by a successful-appearing persona.

What, then, are the basic tasks that confront the analyst in this variegated spectrum? Certainly, they include getting a sense of the difficulties that bring the person to analysis and some surmise of the core personality as well as the formal classificatory diagnosis. Another responsibility is arriving at a working hypothesis as to whether the direc-

ROSE SPIEGEL • Fellow, Training and Supervising Analyst, William Alanson White Institute of Psychiatry, Psychoanalysis and Psychology, New York, New York 10023 and Consulting Psychiatrist, Saint Luke's-Roosevelt Hospital Center, New York, New York 10025.

tion of appropriate therapy for the patient is psychoanalysis or somewhere in the range of psychotherapy. Which general approach would
meet this person's most pressing immediate need? Which would be
within his capacity for enriched communication and development of
potentiality? One analyst in supervision presented a very basic question
that had preoccupied him—namely, how does psychoanalytic theory
connect with psychoanalytic technique, an issue that will be addressed
later.

At this point, let us see what distinction can be made between
psychoanalysis in its variations and the numerous reported varieties of
psychotherapy, many of which have their linkage to psychoanalysis and
share overlapping goals, in spite of significant differences. It seems to
me that the fundamental difference is that in psychoanalysis the deep
objective goes beyond the relief of distress and symptoms, or the prac-
ticality of problem solving, though both are included. Psychoanalysis
also includes and emphasizes the cultivation of "know thyself" as a
goal, value, and experience worthy in itself. In that sense, all psychoanalysis is existential. The task of "know thyself" includes the emergence of some aspects of the Unconscious into awareness, though no
one can know all. Indeed, that emergence is only one tool of self-knowledge, which includes other foci of attention—the recognition of the quality of one's relatedness by means of "selective attention." On the other
hand, the stress on the surfacing of the Unconscious into awareness,
hopefully by means of free association in the classical sense, has brought
with it vulnerability to evasive, self-deceptive discursiveness—that is, to
faulty communication with oneself. One concern of neo-Freudians is
how to aid this surfacing—the communication with the self in the analytic situation with the analyst. The task is to assist authentic self-report-
ing—to become both more subtle concerning what is subsumed by "free
association" and broader concerning the vastness of what is subsumed
in communication.

Psychoanalysis cultivates reanimation of past experiences, both as a
deepening of self-awareness and as a digging for the roots of how one
has become the contemporary person. On the whole, though not exclusively, the psychotherapies address *the here and now* both as source of
information and goal for problem solving. More characteristically, the
authority relationship moves from therapist to patient directively, while
in psychoanalysis the ideal is to have the patient mobilize his or her own
resources both for awareness and emerging with solutions. This admir-
able ideal as well as the ideal of true free association carries the danger of
the analyst's taking on the posture of passivity in regard to the patient's
communication, both in terms of his or her own ongoing reflection as

well as in the explicit interaction and communication with the patient, in the overly relaxed expectation that the latter's verbal flow on the couch will ultimately and automatically solve all.

About the Supervisory Interaction. Not withstanding the "noise" concerning the analyst's inevitable anxiety about evaluation in the formal institutional training program, the supervisor will hopefully contribute skill, experience, a conceptual approach, and often a more profound outlook for which supervision offers a domain for expression. Sullivan saw the analyst as a person with expertise and skill in this field of endeavor but who is not equipped with sacrosanct qualities—all of which applies to supervisors. Hopefully, light is shed, perhaps a Socratic question stimulated, and the analyst's anxiety is not avoidably increased. The analyst develops awareness of his or her individual patterns of response, including the countertransferential. With the variety in supervisors, the analyst encounters a variety of concepts, styles, and needs to shape a personal style. Given this variety in supervisors, it is striking how often they share a common impression of the particular analyst-in-training.

It is the function of the supervisor to discern the patient through the analyst's reporting. Though at times omissions in description occur, it is amazing how one experiences the gap, fills in the missing theme, and, on hunch, plays it back to the analyst. Often the patient in this network of communication either comments that another element had been added and, almost as though having overheard the supervisory session, produces material as if taking off from that session—a matter of a three-way common network. At times when I have met with an analyst's patient in consultation, I have been impressed with the clarity and discernment of the analyst and how challenging the difficulties were.

Another function appropriate to the supervisor is to contribute through his or her own life experience and maturity, though it is not necessarily the case that the greater and deeper range of experience is on the side of the supervisor. A common experience in supervision is that different analysts evoke different emphases, depending both on the problems of the patient and on how the analyst is relating.

For example, Dr. A., an analyst of Latin American birth, was in a quandary about his patient—a young woman 28 years old, of Orthodox Jewish origin, who was a vocational therapist and who had numerous difficulties. Though Dr. A. went on to describe these, he also stated that what he wished for from supervision was to solve an issue distressing him—the distinction between psychoanalysis as a technique and as a theory. As interesting and valid as the issue is, his anxiety and preoccupation with it blocked him from receptivity to what the patient was about and what she was conveying.

Clinically and on a parallel track with the concern of Dr. A., the patient was troubled about her work relationship with her director and about a frustrating, constricted relationship with a man who offered no hope of marriage. Stemming from her intricate family relationship was a deep depression about being less attractive than her younger sister. She had made some comments about not knowing why she was in therapy, which, on that particular occasion, was difficult for the analyst to address. However, when she reported her despair about not having children because she believed age 30 was the turning point for fertility and because she was not yet married, the analyst was helpful in pointing out what she actually knew—namely, that there is not a sudden cut off point for fertility and childbearing. He also helped her in her depressive anxiety about her father, who was terminally ill with cancer and in preparing herself for the ultimate separation. In general, Dr. A. was distinctly helpful if there was a clear problem for solution, with distinct objective information.

On the other hand, the patient's dreams were not addressed. There was no communication about feelings, nor about her visual imagery and metaphors that occasionally were bizarre. The challenge in supervision was to help the analyst solve the issue of theory and technique, but, more importantly, to consider whether one unrecognized function of this issue was to serve as a smokescreen between him and the patient.

It seemed to the analyst that technique involved simply getting information. Beyond that limited requirement I suggested that *psychoanalysis* was the label for a package, a conglomerate of processes that include the patient's emotions, recollection, and interpretation of his or her experience. *Technique* involves recognition of the elements included in the psychoanalytic view, drawing inferences, and offering occasional interpretations. It goes beyond information-getting in that it implements recognition of what transpires. Thus, "theory" and "technique" are not intrinsically disparate. The following suggestions that I made served to link a theoretical approach with some how-to suggestions to free the analyst for fuller and more uncluttered receptive communication with the patient.

First, I suggested that he help the patient develop greater awareness of her own need by helping her focus on goals in therapy—that is, to find her own self-hood in terms of her needs and wishes and in her communication and relatedness with her self. *Second*, I suggested that the problem in methodology was how to help the patient communicate in the analytic setting, and how he might deepen his communication with her. The method begins with the development of the therapist's awareness of the patient and her fluctuations, thereby freeing the analyst of preoccupation with methodology and technique. This required his going beyond the standard "objective" observing of the patient, instead allowing himself to receive impressions and feel the impact of the patient. This entailed a kind of receptiveness suggestive of the openness of meditation.

The patient was to be helped to distinguish between what she experienced and how others responded. Where one can, one should confirm experiences and interpretations with the patient, offering what Sullivan termed *consensual validation*.

I find it important in understanding the patient to recognize his or her range of communication. Some dimensions in this range include the openness to self-perception, whether of body experiences or affects and emotions; the ability to recall and perhaps reanimate the past, as opposed to total emphasis on the here and the now; any tendency to denial or to distort reporting of past and present events and experiences; the ability to recall and report dreams; the richness of dream imagery; and the ability to deal with abstractions versus being overly concrete. Is there a paucity of descriptive language, a tendency toward obsessionally meticulous, tedious detail? Is there a tendency to be simplistic in language? (For example, is there a tendency to express a range of negative emotions by a repetitive pattern of angry, debasing terms from the genital or excretory bodily zones?)

Another helpful approach to understanding the patient is through his or her personality type or the diagnostic category. This is often expressed in a characteristic style of language and communication. For example, Sullivan ascribed obsessional communication to power struggles in early parent–child interaction expressed in language maneuvers rather than to the Freudian emphasis on anality.

In verbal exchanges in analysis, the analyst's own verbal obsessional propensities are often aroused because of the analyst's own investment in being recognized as *right*. Verbal communication between two people with this propensity unhappily obscures communication of emotions other than frustration, mounting resentment, and even rage—a situation that Clara Thompson once characterized as *having hold of an electric wire and being unable to let go*. As I well know autobiographically, this calls for a degree of self-knowledge on the analyst's part and an ability, so to speak, to step back in the communication rather than forward into it.

Another called-for and often difficult achievement is for the analyst to find the patient's developmental level of communication and, for the time being, to accept it. Generally, a more opportune time arises for the patient to gain insight into his characteristic patterns and the ways in which they handicap him.

The preceding is essentially what was offered Dr. A. over some supervisory sessions to address the issue of theory and technique with the aim of helping in the recognition of the patient and in furthering communication rather than as a free-floating abstraction. An additional inner burden that impeded his functioning with the patient concerned anxiety of another kind. Dr. A. was highly intelligent, sensitive, with a keen sense of responsibility, which was expressed as a preoccupation with "What mistakes did I make? What did I do wrong?" It even impeded his reporting what had transpired in sessions. He was also very concerned with not making formulations to the patient that in any way might be construed as an attack on her self-esteem. For instance, the patient, who was distressed by her body image, had been told by her director and her patients that she often made exaggerated body movements that were disturbing to them. In Dr. A.'s session with me, it became clear to both of us that he was "resistant" (his word) to actively helping the patient develop understanding of the significance of these movements, because, he thought, this would be experienced by her as his siding with the "attackers." At times, in his anxiety and guardedness, Dr. A. would take the passive position of "not understanding" what I was saying. For instance, in discussing how he might address the patient without setting it up as hostility or attack, I said, "It depends on how it is said." He responded, "I don't know what you mean." As we explored it, he was able to be more understanding of his tendency to back off. He became more communicative. Such are some of the nuts and bolts involved in the supervisory alliance and collaboration.

There has been some description in the preceding account of the analyst's subjective experiences that got in the way of understanding what was going on in the patient and himself. One further variety of interference with analytic communication was the analyst's aversion to the manifestation by the patient of emotion or powerful mood states, even to the point of not addressing the patient's dreams. This aversion was characteristic of Dr. A. for a while, and also of another analyst—Dr. B.

Dr. B.'s patient was a young man of 28, an art historian who was concerned with a final decision about his career, a lack of self-assertiveness and self-esteem, and a constricted relationship with his girlfriend. On one occasion the analyst canceled a session because of personal-professional business. The patient, who was a little younger than the analyst, reported a dream in which there had been a very urgent reason for him to phone the analyst for an extra session, but he had decided against it. The analyst, as he described it in the supervisory session, did not inquire about the urgency nor about the decision not to phone. As it was, he settled instead for discussing with the patient the latter's thought that his friend, who had five sessions weekly rather than his three, must be faring better than he, while his girlfriend, with one session weekly, must also be progressing much faster than he. In other words, however much he got, he would be underprivileged, and nothing could fare well for him. This the analyst recognized and shared.

The analyst himself needed a rather low-keyed atmosphere, in which there was discussion *about* emotion, rather than the actual surfacing of it, that might indeed evoke reproach of therapy, as had happened. Through discussion in supervision, the analyst recognized his personal need for avoidance of emotion and soothing the patient away from it, as something to address in his own analysis.

Such flight from recognition of the patient's emotion or the almost unaware directing the patient away from it may be an unconscious negating of the patient—a distraction from the task of recognition that arises from the analyst's private need. And yet, there are occasions when the anxiety, rage, or depression of a patient are so painful both for the patient in the experience, and for the analyst to witness and empathize with, that the analyst feels unable to help. At this point one longs to assuage the painful experience in behalf of the person's staying psychologically intact.

Dr. C.'s patient, a young woman of 27, came to analysis because of a block in her goal of creative writing, distress with her marriage, and waves of anxiety. She presented a number of challenges to the analyst, some of them painful. Her style of communication in the analysis was commandeering and brooked no comment, which was experienced as gross interference. Her style was of a highly structured narrative that must run its course. The taped interviews revealed also that she moved in a rather tangential pattern, without direction into depth or the underlying feelings or motivations. The analyst felt he could get no handle on communication. The distress with the marriage turned into divorce proceedings. It was difficult to be clear as to who got the disengagement going. Her reporting never clearly established the old newspaper criteria of *who did what to whom.*

Meanwhile, she had given a rest to her concern about writing and had taken up another vocational skill—namely, gourmet cooking in a restaurant. She later reported to her analyst how she had been victimized by another woman chef, and that she had gotten summarily dismissed in connection with that situation. The missing "Chapter 1" turned out to be that she had given the manager of the restaurant a time ultimatum about a raise and about the other woman's assignment. By the logic of the manager's not meeting her demands about her scheduling, she was out of the job. That is, her aggressive attempt having failed, she experienced herself as victim and so presented herself to the analyst. This raises the intricate issue of reality testing, subjective truth, lying to oneself and others, and confabulating (see Kovar, 1974).

To recognize the person within the patient required further inquiry to ascertain where the incident really began and to recognize also her attempt to manipulate and in a way to rewrite history. The analyst's task, despite the patient's attempt at hurtful behavior to the other employee, still called for linking this to necessities of her developmental past. That is, the patient was the youngest child and the only girl in a large family who found a place for herself by her brightness and precocity in competition with the older siblings. The analyst was caught between the recognition of tampered values and of helping the person reveal the formative circumstances for this aggressive defense. All of this with the avoidance of unwitting collusion with the patient's neurosis—the omission of how it all started in a particular incident.

I have found a wide range of accuracy, freedom of distortion, and manipulation of purported facts by patients. With some, I have had validation that the description is appropriately complete both for the span of time and the events. With others, I have found significant omissions that lead one to draw incorrect inferences, and finally the ultimate in persuasive confabulation.

This range of accuracy in describing and offering "information" I designate as *the credibility of the patient* (as my association to the legal term *the credibility of the witness*). Again, one task in analysis is to help the patient bring to light what gave the impetus to this twist. As I see it, one important supervisory task is to help the analyst search for the person within the patient, and in this search the person's patterns of communication offer one road, if not the royal one.

THE USE OF THE COUCH

An important issue that arises in psychoanalysis is the *role of the couch:* What criteria should be met for the patient's taking that position? Some analysts in supervision have made such diffuse comments as, "I wanted to know what it would be like to have a patient on the couch" or, "the patient one day decided to lie down." Patients themselves attach various interpretations to this *ceremonial* (to use a term of Freud's).

The "couch" has a mystique, which was originally symbolic of Freud—the founder of psychoanalysis—and then it was generalized. For a while there was a pervasive sense, first, that the "couch" was solely the entitlement of Freudian analysts; and second, that its use is based on the diagnosis of neurosis, analyzability, and the ability to free associate. On the other hand, it was believed to be dangerous to the patient if a psychosis exists or is suspected of being present. Understandably, patients have inferred—of course not necessarily correctly—that if the couch is not recommended, then such a condition exists.

The procedure of some neo-Freudian analysts in regard to the couch has evolved as follows: Since the therapist–patient relationship itself is actively interpersonal, with the former the participant observer, the more symmetrical seating arrangement, with the option open of looking at each other, tacitly declares this interaction to be operative. It also implies a more democratic authority relationship. Actually, there is neither rigidity nor uniformity among non-Freudian analysts.

As will be presented, beyond these polar opposites is an appropriate and productive use of the couch that reveals meaning for specific patients in terms of communication and transference.

To begin at the beginning—Freud spelled out his rationale for the use of the couch in 1913 in his paper "Further Recommendations in the Technique of Psycho-Analysis":

> A word must be said about a certain ceremonial observance which concerns the position in which the treatment is carried out. I hold to the plan of getting the patient to lie on a sofa while I sit behind him out of his sight. This arrangement has an historical basis; it is the last vestige of the hypnotic method out of which psycho-analysis was evolved; but for many reasons it deserves to be retained. The first is a personal motive, one that others may share with me however. I cannot bear to be gazed at for eight hours a day. . . . Since, while I listen I resign myself to the control of my unconscious thoughts I do not wish my expression to give [the patient] indications. (p. 354)

Then, rather petulantly, Freud notes "that many analysts work in a different way," and he proceeds to describe how he instructs the patient in the art of free association.

It is this "personal motive," often patronizingly referred to, that is based, I believe, on a misinterpretation both of his subjective experience and what was transpiring between him and his patient. These bear a broader but unrecognized significance concerning communication between patient and analyst.

The views of various analysts of distinction are thought provoking. Frieda Fromm-Reichmann discussed the use of the couch in a neutral tone, and she raised some question about Freud in the vis-à-vis position, but she did not spell out what does make the couch "advisable" or when it facilitates treatment. In "Recent Advances in Psychoanalysis" (1949, pp. 96–97), she wrote the following:

> Many psychoanalysts allow patients to sit or to lie down, whichever may seem to work best with each patient. With some patients this may be decided upon at once for the entire course of treatment; with others, changes of position once or repeatedly may be advisable during the course of treatment.

In "Psychoanalytic Psychotherapy with Psychotics" (1943, p. 133), discussing schizophrenic patients, she said that "sitting behind the patient in the beginning of treatment . . . is too unreal, for the psychoanalyst is the bridge to external reality."

Fromm-Reichmann continued:

> It is beneficial and relaxing for *some* neurotic patients to lie on the couch in the classical manner; it may be quite the contrary—and artificial—for *others*, depending on their habits and life-histories. Accordingly, that position is recommended which allows the patient and analyst to look at each other whenever the patient desires.
>
> Seated behind the patient, the psychoanalyst may, or may not listen; the patient's thoughts may, or may not, "wander away" ["free associate?"] from the interpersonal relation with the invisible, silent physician.[1] (p. 133)

Further along in this section, she made a comment that I believe involves a misunderstanding of Freud's experience:

> Freud remarked that *he* could not endure to have patients gazing at him for eight hours. This suggests a change in the eight-hour system rather than the maintenance of invisibility for those who share Freud's feeling. Personally, I have found the ten- or fifteen-minute interval between interviews most helpful. (pp. 133–134)

Since then, books dealing with psychoanalytic therapy take the couch for granted. However, John Klauber in his "Psychoanalytic Consultation" (1972) made a refreshing exception to the use of the couch, which is as follows:

> Whether the patient sits or lies or takes a walk around town like Gustave Mahler is to some extent peripheral. . . . Clearly a patient may receive more psychoanalysis (in the sense of analytic understanding) by sitting in a chair

---

[1] I have been unable to find any discussion by Harry Stack Sullivan on the use of the couch in any of his writings nor in Patrick Mullahy's interpretations. In his book, *The Psychiatric Interview* (1954) Sullivan stated his discontent with the patient's ability to respond to being asked to "free associate," finding it more fruitful to ask about "marginal thoughts."

twice a week opposite . . . to someone who understands him easily than by lying on a couch five times a week talking to an analyst who has difficulty grasping the continuity. (pp. 108, 111)

Incidentally, it is interesting that the working assumption is—if it is twice-weekly therapy, the patient faces the analyst; if it's on a four- or five-times schedule, it's the couch.

The assumption that if the analysand just goes on talking and "free associating" long enough "on the couch," all will in due course surface—the trauma, the defenses evoked, and the analysand's insightful recognition of the psychopathology, which will then be resolved and be aided by timely interpretations. Some analysts have turned this into a sanction for passivity, in which they make no parallel inner commentary nor reverberation from their own experience that is responsive to the patient's communication. This is a different issue from whether at that moment the analyst will communicate verbally. It is that parallel empathic, reflective inner commentary that Freud referred to in the previously cited quotation. It is that inner passivity that is challenged in Sullivan's concept of *the analyst as participant observer*.

In short, the Freudian working assumption is that the use of the couch facilitates free association for the patient, and for the analyst it secures freedom from feeling inhibited by the patient's gaze.

However—perhaps with one exception to be mentioned—there prevails a disregard of one aspect of the patient–couch relationship that has therapeutic significance, namely, its meaning to the patient. The meaning involves the belief system and expectation that the patient brings regarding the significance of the couch as well as transferential elements in the patient–couch relationship.

To illustrate: By her own decision, Dr. A.'s patient reclined on the couch 10 months after beginning analysis, and thereafter she occasionally sat up. Her expressed fear was that she would not be listened to if she was not connecting with him visually; that he would not be paying attention. On the other hand, she felt that the position would enable her to relax and allow more free-floating thoughts. She did indeed permit primary process material to surface—her hidden terror of men as being brutal and aggressive, reveries having the imagery and symbolism of dreams, sad feelings of self-doubt about herself as a desirable woman— all this amply fulfilling Freud's promise.

Now for the transferential implications. The patient's apprehension about being ignored stemmed from her situation within a family with three children. She was the middle child, and she had a father whose absentmindedness she had tried to penetrate as a youngster on walks with him. Her mother was absorbed in impressing the neighbors with a properly conformist daughter, but without the faintest interest in her as a young woman and person in her own right.

One of the analytic tasks she accomplished was distinguishing between the family mode of tuning her out and her analyst's sensitive, caring interest in her. Not only did he address with her the psychogenesis of her defensive disturbances, but he also helped her with her anticipatory grief about her father's terminal illness, her developing self, and her fulfillment as a woman. It was the analyst's exploration with her of her ambivalence about trusting his involvement and participation that led to the opening up of her basic distrust arising from her family's self-centeredness.

It is interesting that it is in Winnicott's article "Fragment of an Analysis" (1974, p. 662) that the couch itself was noted as having transferential meaning. "Satisfaction of the need to be held by the analyst [was] represented by the couch."

The experience of Dr. B. with his patient was reminiscent of Freud's discomfort. After several months of analysis, the patient spontaneously reclined on the couch. Dr. B. felt it freed him from having the patient dependent on his facial expression. "I don't have a poker face. If I'm puzzled about something, I don't have to watch my face. The guy takes the authority into his own hands on the couch."

Several months later, a transferential dimension emerged concerning the couch. The patient revealed that he used to scrutinize the analyst—only a few years his senior—searching competitively for some superior quality and matching himself as the presumed failure, as he had done with his older brothers. It is interesting, that before this transference was clearly stated, the analyst had experienced only unidentified emotional discomfort. For a while, the analyst maintained that he was *not* transferentially the patient's older brother. For countertransferential reasons, he saw himself instead as being transferentially the patient's father. It was through examining the countertransference that the patient's experience was accepted and explored. It is interesting that emotional experiences were in process in each before either patient or analyst could identify them and their basis, and only later could they translate them into language.

Dr. C.'s patient used the couch situation to control communication, both to keep the analyst in his place, so to speak, and to soar into her narration. Her verbal style was almost that of creatively unfolding a short story, and was not to be touched by her analyst. After several months, Dr. C., in discerning some of the authentic intrapsychic and interpersonal themes both in this material and in dreams, enabled her to engage more in self-exploration instead of in the deft, defensive, impenetrable presentations.

The range of responses to the couch is interesting; for some patients it means trust and acceptance; for some freedom for communication; and for others distancing and resistance. What has also been overlooked is the occasional contribution of the analyst to problems in communication in the vis-à-vis positions, as will be noted with Dr. D. and Dr. E.

Dr. D. observed that "my previous supervisor suggested that the patient be on the couch, because she was waiting for me to react. And on the couch, she does not look at me."

The patient being presented in supervision with me had taken the initiative in a lengthy discussion about being on the couch. First, she said that it would indicate she was accepting being in analysis with Dr. D. because analysis "is done on the couch." Second, she said that she wanted to make the decision herself and not have Dr. D. make it for her. She felt, however, that being on the couch would please Dr. D. It was her impression, as it was Dr. D.'s, that going on the couch would bring her closer to the unconscious and to free association. Dr. D. wisely exerted no pressure, and awaited the patient's timing for the decision that in due course was made in its favor.

Now Dr. D., in the supervisory situation, was depending, almost in the literal, etymological sense of "hanging on to" my face, sometimes for some indication of approval or for a kind of closure, whether verbalized or by my expression, before the presentation could continue, and which I experienced as pressure (again the experience reminiscent of Freud's). I found myself tempted to keep my face blank to hold off the pressure, not so much because of discomfort as because of obstinacy. I soon drew attention to our nonverbal interplay. Not surprisingly, it turned out that this was transferential from early experience with the grandmother—the central authoritative person—and this role had been assigned to me in our supervisory experience. The analyst became aware that she tended to use this interplay by facial expression, from which, as a nonverbal pressure of communication, the couch freed the patient. It became easier for her to delve into herself, to communicate with herself.

Briefly, Dr. E.'s patient began analysis three years ago, at first sitting facing each other. At the suggestion of the then supervisor, the switch was made to the couch in order to have less eye contact, and therefore "you'll be much more comfortable." Actually, Dr. E. believed it was because of her own pressure for facial expressive interaction. The patient at first said she was afraid and then observed that this is part of the analytic pattern—that you come three times a week and lie on the couch. Dr. E., in the work with her patients, developed an easier, more listening, unpressuring style.

In our supervisory situation, Dr. E. was, in her anxiety, at first extremely rushed and hyperactive in gesture and facial interaction with me. She waited with bated breath for either facial or verbal response from me. Out of our discussion emerged the prototypic experience with a demanding mother, who gave approval reluctantly, and the young daughter who would wait in breathless alert silence, gazing at her to read her response.

This discussion of supervisory experiences underscores how variegated and open-ended is communication within the psychoanalytic situation. I have also tried to show how the use of the couch is an important element in the communicational field of psychoanalysis and supervision.

REFERENCES

Freud, S. On beginning the treatment (Further recommendations in the technique of psychoanalysis, I). In J. Strachey (Ed. and trans.), *The complete psychological works: Standard edition* (Vol. 12). London: Hogarth Press, 1958. (Originally published, 1913).

Fromm-Reichmann, F. Psychoanalytic psychotherapy with psychotics: The influence of modifications in technique on present trends in psychoanalysis. In D. M. Bullard (Ed.), *Psychoanalysis and psychotherapy: Selected papers of Frieda Fromm-Reichmann.* Chicago: University of Chicago Press, 1959. (Originally published, 1943.)

Fromm-Reichmann, F. Recent advances in psychoanalysis. In D. M. Bullard (Ed.), *Psychoanalysis and psychotherapy: Selected papers of Frieda Fromm-Reichmann.* Chicago: University of Chicago Press, 1959. (Originally published, 1949.)

Klauber, J. Psychoanalytic consultation. In P. L. Giovacchini (Ed.), *Tactics and techniques in psychoanalytic therapy.* Science House, 1972.

Kovar, L. The pursuit of self-deception. (Review of *Existential Psychology and Psychiatry,* 1974, *12,* 136–149.) *Existential Psychology and Psychiatry,* 1974, *13,* 32.

Sullivan, H. S. *The psychiatric interview.* New York: Norton, 1954.

Winicott, D. W. Fragment of an analysis. In P. L. Giovacchini (Ed.), *Tactics and techniques in psychoanalytic therapy.* New York: Jason Aronson, 1972.

15

Educational and Clinical Pitfalls in Psychoanalytic Supervision

MILTIADES L. ZAPHIROPOULOS

Psychoanalytic supervision as one of the three basic categories of requirements for psychoanalytic training has remained constant for almost 60 years. The other two categories—the so-called training analysis and assorted course and clinical seminars—have also continued to be an integral part of psychoanalytic training. However, with the development of variable jurisdictional bodies and the proliferation of training institutes, there seem to have been more modifications regarding these other two categories, and fewer changes in psychoanalytic supervision as these pertain to the teaching and learning of the therapeutic aspects of psychoanalysis as well as to the evaluation of progress in training of the psychoanalytic candidate.

I shall mention only a few of the modifications in the training-analysis requirement and its implementation. These include aspects of frequency of sessions and overall duration of the training analysis, the extent to which it is prescribed as a prerequisite to beginning course work or supervision, the training analyst's participation or not in the evaluation of progress in training of the candidate, factors entering into the appointment of training analysts, and even the consideration of retirement of training analysts. Of lasting and shared importance is, of course, the almost general prohibition for the training analyst to be or to become the analysand's supervising analyst, at least for the fulfilment of the requirement of supervised analysis. As for the category of courses and seminars, curricula have had to be modified, if not radically, at least in regard to chronology and emphasis.

MILTIADES ZAPHIROPOULOS • Director of Training, Fellow, Training and Supervising Analyst, William Alanson White Institute of Psychiatry, Psychoanalysis and Psychology, New York, New York 10023 and Associate Clinical Professor of Psychiatry, College of Physicians and Surgeons, Columbia University, New York, New York 10027.

Compared to the previously hinted at evolution, the category of analysis under supervision seems to have remained almost unchanged. In most instances, psychoanalytic institutes continue to require supervised work with a minimum of three supervisors and a total of four different patients for a varying number of hours as specified by the institute. Supervising analysts are so appointed and accredited by the particular training institution, and candidates are permitted to make their own choice from the official roster. Assignment of a particular candidate to a particular supervising analyst may be made by a training or educational committee—usually in cases where there is considerable conflict or discrepancy in reports of progress between or among supervising analysts. Rarely is credit given for supervision with an analyst not accredited by the candidate's institution. Occasionally, supervising analysts may be accredited by more than one psychoanalytic institute and thus are available to candidates in different institutes. Generally, it is conceded that the model of psychoanalytic supervision instituted by the Berlin Psychoanalytic Institute in the middle 1920s and 1930s, with some sprinkling of Viennese and Hungarian stipulations, has been adopted and continues to prevail close to three-score years later.

In this essay I shall consider that supervision is a presumably valuable necessity and instrumentality in the development of resourceful psychoanalysts. In that context I shall state some impressions and raise some questions as to educational and clinical aspects that may constitute potentially problematic areas in psychoanalytic supervision. By extension, and to a variable extent, these observations may prove applicable to psychoanalytically oriented psychotherapy as well, although this is not going to be the focus of my inquiry. These problematic areas are composed of the following:

1. The questionable equation of teaching and learning
2. The tenuous aspects of a transmissible body of knowledge
3. The difficulty in bringing similar or dissimilar assumptions about psychoanalytic supervision into alignment or integration
4. The attendant vicissitudes regarding roles, processes, and contents

Although a number of questions pertaining to the preceding areas may remain unanswered and—preferably and probably—should continue so, I shall make some attempts at clarifying the more effectively contributory elements of psychoanalytic supervision both to the candidate's training and to the patient's welfare, not to mention the inevitable corollary of the supervising psychoanalyst's concerns and morale.

TEACHING AND LEARNING

In raising the question whether teaching and learning can be equated, I have in mind several kinds of experiences and concerns. Having had the opportunity on one occasion to glance at a report of one of my supervisors after I completed my psychoanalytic training (this was at a time when, in my particular institute, copies of such reports were not routinely given to candidates), I was struck by her statement that I did not seem to want to be taught, but that I could and did learn. Interestingly enough, my experience with that supervisor, who also said that she could trust me to work well with patients having varying degrees of psychopathology, was that she would not tell me what to do or not to do and, in fact, she did not say much of anything except to raise questions in my mind as to what I was doing or trying to do with my patient. In due time, my ruminations about unresolved narcissitic tendencies yielded to an understanding of her observations in terms of differing cognitive styles and their contribution to teaching and learning. Also, I became aware of such understanding in my work with my supervisees, which allowed me to modify my approach to them in ways that could facilitate their learning rather than vindicate my teaching.

References to the questionable equation of teaching and learning, or to the nature of teaching in psychoanalytic supervision are not lacking in the relatively meager literature on psychoanalytic supervision. They seem to span a long and tortured path of evolution reflecting educational and clinical concerns in the broader sense as well as specific matters of creativeness, responsibility, and ethics. This is not surprising in the light of the more or less agreed upon raison d'être of supervision in its various aspects.

Educationally, psychoanalytic supervision serves two purposes that we hope are affirmatively and conjunctively interconnected. The basic aim is to enhance the development of the candidate's skills in dealing psychoanalytically with patients. These skills should reflect both the candidate's natural propensities and abilities as elicited through the selection process leading to his or her admission to the training institution and as honed by the candidate's personal psychoanalysis and course and seminar instruction. A corollary aim is the ongoing evaluation of such developments—a monitoring process of the way and the extent to which the aforementioned premises and promises appear to be on the way of being realized and fulfilled. Since the task of psychoanalysis as therapy is a complex and demanding one, the supervisor as teacher and evaluator would often tend to be looking for a degree of superior achievement as the acceptable minimum on the part of the candidate.

This may prove to be as exacting for the supervisor as it is for the supervisee. One possible but not infrequent effect is for the supervisor to become particularly focused—at times essentially or exclusively—on one of the specific aspects of analysis such as the interpretation of transference, of dreams, the recovery of early memories, the awareness and use of countertransference, or anything else he or she considers to be his or her own area of proficiency and, as such, a hoped for and presumably objective assessment of his or her teaching success with the supervisee. The latter may respond to this in a complying or resisting way—neither of which accrues to a learning process. In either case, the supervisor's evaluation may interfere with the candidate's progress and with the work of the training or educational committee in that regard. Glowing or scathing supervisory reports more often than not prove to reflect overly zealous teaching rather than the painstaking trial-and-error acquisition of experience and the gradual growth on the part of the analyst-in-training. The previously etched predicament can, of course, be compounded by a candidate's wish to be taught, spoon-fed, or molded, rather than learn the hard way.

Another area of potential difficulty pertains to the supervisor's anxiety as teacher and evaluator of a candidate whose training analyst is experienced as a competitor or a critic. This may be outside the supervisor's awareness or partly within it and dealt with by varying rationalizations. It is more likely to exist in instances where the training analyst is not required or is actually forbidden to participate in the evaluation of the candidate's progress and the supervisor's responsibility is greater. Occasionally, this difficulty may take the form of the supervisor's teaching unwittingly seeking to have the candidate unlearn what he or she has derived from the training analysis—especially if actual or assumed theoretical differences with the training analyst exist.

If the supervising analyst was part of the selection process for admission of a candidate to the institute, an additional vested interest in such candidate's proving teachable may constitute a pitfall. The supervisor's efforts and expectations may become burdensome, or they may constitute an interference with the candidate's individual learning process.

Another caveat applies to the degree to which a supervising analyst proceeds as a teacher of theory—general or specific—in the process of doing supervision. This may prove problematic on two accounts. One is the supervisor's predilection for such teaching and the ensuing carryover from course instruction to supervised analysis. The second is the extent to which the supervisor tends to fill in gaps in theoretical knowledge as elicited in the legitimate assessment of such knowledge within the supervisory context.

Clinically, the concern with responsibility for the welfare of the patient presented in supervision is both an unavoidable reality and the subject of a delicate balance. As in medical practice, and even more so, the learning of psychoanalysis as a therapeutic modality reflects its dual nature as an art and a science. Neither aspect can be said to be equally applicable at any given time by any particular therapist with any individual patient. It follows that there is no uniform way in which these can be taught, although there has to be continuous and unrelenting assessment of the way in which they are used by a supervisee in dealing with a patient entrusted to his or her therapeutic function.

Gross incompetence on the part of a candidate as elicited in supervision can be found to account for either harm to the patient or for lack of progress or improvement in the analytic undertaking. The supervisor may be tempted to take over the patient's analysis by becoming overly didactic and virtually prescribing topical interventions in session after session, with anxious concern and repetitious checking as to how much or how well they are heeded by the candidate. When the latter is particularly suggestible or obedient, apparent learning seems to take place—at least temporarily—thus diminishing the supervisor's frustration and reassuring him or her about the patient's welfare. Sooner or later the lack of real gains in the clinical situation may result in renewed efforts at technical teaching or in the supervisor's giving up altogether. In the latter case, both candidate and patient are abandoned, and the supervisor's sense of responsibility shifts essentially if not exclusively from that of a concerned clinician to that of a righteous educator who has been failed.

The previously outlined predicament may be at least partly avoided if three factors often contributing to observable incompetence are identified and assessed. First, is the candidate's training thus far the kind that may have taken place in such a way as to minimize his or her use of personal initiative, imaginative curiosity, and unhampered judgment in situations where heavy clinical responsibility is experienced. In such instances, the candidate needs help in unlearning the faulty pattern rather than have an alternate limiting teaching imposed. Second, any unresolved or insufficiently dealt with personality difficulties that interfere with the full and proper use of the candidate's talent and personal resources need to be recognized and acknowledged. There should be no attempt to remedy them within the supervisory process because such effort would only complicate matters and confuse the candidate. Rather, the supervisor should help the candidate to work out the problem with his or her training analyst, even if it means returning to analysis after this had been terminated. Third, if the preceding two factors do not seem to apply, the possibility of the candidate's lacking any talent or abilities for doing psychoanalysis may have to be explored, his or her motivation for entering the field clarified, and a realistic and often relief-producing decision to resign from the training program can be reached.

If the supervising analyst succeeds in avoiding becoming the candidate's or the candidate's patient's analyst, there still has to be some ongoing awareness of his or her participation in and contribution to the supervised analysis. Pragmatically, the merit of such awareness cannot be overstated. It is necessary in order for the supervising analyst to continue to foster truly the individuality and the appraisal of differences in his or her supervisee's analysis of the patient. Presuming or pretending noninvolvement or noninfluence is likely to result in covert control of the supervised analysis. The difference between intent and goal of supervision on the one hand and the actuality of incidental processes in the supervised analysis, on the other, has to be kept clear throughout.

A TRANSMISSIBLE BODY OF KNOWLEDGE

In speaking of the tenuous aspects of a transmissible body of knowledge in psychoanalytic supervision, I am referring to a category that has been considered as one of the requirements for a profession and how it fares in this case. Psychoanalysis is more of a heuristic enterprise than an exercise in knowledge. We have theories—general and specific—of lasting value or of current importance or concern. To the extent that we learn to know what they are and that they are theories, we owe to ourselves and to those we teach to recurrently, if not constantly, be aware of their influence on our work and of the more or less conveniently chosen uses to which we put them.

However, theory is all gray but the golden tree of life grows ever green, as Goethe had Mephistopheles put it to Faust. Or, as Mach suggested, theories are like leaves that fall off after having allowed the tree of science to breathe. One is not likely to learn much about human beings, by way of psychoanalysis or otherwise, if one adheres unwaveringly to a theory, no matter how persuasive or sophisticated the latter and no matter how attractive the illusion of definitive or final truth may be. I am not suggesting that theories should never be developed, held, or examined critically, and even experimented with responsibly. As a matter of fact, I believe that we would be lying to ourselves if we maintained we did not have any. I am only saying that theories cannot replace or supersede experience—actual or potential. Oppenheimer stated that the "sense that the future is richer and more complex than our prediction of it, and that wisdom lies in sensitiveness to what is new and hopeful, is perhaps a sign of some maturity in politics" (p. 53). And Feigl (1953) indicated that "it is a sign of maturity to live with an unfinished world view" (p. 13).

Psychoanalytic literature dealing with the teaching of technique appears to reflect two attitudes. The older one is minimizing if not altogether avoiding the idea that technical considerations constitute a transmissible body of knowledge. Basically, it suggests that whatever accrued to the theories of psychoanalysis can be understood only in terms of the actual experience of being analyzed and of doing analysis. Freud and his early disciples and colleagues never really abandoned this position. They encouraged all those interested in psychoanalysis to find their way by observing a rather simple, fundamental rule—by avoiding "wild analysis" and by seeking out historical data and their vicissitudes. The probable development of a *transference neurosis* and its resolution was a consummation to be sought and found. The recovery of repressed memories, making the unconscious conscious, broadening the less conflict-bound functions of the ego, and an eventual gain in insight were goals to be achieved through the analysis of the transference. In due time, the development of interest in the countertransference and its evolving definitions became a new dimension in the process of doing psychoanalysis. In the light of this early attitude, psychoanalytic supervision was essentially the monitoring of the extent to which the candidate's own analysis had succeeded and, possibly, the way in which basic theoretical concepts were integrated.

A newer attitude regarding the teaching of technique appears to reflect varying responses to theoretical deviations *or* developments—the latter usually arising out of therapeutic dissatisfaction or despair. A conservative element in the psychoanalytic community chose to believe that such a state of affairs represented inadequate resolution of intrapsychic conflicts and was due to inadequate training. For this group, the tightening of training requirements led to a more rigid and exacting application of theoretical tenets to both the training analysis and the psychoanalytic supervision. The ensuing theory of technique became the presumably transmissible body of knowledge, and the failure to show an adoption of it became a transgression. Interestingly enough, and not unexpectedly, a similar preoccupation with transmissible techniques developed among those whose new approaches to psychoanalysis as therapy, which were apparently more rewarding, were thought to justify and vindicate their divergent theoretical formulations.

It is my contention that any transmissible body of knowledge in psychoanalytic training is best conveyed through course instruction. Also, varying degrees of success in that enterprise should be properly checked there. As mentioned before, the supervising analyst as well as the candidate will become aware from time to time of whether the goal of instruction has been achieved. Usually, this comes up incidentally and, I trust, heuristically in some extrapolations from the supervisory process. Since theory is taught, it makes sense to trace the use of it in actual analytic work including instances, reasons, and effects. It may be useful also to assess what of the analytic experience becomes integrated with theory. However, it would be onerous to undertake the teaching of theory or the filling of gaps in it as a direct part of a supervised analysis. The candidate may be encouraged to fill such gaps on his or her own or to be referred back to the appropriate resources. More often than not, it is didactic propensity or preoccupation with orthodoxy that tempts the supervising analyst to resort to theoretical teaching directly and demandingly. If the supervising analyst in his or her capacity as therapist does not rely essentially—let alone exclusively—on the use of theory, to require this when doing supervision would constitute betrayal of oneself and others. Rather, it is the exploration of the candidate's experiencing of the analytic encounter that deserves to be the task of the supervisory process as an evolving one.

ASSUMPTIONS UNDERLYING SUPERVISION

Although supervision has remained an almost unchanging requirement of the training in psychoanalysis, the assumptions underlying it may be similar or dissimilar as regards any and all concerned. Pragmatically, these are composed of the patient whose analysis is being supervised, the candidate who is entrusted with that analysis, the candidate's supervising analyst and, by extension, the candidate's training analyst, the candidate's other supervisors, and a training or educational committee. Perhaps, one might add the remainder of the student body and of the faculty of the institute for good measure and for their, at least, peripheral or collateral contributions to the assumptions.

I am not aware of any specific studies referring to the patient's point of view in regard to supervised analyses. When the patient is obtaining analysis through the clinical services of a psychoanalytic institute, it becomes common knowledge that the person conducting the analysis is an analyst-in-training and that the analysis is supervised by a senior analyst. When the patient is referred to the analyst-in-training directly or by an outside source, it is possible that no such awareness exists, though it may develop at some future time. There are varying opinions and practices as to what the patient should be told or not be told, even when the candidate or analyst-in-training has pledged to the institute that he or she will not represent to the public that they are psychoanalysts until permitted to do so. Conceivably, there are no particular assumptions on the part of the patient who has no idea that the therapist receives supervision of the work in which they are mutually engaged. This fact remains, however, as a part of the candidate's concern and any attendant assumptions.

When the patient is fully cognizant of the status of the analyst-in-training, it is necessary to keep in mind the probability of a number of assumptions that rightfully become part of the supervisory situation as well as contaminants of the analysis itself. It is a relatively simple matter if the patient assumes both that the analyst-in-training is inexperienced and that the supervising analyst serves as a safeguard or a saving grace, although this may accrue to foreseeable transferential and countertransferential developments not always recognized as soon or as often as they occur. It may be more complex if the patient develops an institutional transference parallel to the one that the candidate has. This has been noted particularly in two areas. One is that of the financial arrangements when fees are paid to the psychoanalytic institute directly by the patient or indirectly through the candidate. Often, either patient or candidate or both tend to avoid the transferential aspects of financing in the analysis for a long time. It is usually after the patient transfers into the candidate's private practice when these become an issue—suddenly and bitterly. To the extent that the supervising analyst has remained unaware of the situation, whether through some sharing of the institutional transference or otherwise, the situation may become further complicated before a resolution is in sight.

The second area parallels the first and has to do with the patient's reliance on the institution as a nurturing agency as well as a court of last resort. The patient may thus pit the institution, and at times the supervisor, against the analyst-in-training, using them as presumably adversarial parental figures. Or the patient may enter a comparative and competitive vying with the candidate vis-à-vis the institution in instances of threatened dependency or felt separation and abandonment as when transferring to the candidate's private practice. Failure by the supervising analyst to be aware of such pitfalls and to alert the candidate about them is likely to add to the more obvious complications of supervised analysis.

Such complications may reflect the candidate's assumptions about supervision and the ways in which they collide or collude with those of the supervisor. The growing bureaucratization of psychoanalytic education and institutionalization of some of its training aspects seems to have paralleled developments and trends in the field of education in general. Technological emphasis is but one of the results, both as an expectation and a requirement with varying degrees of agreement or conflict. Concerns with proving effectiveness and managing cost containment have contributed to the paradoxical proposition of acquiring foolproof know-how at any cost. Without entering into invidious comparisons, psychoanalytic educators observe apparent, if not conspicuous, differences in motivations for and approaches to psychoanalytic training among applicants in the last 10 or 15 years as compared with those of previous generations. The acquisition of psychoanalytic skills as only part of one's professional armamentarium may be more evident among psychiatrist applicants than among psychologists, but it is hardly exclusive with the former. Broader and continued curiosity seems to suffer by comparison to the achievement and mastery of technique. The latter preoccupation naturally enters into the assumptions with which analysts-in-training enter supervision and voice their wishes for an ideal patient who will fit successfully the technique they hope to acquire or to display. To some extent this may reflect or coincide with parallel preoccupations on the part of the patient who may also be seeking easy solutions to problems, with lessened expenditures of time and money.

Similarly, the supervising analyst's possible preoccupation with "training" the candidate in a particular and favored way of doing analysis may compound the predicament. At times, and fortunately for a time only, the result may be a fool's paradise for all three concerned. More often than not, similar preoccupations are likely to result in respective dissatisfaction for at least one member of the triad (patient, supervisee, and supervisor) who feels betrayed in the process. That this constitutes a vindication of the basic proposition that psychoanalysis needs to remain a heuristic enterprise may prove of little solace to all concerned, unless they learn to mend their ways by clarifying their assumptions and misconceptions. When such assumptions are not shared, a different set of difficulties may develop, and this will need to be identified and dealt with. The candidate who feels deprived of spoon feeding or of demonstration of technique may react with passivity and unavailability in both the clinical situation with the patient and the educational one with the supervisor. The unspoken expectations based on the candidate's assumptions about supervision, once recognized, will help avoid acrimony and hectoring. Also, disabusing the candidate of notions that would contribute further to the regressive elements attendant to supervision may open the way to enhancing the development of autonomy and to the acquisition, rather than usurpation, of wisdom.

A final caveat, often referring to remnants of earlier educational experiences, has to do with the supervising analyst's evaluative function as perceived by the candidate. There is no question about the supervisor's participation in assessing the candidate's progress in training and in deciding his or her readiness for graduation or the need for probation or the validity of continuing with psychoanalytic training. It may become necessary to emphasize the element of the common pursuit of excellence in a highly complex enterprise so as to maximize the collaborative aspects and minimize the adversarial ones. Thus, the supervisor-evaluator can be seen not as a seeker of what can be found wrong with the supervisee, the better to judge and condemn him or her, but rather as a catalyst for the supervisee's freer and more effective use of his or her abilities as they are liberated through the personal analysis and as they are honed by the continued self-observation of what goes on between the analyst-in-training and his or her patient. In this sense the supervising analyst may "mediate" but surely will not conduct the patient's analysis, and the supervisee may come to experience the supervisor as a rational authority rather than as an irrational one.

As for the supervising analyst's assumptions about supervision, many of them are subsumed in what I have stated so far. To amplify and refine some of the points of concern the following considerations are in order. Does the supervising analyst assume that the supervisee's selection of him or her is based on the supervisee's awareness of and agreement with the supervisor's view of himself or herself as a clinician, a theoretician, and a teacher, let alone as a person? Does such an assumption get checked out to begin with or at least from time to time, or is it left unexamined and thought of as corroborated by the supervisee's deferential stance?

If the previously mentioned tendencies constitute one of the most insidious forms of countertransference in working with a patient, what is the likelihood of their not becoming an obstacle to the development of autonomy in a supervisee? Also, what are the chances of the supervisee's patient obliging both supervisee and supervisor under such conditions? In the more fortunate instances, the patient's dreams or even direct productions may serve to alert the supervisee–supervisor dyad and to avert prolonged impasses, provided proper attention to them is forthcoming. In another vein, there is a possible problem in the supervising analyst's occasional assumption that the supervisee has already worked out characterological difficulties that might interfere with his or her work with patients as well as with the supervisory situation. In this regard, if the supervisor fails to consider the supervisee's level of experience within the training program, there may result an inadequate assessing of the latter's performance as compared with his or her potential.

Additional assumptions need to be considered regarding interactions of the supervising analyst in the role of evaluator with the candidate's training analyst, other supervising analysts who work or have worked with the candidate at some point, and any other faculty or even peer judgment that may be brought to bear on the training or educational committee's deliberations. In institutes where the training analyst is allowed or required to participate in the evaluation of the candidate's progress in training, the former may assume he or she has an advantage over the supervising analyst. The question of who is assessing what can easily be raised but not necessarily answered with either equanimity or equitability. In such instances, the candidate may view the training analyst as either an advocate or a betrayer of his confidences and, conversely, may view his or her supervising analyst as either a judgmental critic or a redeeming avenger. If these are distortions, presumably they could be as analyzable as the rest of transferences are supposed to be. If they are more or less valid perceptions of the actual assumptions of the training analyst, they may create a problem for everybody concerned, with the additional complication of repercussions that remain unanalyzed, unless the supervising analyst assumes the role of the training analyst, which is highly undesirable, or until a clarification takes place between training and supervising analysts about their respective contributions.

When the training analyst is excluded from any participation in the evaluation of the candidate's progress though made privy to the reports of supervising analysts and the discussions of the educational or training committee, possible problems may arise if the training analyst proceeds with the assumption that any difficulties on the part of the candidate in conducting psychoanalyses will be taken up by the supervising analyst directly and that the training analyst need not become involved in approaching those issues with the candidate as long as the latter does not broach them in his or her analysis. Such issues might reflect characterological factors resulting in repeated countertransferential interferences with the analysis under supervision. They can also represent transferential developments in the supervisory situation that can hardly be resolved analytically within that situation.

It makes sense that the confidentiality of the candidate's analysis be preserved through the training analyst's not exposing it to others by not participating in the candidate's evaluation at any time. However, because the candidate's personal analysis is a stated requirement of his or her training and because the collateral information about his or her performance in supervised analysis is conveyed to the training analyst, it makes sense as well that the issues arising be taken up in the candidate's analysis. A corollary to the preceding would suggest that the supervising analyst should not always assume that the candidate will be clear enough about interfering factors so as to look into them forthwith in his or her analysis before the training analyst has an opportunity to hear about them. In such instances, the supervising analyst could at least lead the candidate to consider the matter of taking the issue back into his or her own analysis, if not altogether suggest the same.

Any further assumptions under this rubric will have to be considered as matters of the ways in which supervising analysts are viewed within a particular institute, both in the experience or assessment of their contributions and in the "grapevine" rumoring or lore among the candidate group. The tendency is to think of certain supervising analysts as tough and of others as tender. Multiple misconceptions can ensue with attendant corroboration or disappointment affecting all concerned and resulting in rather spurious elements of predictability or reliability. It is not surprising that the effect of such assumptions is temporary confusion or, worse, lasting suspicion, which at times undermines the work of the supervising analyst and interferes with the progress of the candidate under supervision.

Role, Process, and Contents

The previously mentioned considerations, insofar as they enter the supervisory situation are bound to involve matters of role, processes, and contents. It is probable that the psychoanalytic literature has been more explicit in regard to these concerns than otherwise. Therefore, only a brief review appears to be indicated at this point, which essentially highlights the matter of potential pitfalls.

As with everything else in psychoanalysis, there may be no universal agreement about the role of the supervising analyst. However, there is little disagreement that this role is both educational and evaluatory, and is concerned with both the candidate's development and the patient's welfare as natural concomitants to psychoanalytic training and requisites for psychoanalytic competence. As a matter of personal and significant preference, I have opted for and adopted the wording of *supervised analysis*, as conceived and commented upon by Helene Deutsch close to 50 years ago, as being still applicable. In this sense, as already indicated, the supervising analyst undertakes and pursues a multiple task. He or she has the advantage of personal experience not

only in doing analysis but also in being aware of what has contributed to
his or development as an analyst. This should encompass his or her own
experience with a personal analysis and with varying uses of supervision as well as the awareness of the appeal of lasting or ephemeral
theoretical and technical representations, acquisitions, adoptions, revi-
sions, and rejections.

Also, this should be an ongoing process in order to avoid the im-
position of ensconced stances or fleeting notions on the candidate. Otherwise, the supervising analyst is at risk of becoming a proselytizer for
an old faith or a new belief. Conversely, the supervisee is at risk of
having to develop into a docile disciple or an opportunistic zealot. To
use the supervisee so as to vindicate a presumably desirable or definitive
approach, theoretical or technical, that has left the supervising analyst
frustrated but stubborn is not only irresponsible, but it most likely will
not succeed. On the other hand, if the supervising analyst knows of
approaches that seem generally workable though he or she finds it difficult or impossible to use them personally, there may be good reason to
encourage the supervisee in their use, particularly if evidence that this
would be helpful to both the supervisee and the supervised analysis is
forthcoming in the supervisee's presentation and that such approaches
suit the supervisee's style. The significant consideration in such situations lies in discerning between obtaining vicarious fulfillment of the
supervising analyst's preoccupations and experiencing satisfaction resulting from the development of competent autonomy in the supervisee.

I have already mentioned or hinted at some of the processes to be
anticipated in the supervisory situation from the point of view of dis-
junctive rather than conjunctive interaction—both from an educational
and a clinical vantage point. An increasing concern with and documentation of a "parallel process" between what takes place in the analysis
involving the patient and the analyst-in-training and what gets reported
or transpires in the supervisory situation with the analyst-in-training
and the supervising analyst has been the subject of a number of recent
communications and ongoing research. It is more than probable that a
similar concern within the supervisory process would not be out of
order. Depending on a more or less tacit understanding that becomes
established between the supervising analyst and candidate, more often
than not based on the concept of their respective roles, the candidate
may end up carrying over to the analytic situation with the patient a
series of interventions that are not always pertinent to the latter's needs
or those of that particular analysis. Most supervising analysts have the
experience of a candidate's emulating something they say or even

vaguely suggest, out of order or out of synchrony. At times this represents a concept not agreed with or not understood. At other times it may be a matter of the candidate's resenting an obvious insight offered by the supervising analyst without full awareness that it follows on what the candidate had presented but had missed on a certain level. The bird's-eye view afforded any supervisor offers an advantage that is often misconstrued as superior, if not supercilious, knowledge rather than as a pragmatic edge. However, if the supervising analyst has a vested interest in the righteousness of the approach that the candidate adopts in an overestimated way, the patient may be actually lost out of sight in the process and blamed for any ensuing lack of expected—if not exacted—response. Multiple recriminations may develop that can wreak havoc on the patient's progress, the supervisee's learning process, and the supervising analyst's effectiveness as both teacher and evaluator.

Whatever contributes to or reflects the lack of clarity in roles and the unawareness of covert processes, as partly stated before, does also suggest potential pitfalls in the way contents are determined and used in the supervisory interaction. Although it might be of remarkable significance, the parallel between what the supervisee chooses to present in a supervisory session and what he or she elects to pursue with the patient in any given analytic session—out of the wealth of material available—is not likely to be sufficiently identified and assessed, let alone researched. There is simply not enough time for it, if only because of the discrepancy between analytic hours and supervisory ones. The use of tapes offers some advantages and some disadvantages in that regard as does the presentation from notes that are taken during an analytic session or after it. Whatever remedies for this state of affairs different supervisors have devised, based on their respective experiences, may be easily flawed by consistency that becomes rigidity and repetitiousness that results in triteness. At best, the supervising analyst can only rely on listening to the supervisee as he or she would listen to a patient—with all ears and on all levels—and also on clarifying and helping to amplify the way that the supervisee does or does not listen to his or her patient, which, indeed is not an easy task.

OVERVIEW

I have tried to sketch a series of potential pitfalls in psychoanalytic supervision as required and carried out in officially conducted psychoanalytic training. I have confined these to the educational and clinical aspects because psychoanalytic supervision is a teaching and evaluative endeavor concerned with how well a candidate can be prepared to conduct psychoanalysis, which is itself at best a continuously heuristic enterprise in its clinical and therapeutic exercises. In that sense, the paradoxical would seem to outweigh or supersede the orthodox and any diminution—let alone disregard—of this uncomfortable fact means borrowing trouble or courting disaster. If we learn how to live with this set of contradictory propositions, we may be able also to manage to deal with the inevitable conflicts of interest that arise from them.

Just as it is impossible to teach the unteachable, so too is it impossible to abdicate our responsibility for facilitating the learning of it by those whom we invited to come to us and who are in a position to commit themselves to it. If we think that we can help our patients to develop their autonomy as human beings, thus becoming as free as possible to choose how best to use what they are capable of, we should be able to do so with our supervisees who have the added advantage of their own analyses and some potentially useful accumulated experience in the way of testable hypotheses. Obvious as the risks and the pitfalls may be, if we lose sight of the paradox while opting for the presumably more comfortable orthodox, we need to keep them in mind with the same vigilance as all preservation of freedom and pursuit of truth requires.

As supervising analysts, once we allow imaginative curiosity to prevail over indolent orthodoxy, we can foster the development of the former in our supervisees. If they prove themselves incapable of learning it, we may have to cease and desist from proceeding with any further teaching lest it become indoctrination. We may cultivate discipline instead of collecting disciples. And, in the long run, we will have rendered our best service to everyone concerned if we shall have contributed to the development of creative originals instead of insipid clones.

REFERENCES

Bernfeld, S. On psychoanalytic training. *Psychoanalytic Quarterly*, 1962, *31*(4), 453–482.

Bromberg, P. M. The supervisory process and parallel process. *Contemporary Psychoanalysis*, 1982, *18*(1), 92–111.

Caligor, L. Parallel and reciprocal processes in psychoanalytic supervision. *Contemporary Psychoanalysis*, 1981, *17*(1), 1–27.

Deutsch, H. On supervised analysis. *Contemporary Psychoanalysis*, 1983, *19*(1), 59–67.

Dorn, R. M. Psychoanalysis and psychoanalytic education: What kind of "journey"? *The Psychoanalytic Forum*, 1969, *3*, 238–254.

D'Zmura, T. L. The function of individual supervision. In F. H. Hoffman (Ed.), *Teaching of psychotherapy*. Boston: Little, Brown, 1964.

Ekstein, R., & Wallerstein, R. S. *The teaching and learning of psychotherapy*. New York: Basic books, 1958.

Feigl, H. The scientific outlook: Naturalism and humanism. In H. Feigl & M. Brodbeck (Eds.), *Readings in the philosophy of science*. New York: Appleton-Century-Crofts, 1953. (Reprinted from *American Quarterly*, 1949, *1*.)

Fleming, J., & Benedek, T. Supervision: A method of teaching psychoanalysis. *Psychoanalytic Quarterly*, 1964, *33*(1), 71–96.

Fleming, J., & Benedek, T. *Psychoanalytic supervision*. New York: Grune & Stratton, 1966.

Frijling-Schreuder, E. C. M., Isaac-Edersheim, E., & Van Der Leeuw, P. J. The supervisor's evaluation of the candidate. *International Review of Psycho-Analysis*, 1981, *8*(4), 393–400.

Gediman, H. K., & Wolkenfeld, F. The parallelism phenomenon in psychoanalysis and supervision: Its reconsideration as a triadic system. *Psychoanalytic Quarterly*, 1980, *49*(2), 234–255.

Gitelson, M. Problems of psychoanalytic training. *Psychoanalytic Quarterly*, 1948, *17*(2), 198–211.

Goin, M. K., & Kline, F. Countertransference: A neglected subject in clinical supervision. *American Journal of Psychiatry*, 1976, *133*(1), 41–44.

Kubie, L. S. Research into the process of supervision in psychoanalysis. *Psychoanalytic Quarterly*, 1958, *27*(2), 226–236.

McLaughlin, F. Addendum to a controversial proposal: Some observations on the training analysis. *Psychoanalytic Quarterly*, 1967, *36*(2), 230–247.

Michaels, J. J., & Schoenberg, M. L. Some considerations of a retirement policy for training analysts. *Psychoanalytic Quarterly*, 1966, *35*(2), 199–216.

Oppenheimer, J. R. *The open mind*. New York: Simon & Schuster, 1955.

Pollock, G. H. Historical perspectives in the selection of candidates for psychoanalytic training. *Psychoanalytic Quarterly*, 1961, *30*(4), 481–496.

Roazen, P. Introduction to H. Deutsch's "On supervised analysis." *Contemporary Psychoanalysis*, 1983, *19*(1), 53–59.

Schneider, K. The use of patients to act out professional conflicts. *Psychiatry*, 1963, *26*(1), 88–94.

Searles, H. F. The informational value of the supervisor's emotional experiences. *Psychiatry*, 1955, *18*(2), 135–146.

Searles, H. F. Problems of psychoanalytic supervision. In J. Masserman (Ed.), *Science and Psychoanalysis* (Vol. 5). New York: Grune & Stratton, 1962.

Spence, D. P. Psychoanalytic Competence. *International Journal of Psycho-Analysis*, 1981, *62*(1), 113–124.

Zaphiropoulos, M. L. An appraisal of H. Deutsch's "On supervised analysis." *Contemporary Psychoanalysis*, 1983, *19*(1), 67–70.

Author Index

Subject Index